THE HEALING MIND OF MAN
ARISE & SHINE

The importance of the mental and spiritual levels in the healing and life of man.

THE HEALING MIND OF MAN ARISE & SHINE

Volume V, "Man" Series

Bernard Jensen, Ph.D.

Bernard Jensen, Publisher

This book is intended for use as an information source. It is not intended as advice for self diagnosis or a prescription for self treatment. It is hoped that the information contained herein will stimulate thought and encourage the adoption of a beneficial lifestyle.

FIRST EDITION

BERNARD JENSEN, Publisher
Route 1, Box 52
Escondido, CA 92025

Library of Congress Card Catalog Number 84-080045
ISBN 0-9608360-3-9

Dedication

This book is dedicated to a dedicated woman, my wife Marie, who has meant so much to me in sharing many of the experiences described in these pages.

I express great appreciation for the Love I have received, for the Love that has so generously been given and to the Divine that has so generously poured this Principle, this Divine Spark, into the heart of every human being. May we get better acquainted and cultivate this budding Divinity within so that it will not exist as a stranger. This is what a devoted mother taught me. This all comes as a soft spoken word.

—The Author

Biography

Bernard Jensen, teacher, lecturer and author, has traveled in over 55 countries, published over 32 books and describes himself as "a seeker on the path." He has received awards and honors from many nations for his contributions to iridology, wholistic health and international goodwill. His recent books, ***The Chemistry of Man*** and ***Food Healing For Man***, have been well received by thousands of readers concerned with their health and wholeness.

In over 50 years of experience with patients and sanitariums, Dr. Jensen has developed a deep appreciation for the role of the spiritual and mental dimensions in health and healing, a role seldom explored by health care professionals. "Within limitations, we understand what we can do at the physical level to encourage healing in the human body," he says, "but we are only beginning to understand what spiritual and mental resources we can go to for assistance."

Dr. Jensen discovered that principle at the age of 20 when his health suddenly failed and he was given limited time by his doctor. It was a Seventh Day Adventist doctor who taught him that nutrition and health had its spiritual side and who put him on the diet that possibly saved his life. But it was V. G Rocine who so inspired Dr. Jensen that he began what became a lifelong study of the relationship between the spiritual, mental and physical activities in man.

Dr. Rocine was a brilliant Norwegian homeopath who had a dramatic flair for teaching, writing and lecturing. He taught that the spiritual came before the mental and physical, and that it was necessary to go into the Great Within and communicate with the Divine Presence to bring out healing.

"Eventually I not only overcame my physical problem, but nerve depletion and a habit of stuttering and stammering too," says the Doctor. "Rocine and I were friends for over 20 years after that, and he considered me his top student. In turn, I passed along what I learned to my own patients.

"At that time, the idea that unforgiveness, resentment and resistance contributed to the development of chronic disease was so new that many people had difficulty believing it," Dr. Jensen recalls, "but we proved it. Those who gave up resentment and eliminated their hostilities turned their lives around, found a new and higher path. They left their diseases behind. I have seen a great many healings that most people would term miraculous."

Dr. Jensen has met and talked with Sri Aurobindo and Sai Baba, two of the great spiritual leaders of India, and has studied both Eastern and Western spiritual philosophies.

Brought up in one of the traditional denominational churches, Dr. Jensen knew and studied with several renowned spiritual teachers of the 20th century. "I studied with Krishnamurti in Ojai, California," he recalls. "In London, I used to meet with Glen Clark in Trafalgar Square where there were more pigeons than people." He studied with Dr. Ernest Holmes, founder of the Church of Religious Science, and Emmet Fox, a prolific writer and well-known lecturer on metaphysics. Yogananda, founder of the Self Realization Fellowship, lived not far from his Ranch in Southern California.

The Healing Mind of Man is adapted from a series of 30 talks given at the Ranch to groups of patients on Sundays by the Doctor. Much of it is biographical, never before published. Dr. Jensen is now retired and his current activities are limited to teaching, lecturing, traveling and research.

At the age of 76, Dr. Jensen earned his Ph.D. degree from the University of Humanistic Studies in San Diego, California, climaxing a lifetime of study, work and teaching in the healing arts.

Foreword

This book is a collection of my Sunday talks, originally given before groups of patients at my Ranch. The contents are presented for those who desire to come alive, to attain a higher consciousness and to serve in the *Light*. We live in Enlightenment.

In over 50 years of practice in the art of healing, I have treated more than 350,000 patients. I have learned that there is much more to healing than simply treating the physical body. There is a spiritual aspect of healing. There is a mental aspect of healing. To become a whole and healthy person requires peace, harmony and balance at the spiritual, mental and physical levels.

The series of talks transcribed and presented here is designed to awaken you from your present state of consciousness, to teach you how to lift yourself from present ill health, disharmonies and poor economic status to a realization of your true birthright—the life more abundant.

As you walk the higher path, you will begin to release your worries, anxieties, depressions, fears, physical ills and mental snarls to be filled instead with peace, harmony, love, joy and that exuberance of life that comes only to those who learn to overcome. It is closer than you think. There is a wonderful person inside you just waiting to bloom and come forth.

In the pages of this book, you will learn to let your light shine. You will learn to go to the Upper Room, the secret place of the Most High, where you will grow and develop. It is in the Upper Room, the deepest place within, where you meet with the God Presence and come forth in a new state of beingness. This is very simple—but it isn't easy. You may have tried the quick and easy ways, but they didn't work, did they? That is because the quick and easy ways cannot touch the deepest inner self. This is the aspect of your life that must be touched and awakened before meaningful change can take place, before the deep healing can take place, before you will learn to see all things anew.

It is my privilege to offer you the means for this awakening. The rest is up to you.

A good starting point is to realize that without spirit, the body is nothing. *It is the spirit that quickeneth; the flesh profiteth nothing,* it has been written. Most medical treatment deals only with the physical level. Most psychiatric treatments deal only with the mental level. But if the problem is at the spiritual level, these treatments won't help you. You will have to go deeper.

The origin of most physical problems is in the mind. The origin of most mental troubles can be found in the failure to seek and follow spiritual truth. Where does spiritual truth come from? Spiritual truth comes only from the God Presence. To change your life, you must learn to go to the Source of Life. There is no disease or disharmony at the level of the God Presence. There is no disease or disharmony at the level of spirit. We must go to the Great Within so that what comes forth from your Deeper Self will be felt by every cell in the body. We live on what we give forth.

Now, we will be spending a good deal of time in this book talking about the physical and mental levels of the person. It is important to see how these levels interrelate with one another and with spirit. You will need to understand these things because I believe that the spiritual principles must be applied at both the mental and physical levels.

There is an obligation on the part of the teacher to make sure he has done his best to reach the student. There is, in turn, an obligation on the part of the student to seek and reach for the higher values in life. *I believe that the best teacher is the one who inspires his student with the desire to teach himself.*

This book deals with the knowledge, wisdom and experiences I have gathered in my travels all over the world. I feel that every religion has something good to offer. Many religions teach love, tenderness and care for one another.

The basis of all good religions must be that we are our brother's keeper, that we must share with one another, that we are on this planet to serve others as well as to take care of ourselves. We can't feel good unless those around us feel good, too. The moment the other person becomes happy, we do too.

It doesn't matter to me whether a person is a Hindu, Moslem, Buddhist, Taoist or Christian, we have to deal with the divine innate nature of each one. My obligation in this book has been to present the truth as I see it so it is acceptable to anyone or any religion. I feel it is important to be a truth seeker.

My main object in this book is to state that we should be getting along better in our human relations. There are too many walls, fences and other barriers that keep people from each other. Yet, in every country I have visited, I find that a smile goes far in breaking down barriers. When people know each other deeply, they live in greater harmony, a greater willingness to share with and help one another.

I have not attempted to present the teaching of any particular religion, sect or cult as better than any other. Rather, I have tried to draw from the well of wisdom of the humanities. All people need upliftment and tender care as far as the mind is concerned.

Although I was raised in a Christian family, I realize we must all get along with one another. If there is anything in a religion that prevents us from helping others, lifting others, that religion is lacking. We are our brother's keeper in our attitude.

The Healing Mind of Man is intended to be universal in application. I feel its principles should be known in our educational system, homes, places of employment. We should be aware of mankind's needs and hungers so we can respond to them. We should all go to the highest pinnacle of love for the highest good of one another.

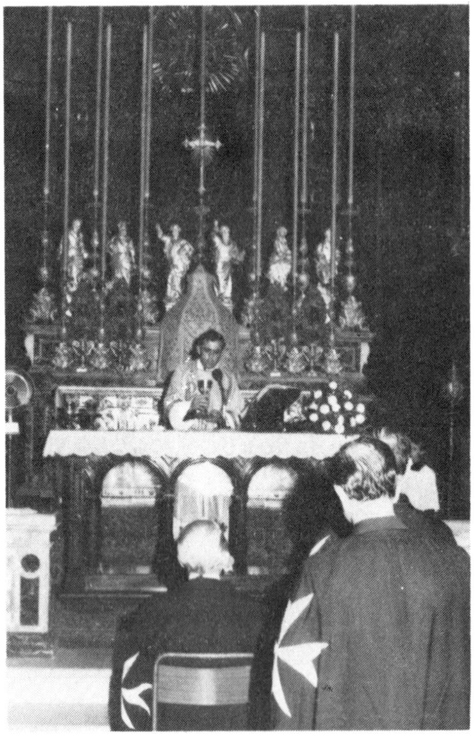

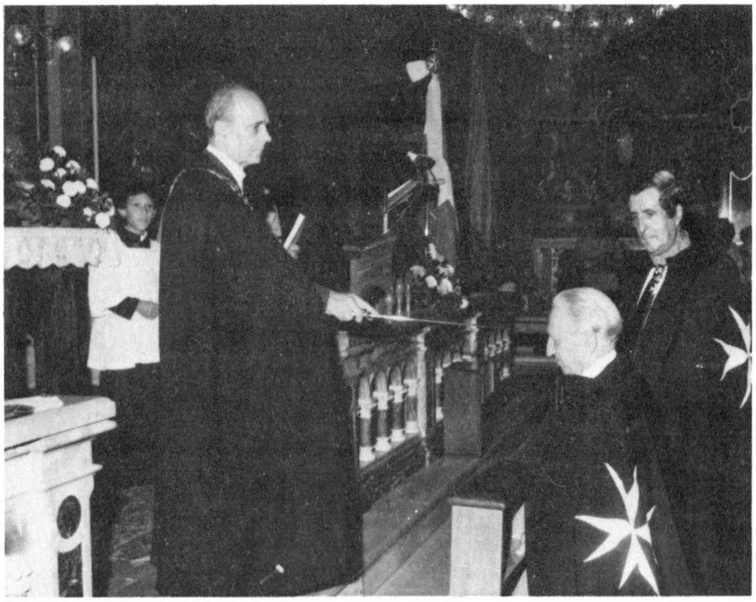

Left: The knighting of Dr. Jensen took place at the beautiful Basilica of Our Lady of the Victories, the Basilica of Xaghra on the Island of Malta, September 7, 1984. Right: Grand Prior International, the Marquis don K. Vella Haber, dubs Dr. Bernard Jensen as Knight Commander of the Sovereign Order of St. John of Jerusalem, the Knights of Malta, with Chevalier James Merryfield assisting in the ceremony.

Contents

Chapter 1

I Feel Wonderful! How Do You Feel?

"In the beginning was the Word..." This book may be "the word" and "the beginning" of a new life for you, the dawning of that long awaited change in your life that will help you to inspire all those whom you may contact..."

"I feel WONDERFUL! How do YOU feel?" Wouldn't that make a happy greeting for everyone? Let that be our greeting right now, our personal introduction to one another.

Usually our greetings are so negative that they draw out the poorest response from others, a list of troubles and woes that goes on and on as long as a willing ear is there to listen. In some way *everybody* seems to be in pain today — some physical, some mental — for pain is not only a physical thing, but may also plague us in the mental forms of discontent, resentment and disharmony.

Sometimes we are prone to be TOO honest with our fellowmen. When asked, "How are you?"...as a rule, people will take that greeting as an invitation to tell us all their troubles. But troubles should not be brought to the surface and aired in our greetings to one another. When we talk about our burdens, we may feel temporary relief, but they soon return heavier than ever. There are professional listeners whose business it is to listen to your troubles and to assist you, and they are the only ones with whom you should discuss problems.

Let's Create A Beautiful Carpet Of Words

Let us lighten our load as quickly as possible and then help our fellowman to lighten *his* load. How can this be done? It can be done easily by laying out an inspiring carpet of words to think and walk upon, words that will allow all whose lives touch ours to have beautiful and uplifting thoughts and feelings. As you lay out this inspiring carpet of words, you will bring out the best in others — and yourself. Isn't that worth doing? Like begets like, as the saying goes. Why not bring out the best to discuss and listen to...for your own good?

It is directly to our advantage to recognize that the physical earth we deal with on a day-to-day basis is not the "whole" world. The larger world includes the mental and spiritual activity of man on this earth. The Garden of Eden is still here but we have made a mess of it. Can you see how much better it would be to become a joy-bringer and gloom-chaser, than a poisonous thought-spreader? Living in a world of complaints may be the trend of the day, but finding peace with ourselves and with our fellowman is *essential* for our mental and physical well-being. For example, the liver cannot work properly and the stomach cannot digest its food completely, if these organs are bound up with worry and tension. You can feel better right now by *merely voicing* the idea, **I AM FEELING BETTER.** Try it right this minute. The louder and more joyfully you can say it, the better. Then close your eyes and feel how wonderfully your body responds to what you just said.

If you think about it, you will realize that both tension and relaxation are developed through thought. It is necessary to put the mental attitude in good order *before* the body responds. My years of experience with patients have shown me that happiness and serene thoughts are absolutely necessary for anyone trying to get well. A morbid, blue, dejected person invites constipation, indigestion, poor circulation and a whole host of other ailments.

The Body Responds To Mind And Spirit

"It is the spirit that quickeneth; the flesh profiteth nothing. . ." The Christ shared this insight with his disciples, for He knew that the body responds to the mental attitude. The helping hand is gracious because of the motive behind it. A smile is the end result of what has gone on behind the scenes. In fact, every physical activity has its birth in feeling and attitude, in that subtle quickening spirit that flows through our neural systems before we can so much as lift a finger. The world of feeling is created and expressed in our attitudes; it is rooted within our deepest self.

A man in his workshop may wish to turn out a beautiful table top. He knows that to do this he must carefully shape the edges to make them smooth, bevel the corners precisely right and polish the surface to an exquisite finish. He deals with substance that he can touch, look upon and change with the work of his two hands — a tangible substance. Now let us recognize that within ourselves we have a delicate, intangible substance to work with, a substance that may be expressed as the blues, anger, hatred, fear and despondency. These intangibles exist in a world of feeling where fingers cannot touch nor eyes see. It is in this deep self that we have our beginning, our start in life. It was there before our physical body ever began and it is there that we mold our future. It is here, in our deepest inner self, that we make our present life more pleasant and gracious, or more dejected and unhappy. Yes, there is substance in this world, but it is a fleeting substance, and to shape and polish it nicely requires the proper mental tools — our attitudes.

It is in this feeling world that we can elevate ourselves from fear to courage, from the blues to joy, from sorrow and regret to appreciation and freedom. It is in this feeling world that our health attitude is rooted. Since the body follows the mind, a tranquil mind will permit more harmonious activity in all the physical organs.

Truth, Wisdom and Health Walk Hand In Hand

In ages past, long before the development of the modern lie detector with its electronic gadgetry, the courts of law had a very simple test for discovering whether a man was telling a lie. All they had to do was to place a little flour in his mouth. If he were lying, his digestive juices and saliva would stop secreting. We know that the digestive juices in the stomach and intestines are affected by our mental outlook. I know from personal experience that if the attitudes and personal philosophies of many of the patients who have come to me were straightened out, they would be radiant with health today.

The Mayo Brothers claim that nine out of every ten people who come to them with stomach ulcers have caused the problem themselves through worry, fretting, stewing, love problems or money troubles. These all begin and thrive in the mind. Surely we can become wise enough to know better than to abuse our stomachs by misuse of our mental faculties. By nourishing our mental philosophy with the right thoughts and attitudes, we nurture our bodies and reap the harvest of good health.

It was once very clearly demonstrated to me how a person can destroy himself — in a matter of minutes — by a wrong mental attitude. Two men aboard a barge above Niagara Falls were being towed across the river. Suddenly, the cable snapped! The black hair of one of the two men turned gray in minutes as the barge drifted toward the falls. He actually died of fright twelve minutes later. But the barge never went over the falls! It was stopped by a large pile of rocks! This man killed himself by fearing something that never happened. The mind can be a lethal instrument when wrongly used — and a tremendous power for good when rightly used. We cannot allow ourselves to forget that.

We Live As We Think

Many people today are committing mental suicide. They torture themselves with their thoughts and attitudes to such an extent that their whole bodies suffer from the strain and stress of poisoned feelings. It is necessary for us to find peace within our own minds. We can create a good start for ourselves by not talking about our troubles with other people and by not opening up the path for others to talk about their troubles to us. The best possession you have is your attitude in life. Give the best and you will attract the best from others. Deep inside, we all want to live in an uplifting world.

Let me ask you an honest question. Would you rather be known for the joy you have spread or for the gloomy troubles you have experienced? Too often we are encouraged to tell about our troubles. Can you honestly say you want to hear other people's troubles? Then why should you tell them yours? Too often we only become aware of those loyal, hardworking feet that carry us through life when a shoe pinches one of them. We only become aware of that magnificent nervous system of ours when nerve depletion and nerve acids become so irritating they bring on the ache. But why should we pass our pinches and aches on to others? Your troubles are for *you* to take care of!

Just think, if everybody focused on life's troubles, all we would ever hear about would be mother's headache, father's business problems, the marriage troubles of friends, the ailments of our neighbors and so on and on. We would have every reason to believe there were no happy people in the entire world!

To get the surprise of your life, just try a little experiment the next time anyone says, "How are you?" Dare to say, "I FEEL WONDERFUL!" and mean what you say. Your friend or neighbor will ask, "What has happened to you?" Starting in the mind and in the spirit, you will begin to feel like a new person. A new and beautiful day is waiting to dawn in your life if you will take on this attitude. Suggestion is the most powerful thing in the world, and to consistently suggest to yourself that you FEEL WONDERFUL will cause the entire body to reverberate and readjust itself to this new feeling. You will begin to feel better just because you have given yourself better feelings. Troubles begin to evaporate like mist under a bright morning sun. Physical ailments respond much more easily to treatment if your attitude doesn't hold you back.

Let It Start With You

To bring the best back to ourselves, we must give of our best first. To make this world more wonderful, begin with yourself. The world isn't going to get better when you feed upon idle, troublesome chatter.

You'll see a wonderful world and talk of a wonderful world when you recognize it within yourself first. The beauty of the rose has always been there, but it is only beautiful when you, yourself, take the time to recognize it. Like the rose, we must blossom, open up to the good inside ourselves, so that others may feel and share what is beautiful in our lives. Then we are living!

So often I've heard people say, "I'm just dying to get well." And, do you know what? I believe them. Believe me, these people are using dying ideas and dying mental and physical processes to try to get well. But they are doing more dying than they are living.

One of life's simplest yet more eloquent secrets is this: we can *choose* to feel wonderful. We can develop the riches within ourselves. And we can share these riches with others. To know you have helped somebody get ahead, to know you are able to share, to help someone to a successful venture, is to know that the happiness of others is our happiness, the success of others is our success! This is where we find the true riches in life!

To Lift Yourself, Try Lifting Others

You can never be truly well until you are helping lift other people. You can never be truly well until you are thinking the best thoughts about other people. Anyone who drags on another is down and out. He is living at a lower level. If you want to be on top, you have to raise other people up. Then you are living at a higher level of life. The moment you begin raising other people to greater heights you are accomplishing. . . you are serving. . . you are needed. . . you are indispensable.

Look for your own good in doing good for others. Then you will have something to feel wonderful about. "Thou shalt love thy neighbor as thyself," is one of the great healing truths of all time. In developing this in yourself, you will make the most important discovery of your life. You will find yourself. You will find that inner place where you and God get together and make changes, not only in yourself but in other people. You will find the pearl of great price. You will discover the starting point where man's renewal begins and where the greatest attitudes of life can be used for bettering yourself and your fellowman. Disease and disharmony will fade away because you will be at peace within. If you lose all your money, you have lost little; if you lose your health, you have lost a lot; but if you lose your peace of mind, you have lost everything.

Find Peace and Express It

First, find peace within yourself. Express that — because others need it — then more peace will come to you. The Good Book says, ". . .and His name shall be called Wonderful...." What a powerful word! Let it be in your greeting: "I FEEL WONDERFUL!"

A New Day

This is the beginning of a new day.
God has given me this day to use as I
will.

I can waste it or use it for good.
What I do today is very important
because I am exchanging a day in my
life for it.

When tomorrow comes this day will be
gone forever, leaving something in its
place.

I have traded for it: I want it to be gain,
not loss; good — not evil; success —
not failure. May I not forget the price
I paid for it.

Chapter 2

Arise and Shine

"Arise, shine; for thy light is come..."

Isaiah 60:1

Today we will shine a little light on the lessons we have to learn in this life. Many times I used to talk to patients and students in an old rebuilt barn on my Ranch. That barn was a constant reminder that we can rebuild our bodies just as I had that barn rebuilt into a lovely place where we could come together to share the higher things in life.

We can work on life's lessons in a barn or a cathedral; it is all one to God. God is far more interested in the kind of people who are in a building than the kind of building the people are in. Maybe we can get better lessons out of a barn than a cathedral. It all depends on what you are looking for and what you are looking to. Some of my greatest lessons were learned in very remote, simple places. I studied with Krishnamurti in a cow shed in Ojai, California. It was really an unusual place to get lessons, but I got them anyway. In England, I met with Glen Clark in Trafalgar Square, where there were more pigeons around than people, and yet this is where I got some of my best lessons. There was light in all these places; do you know what I mean? You have to let your light shine, then you can begin to learn your lessons. Then you will be given more light.

Is there any reason why we can't use all things for good? Is there any reason why we can't put our best thinking to work for the good of our health in both the mind and the body?

Health And The Mind

Sometimes you'll be having a discussion with an individual when suddenly you find that the discussion has turned into an argument. You walk away saying to yourself, "That man is sick." Have you ever had that experience?

We have to face the fact that some people are sick in the head. Many people are crippled mentally. A lot of people are just as disturbed and twisted mentally as they are physically.

One of the most difficult things for people to understand is that you can't expect to think sweet thoughts on a sour stomach. By the same token, you can't expect the physical body to function right without the soothing oil of good feelings. Thoughts and feelings have an effect on the physical body, just as the condition of the physical body has an effect on our thoughts and feelings. The two go hand in hand, so to speak.

We go through life, and some people experience the good, while others see every tomorrow as Blue Monday. Can you imagine a whole week of Blue Mondays? Why do we put up with these negative thoughts, these thoughts of sickness? Why do we allow them to control our thinking? We may have heard about this "mind over matter" business, but we don't let it sink in. We go along with sick thoughts until sickness manifests itself in the flesh. A person who says he is sick has captured something in his mind which he then releases to every cell in his body. This is "mind over matter," but it is not working for our good. We need to reverse this type of thinking.

From experience I've learned there is such a thing as mind over matter, and I've observed this process at work in many different ways. I've known people who have managed to think themselves sick and I've known people who have managed to think themselves well. Let's put a little light on this. You know, we sleep through the night, but when that early morning sunlight begins to shine softly through the window, we awaken. When the light comes, we awaken and we arise. We yawn, we rub our eyes and we begin to see.

Thoughts Are Food For The Mind

We are all interested in food. I want to tell you that there is food for the body, mind and soul. It is time we realize that we can't starve the body and have a good mind, and we can't starve the mind and have a good body. There are foods we could eat to remake our joints. But do you think our joints can be affected by what we think? Many a disease has started in the mind. And many a disease has been relieved when a person's thinking was changed.

So it's necessary for us to open our eyes to these things. I don't want you ever to get the idea that carrot juice and vegetables are the cure for everything. By the same token, I don't want you to ever get the idea that all you have to do is think right to have a healthy body. The person who lives on coffee and donuts can't possibly have good health even with right thinking.

Total health must include body, mind and spirit. Total health requires care and attention to the whole person.

I love to watch what happens when people take a worn and weary body, battered just like my old barn once was by the winds and storms of life, and remodel it into a beautiful new temple. I love to watch them fix up the old foundation and floor, then put in a lovely bright-colored carpet, wonderfully soft to walk on. Cheery new furnishings are added to give it that special feeling of home. They make it comfortable. They make it worth living in. I love to watch that happen.

Look For The Good In Others

Let us look for what is right. For the moment I hope I can reach you by sharing some ideas I've discovered in searching for my own good. In a way I've been looking for my own good in the thousands of people who have come to me for help. They have forced me to think this way. They are the leaves of my book. Every patient is a challenge to me, and I like challenges — they quicken me to greater alertness, greater awareness. So I appreciate the many opportunities I've had for learning from my patients. What thousands have shown me — and I hope you can appreciate this — is the fact that we can get rid of sickness. We can get rid of it by remodeling our house. You can make your house so beautiful that you will feel as though you've moved into a new one.

Once when I'd traveled to New Zealand, we had a class of 1,100 people and we couldn't find a hall large enough to lecture in. So we moved into a bar, an old pub, and we lectured right where the usual order of business was serving beer, whiskey and cocktails. We gave out words of life in that place. Many of the people at that lecture returned home with their soul-thirst satisfied from a different type of drink.

As we walk with the soul uplifted and with joy in our hearts, we find virtue in everything we encounter. We change our disadvantages into advantages. There are no stumbling blocks in life if we change them to stepping stones.

How To Rise Above Your Problems

The cure for these problems is found in three beautiful words: "Arise and Shine." To overcome your situation, rise above the problem. How do we do that? It's all very nice to talk, but when we are down, it's terrible to hear someone say, "You have to rise above this." That isn't the time we want advice. We want to be left alone. But we have heard, "Man's extremity is God's opportunity." There is a time when you will find yourself saying, "I am finished smoking." And you are finished. There is a time when you will find yourself saying, "I am done with these foolish things I've been doing. Now I see a new way to go." Then you will drop the old and the new will come about.

Have you ever seen an eagle preening his feathers? The old feathers come out to allow new feathers to come in. We have to preen our feathers. We have to preen our feelings as the eagle preens his feathers.

Wouldn't it be nice to wear joy? Wouldn't it be wonderful to get up in the morning and dress ourselves in happiness and peace and harmony? Just think of how you'd look in them. You'd walk down the street, and everyone would recognize you as the best-dressed person in town!

Some Of Us Need Driving Lessons

How can we rise? We do this just as we'd shift gears in an automobile. We start out in low. We have to get going in life, and that is our first step, our first gear. Then we shift into second and we have higher things to think about. We are gaining real momentum. Then we stick the gear shift into third and we speed right along at a higher level than before. We are in a smooth driving speed. But some of us have been shifting gears and grinding them, and we are only up to about twenty percent of where we should be. There is more shifting to be done. What prevents us from shifting up to a higher level is that we have gotten in the habit of using low gear too much. Once we shift up a few times, we rise to the level at which we are supposed to live. How do we do this?

In India I traveled into a rugged mountain region to see the ancient temples. They had prayer wheels there. A person could put a prayer in one of those brass prayer wheels, and the next person to come along would give that wheel a spin. As it turned, they believed the prayers would go up to heaven. There are many ways to pray, and that is one of the nicer ways I've seen. Prayer is one way to shift to a higher level.

Another way they pray in India is to write their prayer on a flag and hang it up on a clothesline. As a wind comes along, their prayers sail up to heaven. Isn't that a beautiful way? Some people bow their heads and pray silently. Some fold their hands together, and others get down on their knees. Does the system you use matter? I believe that what is essential in prayer is the release of that prayer to God. Whether it is put in a prayer wheel or allowed to sail off with the wind or released from the heart doesn't matter. You have to let go of that prayer. You have to let God have it. You have to "let go and let God." That is the secret of prayer. The next step is to actually begin living that higher level you are seeking.

There are many people who don't seem to realize that to "arise and shine" means to get to that higher level and to *live* that level so other people can see it. At the start, change will take place at the mind level and spirit level. When you give your attention to this level of consciousness, the body just naturally follows along. Then it shows. When you "arise and shine" it shows, because "your light is come," and people notice.

When you give your body a good time by living on these higher levels, you will no longer live in sickness. There is absolutely no sickness in peace and harmony. You can get a very quick healing if you will shift gears, move up to the higher levels and discover the wonderful things that are right there beside you.

"Take No Thought..."

The world is full of wonderful things! A lot of people take thought and try to reason this out. But a long time ago, the Christ said, "Take no thought for your life." This is a hard saying for many people, especially those who believe that keeping their noses to the grindstone is the only way to succeed. "Take no thought." What does that mean? Thinking bakes no bread, as the philosopher said. The necessities of life will be provided to us as we work, but thinking or worrying cannot add or subtract from them.

Capture The Joy Of Living

You may have heard people say, "Life is no good. I go through life, and it's not worth living. I should have died when I was little." I know of these thoughts. Often people may not say it outright that way, but you can tell from the way they live. You can tell from their faces, their postures, the way they walk. Sometimes you can tell from the way they shake hands. The joy of living is missing in them. When I first meet them they lack that "I'm-feeling-wonderful" expression of life. They have allowed the good things in their lives to be destroyed.

Too often we don't let our bodies be moved by what should be moving them — the mind and the spirit. It's the spirit that quickens. The body is simply an instrument that mind and spirit work through.

Society is potentially an instrument for our good, and we should work together for the good of the whole. But society, as an instrument, is no better than what is put into it, what flows through it. If today's society doesn't change, it may destroy the individuals that make it up. The problem is that our society is not yet built on eternal principles. It is built on man's principles not God's principles. Man looks for the short-term gain, the quick profit, the right-now pleasure, the hurried lunch. Man turns his nose up at the treasures of heaven.

As a result, we don't take in the godly foods. Instead we take the processed, polished, devitalized, devitaminized foods into our bodies because we are too much in a hurry to shop for, prepare and eat wholesome foods. But it is time for us to rebuild these bodies — and it is time to rebuild the mind. It's time that we transform. It's time that we transmute. It's time that we move to a higher level of living, and to do that we must arise!

Let's Get Moving Again

The word of action in spiritual work is "arise." It is to get going. It is to get moving. I hear people say, "I'm going to stand pat on this." They aren't going to move. Sometimes we must stand pat on what is right But too often, people are standing pat on certain fears, such as, "If I don't get mine now, I'll never get it." They need to arise. They need to arise because they are short-changing themselves on the mental and spiritual level.

"Unto everyone that hath shall be given, and he shall have abundance," it is written. What does this mean? The person who has risen to the place where he realizes that he is rich in life itself already has the greatest treasure there is. He has risen to a new thought. To him more will be given. If you want to get well, you have to rise out of the old thinking that has brought on your illness, that has caused you trouble for so long. This is food for thought.

If you came to me and said, "I have high blood pressure," I would tell you that for much of your life you've been putting things off until the last minute. You've been doing things always at the eleventh hour. You haven't balanced your life with the right mental and spiritual foods. One lady told me, "I don't like this last minute business — it brings on apoplexy." This is the rupture or blocking of a blood vessel in the brain, what people more commonly refer to as "stroke." And, yes, the lady is right. This last minute business does bring on apoplexy. I know what rushing around does to the mind and I know what it does to the blood pressure. But we have to understand that it started in the mind in the first place. We tell ourselves, "I have to rush to get this thing done," and gradually we get into the habit of doing many things that way. Many people need some new food for their minds. It is starving to death on the old food, and their high blood pressure shows it.

Out Of Sight Is Not Out Of Mind

When we realize our physical problems are brought on by what we have fed into our minds, we have to be wise in the cure we seek. When people take physical problems to a doctor, he can only cure them by getting down to the cause. If a person, these days, has too many fears, his doctor may prescribe a drug instead of spending the time to get at the source of the problem. When he takes the drug, the fears aren't gone, it's just that the drug prevents him from feeling fearful. We don't get rid of flies by swatting them; we get rid of flies by removing the garbage that is attracting them in the first place. The same is true of fears. You have to get rid of that mental garbage that attracts them.

We do not get life, spiritual life, by striving for it or thinking about it. "Take no thought," Christ said, and He meant it. When we have to think or strive for something, it often eludes us. Perhaps the following story will show you what I mean.

The Forest Is Silent For the Hunter

One time I had a very wonderful experience. My dad was a great hunter, and very early one morning we went out to hunt quail in Livermore, California. Of course I carried a shotgun, and the strategy was for dad and the other hunters to walk through the brush along the lower side of the mountain while I remained on top waiting for them to flush the quail in my direction. They were going to force the quail to fly up close to me, and I was supposed to shoot them.

I leaned my gun on a rock and sat there in my hiding place admiring the beautiful sunrise. Did you ever see the sun rise from below a layer of clouds and slowly creep above them? I was watching this lovely scene when all at once I heard the quail. As I reached for my shotgun and started to get up, the quail scattered back down the mountain. So I sat down again and looked at the sunrise. When I sat down, the quail came back up. If I lifted myself above the rock, they would go back down. Each time I reached for the shotgun, the quail would fly down the mountain, but when I lowered the gun to my lap, they would return. I wondered if they were reading my mind. I wondered if they could sense my feelings.

I think there is a feeling, a thought within us that others can feel or determine, just like those quail seemed to be doing. I had never realized this before I went hunting. When you go into the forest with a gun in your hand, you can't hear a sound. Then one bird about 500 feet away goes chirp, chirp, chirp. That is all you hear. It is eerie. You begin to feel funny carrying that gun in your hand. If you tramp through the forest without a gun, you can hear everything. The birds are all singing. But carry a gun, and you won't hear a thing.

A man with a gun never realizes some of the nice things that happen in this world. War and peace are made in the hearts and minds of men. Sickness is also made there. I have sometimes wondered if the two are related. If we are going to change our lives, we are going to have to start with the inside.

There are levels of thinking and feeling that go beyond words. I have a love for people that I cannot explain. Yet even though it goes beyond our human vocabulary, it is no less real.

Things Don't Create Happiness

Too many people believe they would be happier if they were surrounded by certain things in their lives, and if other things were taken away. The other day a patient said, "You know, if I didn't have a mortgage, I would feel better." I'll admit that he might have felt better without the mortgage, but I doubt that he would have been happy to lose the house that the mortgage made possible. If you want the house, the mortgage comes with it. You have to learn to feel good even with the mortgage. In fact, you have to learn to feel good, to feel well, in order to get well. Over the years I have come to realize that things don't create happiness. There are many wealthy people who are sick and unhappy. Happy people think differently from unhappy people. They look at life differently, they talk about life differently. The next time you are around a happy person, pay close attention to the words he or she uses.

Animals try to escape from what they fear. People sometimes do that too, but they also think about their fears. They say in India that 5,000 people died of cholera and 15,000 died of fear just from hearing of the epidemic. Words can be as destructive as bullets. When we have a furious feeling or get into a temper over something, we are fighting the future — we are in constant battle. The other day someone asked me, "How's the battle going?" Each morning some people get up to battle the day. We respond to the words and to the tone of voice in which those words are expressed. Even the expression, "Well, isn't that nice?" can be said with such cutting, insulting sarcasm that it can wound someone's feelings. And our bodies are dragged down by those poor, miserable feelings.

Insecurity, triggered by words, can bring on sickness. Doubt and frustration, diseases that start in the mind and spread to the body, can be caused by words. We grow exhausted and make ourselves vulnerable to illness — because of words.

We Earn Good Health

If we are going to live in constant combat and in constant shock, we are not going to have good rewards. Shall I tell you that good health is a reward? Shall I tell you it comes at the end, after we have done that which is good for us, and not before?

Most people look to doctors for help when they are ill. I am trying to show you there is something beyond doctors that we must get hold of. Doctors may fail you. Then where will you be? You have to have something within yourself to depend on. You have to stop running from fear and insecurity. Look for what is causing them, and change your life to get rid of them.

How many want to run away from joy thinking? How many want to run away from happy thoughts? Someone will say, "Oh, the time goes by so fast when I'm having a good time!" Another will say, "I've been feeling so bad, time just seems to drag on me." I'd like to buy a little time. I need time. My time is too short. It disappears too fast. Why? Because it's happy time I'm spending, and it goes as fast as the nickels and dimes that a boy puts in a pocket with a hole in it. It's joyous time that I have. It's the kind of time where I'm wonderfully tired at the end of the day, and I sleep well.

There is a twist to an old saying. It goes like this: "If you go to bed 'dog-tired,' you've probably been growling all day." Many people are doing just that.

There are many people who have suffered financial ruin. I, too, have had financial losses. But I am wondering if we can't study this spiritually and find that nothing is lost in God's kingdom. Can you see this? There's another way of looking at it.

There is another thing that could possibly save your nervous system. Most people don't realize that the mental faculties trigger off certain glandular secretions in the body. If I told you all the things that result when we trigger off the glands, you would find it hard to believe. For instance, the thyroid gland is the emotional gland, and it reacts to our thinking just as we react to things that have been said to us. In time we can produce dry hair and dry skin. It's possible to speed up or slow down the growth of a man's beard just through the amount of anxiety he experiences.

Our Mind Controls Our Body

So I say this: The body is a very responsive instrument, but the mind determines which way it goes. We are supposed to control the body by what we have in the mind. We have heard of "ears that hear not, eyes that see not." That means we can't be blind and deaf to the lessons of truth and right living, the lessons of God's law, and expect to avoid the consequences. When we have eyes that see and ears that hear, we learn that we are created for happiness. Many people will have to rise to another level before they can know they were created for joy.

We have a standing invitation to go to the higher places in life. Christ did not come to tell us about fear. He was always trying to lift people, trying to free us. He was trying to get us to see things in a different light and from a higher standpoint. He wanted us to extend our vision. He wanted us to go beyond what we see with our physical vision.

Do You Need Spiritual Glasses?

What can you see when you close your eyes? Can you see that everything is all right? Stop and think about this for a moment. We have to extend our senses, extend them beyond the bodily senses. We must go "inside" the physical senses, so to speak, and use the godly senses to know and to sense the spiritual truths.

When he saw Christ walking on the sea, Peter was told, "Come to me." Peter did, but then he started worrying about it and he thought, "It's impossible for me to do this thing!" So, what happened? He sank down, and this is what happens to many of us. We have to look again and we have to see the impossible thing being done. We have to live on both the plane of the possible and the plane of the impossible. The Christ came to tell us, "With men it is impossible; but with God all things are possible." He admitted, "I can do nothing of myself." He could only do what God did through him. God can do anything through us. We find our lives when we lose them. We have eyes that see not and ears that hear not. "I go and prepare a place for you," said the Christ. We don't see that which has already been prepared for us. When the prodigal son was so hungry and miserable and couldn't see a way out of his fix, he returned home to his father.

We have to get away from appearances and the way things look or sound to us. It is written, "Lo here! Lo there! For behold, the kingdom of heaven is within you." Can you look inside? Have you ever looked inside?

Religion comes from the word *religaire* meaning to go back into. It is not "out there." If you don't have the church within you when you walk into the church building, what good is the church to you? The church is only as good as what you have within you.

Jesus was never in the business of fighting anything but untruth. He said, "I am not come to destroy but to fulfill." I can see Him handling the devil but I don't see Him fighting the devil. He just says, "Get thee behind me, Satan." I think He did it very quietly.

Fighting Life Will Kill You

Resisting evil is causing more fatigue today than anything else. Why resist it? Why not just put it behind us where it belongs, and then we won't have to worry about tiredness and fatigue. At the end of the day we will be able to enjoy the time that was meant for us to enjoy — eight hours of recreation. How many times have you heard people say, "I'm so tired when I get home from work, I can't do a thing." And yet those eight hours are meant for your recreation.

Suppose you have been aggravated with the boss and your job. You have been fighting the situation. Work never killed anybody, but fretting over the people we work with, worrying about our work, can wear us out or even kill us. "Come to me all ye that labor and are heavy laden, and I will give you rest," the Christ promised. What is He going to give you? Is He going to let you touch the hem of his garment so you can be healed? The hem of a garment is no different than a statue. Do you think a statue can heal? No. Christ is going to help you rise above your situation, and when you rise above that situation you will touch something else. Then you will find the healing — and you will go about doing healing. You will be shining and doing the healing. When you do this, something wonderful will come back to you.

You have to cast your bread upon the waters before something wonderful comes back to you. We go through life creating that which we really are. We can't expect to attract the good in life if we don't put out our own good.

Learn To Let Your Light Shine

To *let* the light shine is not to *make* it shine. You don't have to make anything shine. Just let it shine! You don't have to make anybody understand. Sometimes a child is whipped to make him understand, but if the right influence were there, he would understand without the whipping. Influence is the gentlest thing in the world. God doesn't whip his children. He doesn't make them do anything. It is a matter of bearing witness to that which is good and then letting it shine. To *Arise and Shine* is the secret.

We have been warned against having ears and hearing not. Too often we just don't listen. Or we listen but don't understand. But then, too often we listen to the wrong thing.

I remember someone saying of a woman, "She could always hear when anything was said against her — even in a crowd." She was listening for it, and believe me she always got it! That which you fear comes upon you because you are looking for it.

An actress heard about a movie producer who was looking for a wonderful singer. One night at the club where she was singing, she thought this man was in the audience. As she tried hard to sing her best, she made so many mistakes that she was terrible. Afterward, she went to her dressing room and cried her heart out. She knew she'd lost her chance at the job. The next night she went back and sang as she usually did. The strange thing was that the producer wasn't there the night she made all the mistakes. He was there the next night. She got the job. The nicest things come to us when we express our real selves.

When Lazarus in his tomb heard Christ's voice calling, "Lazarus, come forth," he just arose and lived in the light again. He didn't live in the dying attitude that had held him in bondage.

"Behold, I stand at the door and knock: if any man hear my voice and open the door, I will come in to him and will sup with him and he with me." But *we* have to open the door.

To extend our vision, we must know that we do not live in this life without bread and still not starve. Yet there are many people who have bread and who are starving to death. I'd be ashamed to be in the position of some people who have money. I heard one lady say, "My husband has a heart of gold — and it's just as hard!"

Our Riches Are Within

It is the richness within that we have to rise to. This is what I wanted to bring you more than anything else.

We have a river of life given to us. Most people will put a bucket down the well with a rope that is too short, and that's as far as they ever get. So, they never drink from the living waters of life.

Many people are running after statues. Many people are running after churches. But I am wondering if we are looking for the right healing.

I can't help but think of an old Buddhist monk I saw over in India. I asked him about their religions, and he said, "There is just one God up there, but there is much activity down here." Wouldn't it be wonderful if all this activity were harmonized into Oneness?

But it isn't. We become obsessed with our status symbols. We are possessed by our possessions. We won't let them go — and they won't let go of us. We don't rise above our possessions. In the Sermon on the Mount Christ warned, "Do not lay up for yourselves treasures upon earth where moth and rust destroy, and where thieves break in and steal." If you released your attachment to these earthly things, you could find that your body would repair and rejuvenate itself. You would become whole again.

Learn To Look Within

We don't realize that the Divine Presence is in the midst of us. We don't realize what healing is until we know that there is a "peace and harmony" way to go.

How about our breath? Many people just think of the breath in their nostrils. They don't realize that when God breathed into the nostrils of man, man became a living soul. Do you realize that the living soul is more important than the air we breathe? If you think the breath in your nostrils is all there is, you have not found the real thing. Spiritual riches are as naturally ours as our breathing, and breathing goes with life.

We must try to rise above this life thing, this breathing thing.

You, Too, Can Rise

The Good Book says much about rising. "I will rise now and go about the city." "He maketh the sun to rise." "And the third day He shall rise again." "Why sleep ye? Rise and pray." "Rise, take up thy bed and walk." "He shall rise again to reign."

"Arise, shine; for thy light is come." What kind of light do we have? To rise to the kind of light we ought to have and let it shine, we have to rid ourselves of our old fears, old thoughts and old beliefs. Then we can come into the new.

I am convinced that we irritate and destroy ourselves by our thinking. If I told you that fifty percent of what you are thinking is causing you trouble, what would you say? According to researchers at a major university, one-third of a person's vocabulary causes destructive effects on the nervous system. Add to this the wrongful or malicious use of ordinary language, and we easily get fifty percent of our thinking as troublesome.

"He maketh a path to shine after him." Don't hide your light under a bushel. Let it shine! Some of us are afraid to let our light shine. Some of us don't have much light to shine with. But, let it shine, so it will light your path.

My mother used to say, "Give a man a light, and he will find his own way." We must have something to shine and to give forth to find our own good in life.

Wouldn't it be marvelous to just notify our face of all our good feelings and to let what we have shine forth? Arise and shine, for your light *has* come! Let your light so shine! His face did shine as the sun!

Positive Thinking Is Healing

We cannot go through life forever repeating the errors that cause unhappiness and sickness. We have to rise to the situation — otherwise we'll stay right where we are. It is very difficult to lift an inebriated man up from the gutter and get him walking. We try and try again. But when he can move under his own power, he finally gets up and goes. There are a lot of people who need to climb out of their stupor. They need to get up and start walking a different life. We can only do that when we arise and shine.

We need to free ourselves. It is time to reorganize our whole attitude, time to recognize and claim all the good that is ours. Unfortunately, we often limit ourselves in the good that we could accept. There is something within us all that knows wonderful things could come to us. That is why people go to yoga classes, change food, change thinking, change directions. That is why we are always looking for something to help us.

Once somebody saw the Christ coming through a crowd and thought, "If only I can touch the hem of his garment, I will be healed." There was only one person in that crowd who had that kind of faith. And when she touched the hem of his garment she was healed. We have to recognize that the Divine Self can change all things. You don't have to take my word for it. Thousands of experiments have been performed that have demonstrated that when the mind is changed, the chemistry of the body changes. Faith can work marvels.

The secret comes when we learn, "Blessed are the pure in heart for they shall see God." If we have resentment, rebellion and anger in our hearts, we don't see God because we can't see through those things. If we can see the pure, then God is right there, and we are seeing Him. God is purity. If we can hold to that and see it in every person and every thing, then we are on the godly path and we are going to have godly things working in us and through us.

This brings to mind a wonderful poem that has always meant a great deal to me:

My Creed

I would be true, for there are those who trust me.
I would be pure, for there are those who care.
I would be strong, for there is much to suffer.
I would be brave, for there is much to dare.

I would be a friend to all, the foe and friendless.
I would be giving and forget the gift.
I would be humble, for I know my weakness.
I would look up, and laugh, and love and lift.

— *Howard Arnold Walter*

This is another level to live in. It is time that we rise to another level of thinking, to another level of acting, to another level of shining. I see it in your face. It is coming already. I'm even afraid you are going to be well! I'm afraid that something good is going to happen to you!

Believe You Can Do It — And You Can!

Let us shine. Let us rise to the occasion. Let us take time out of our busy lives to go back into ourselves. We are interested in unfolding. We are interested in receiving higher thoughts. We are interested in making good lives for ourselves. We are interested in becoming better beings.

We recognize that all good will come to us. Let us recognize that our attunement and our at-one-ment with Him will make a better life flow within us, that God does for us as He does through us. Let us seek the higher values in life, that our life might be worthwhile, that joy and happiness might bathe every single cell of our bodies, that our lives might be bathed with the light that will bring on regeneration and rejuvenation.

Let us stand in absolute joy. Let us show that all is well. "Yea, though I walk through the valley of the shadow of death, I will fear no evil, for Thou art with me."

Let us rise to this feeling. Let us taste this joy. Let us feel. Let us hear. Let us extend our senses so we can hear the still small voice and respond to it. Let us know that this voice will never lead us astray.

Let us arise and shine. Our joy is shining. We wear a garment of joy today. And I see that all is well.

Friendly Voices

If you stand quite still in the heart of the
wood
You will hear many wonderful things;
The snap of a twig, and the wind in the
trees
And the whirr of invisible wings.

If you stand quite still in the turmoil of
life
And you wait for the voice from within,
You'll be led down the quiet ways of
wisdom and peace
In a mad world of chaos and din.

If you stand very still and you hold to
your faith
You will get all the help that you ask.
You will draw from the silence the things
that you need,
Hope and courage — and strength for
your task.

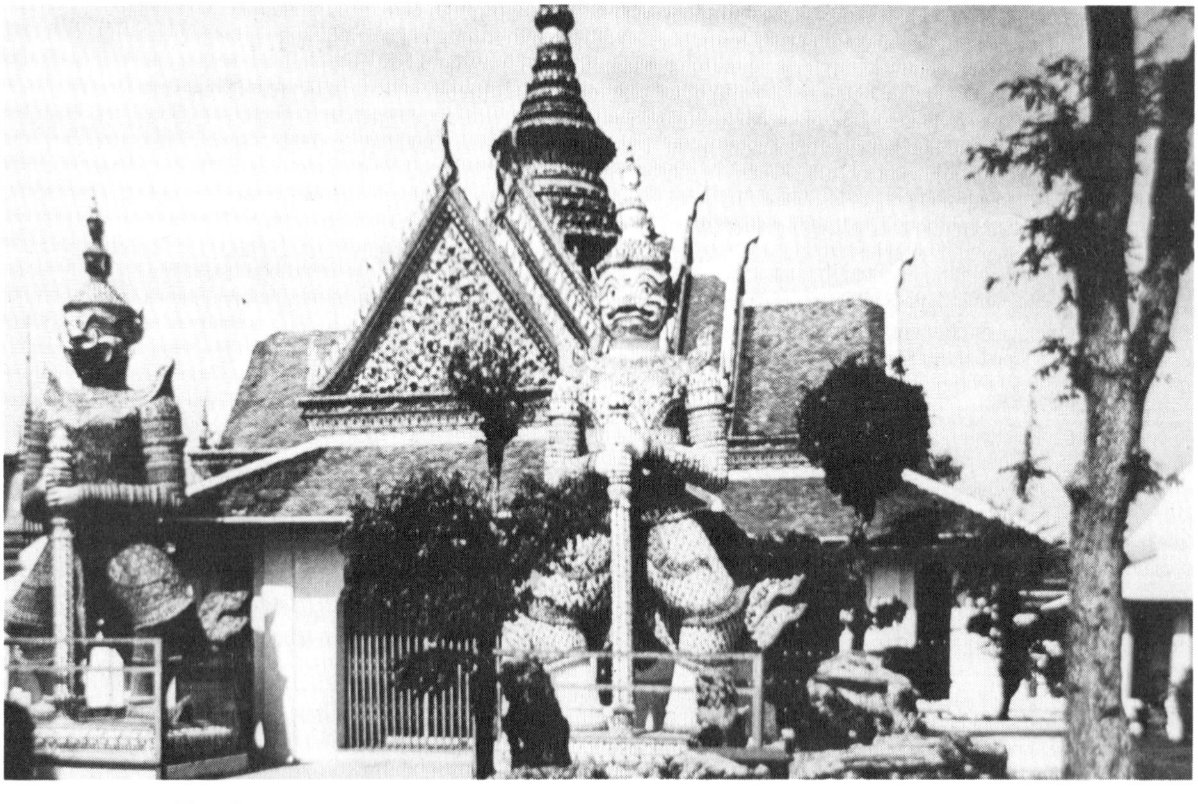

Temple of Thailand. The beauty is just unsurpassed. On the other hand, it is the spiritual thing behind it that tells us what the gesture is and the gesture, of course, is most important. Notice the "guardians of the gate." We also need to guard the gates of our consciousness and our joys.

Chapter 3

The Spiritual Aspect of Healing

If you try to deceive God, you deceive only yourself.

One of the most important discoveries that has emerged from my many years of work with thousands of patients — and from my own life as well — is that there is a spiritual dimension to healing. It simply is not enough to treat the disease; we must treat the whole person. The whole person involves more than body and mind. It is necessary to realize that we must treat the person from the spiritual aspect, too, if we expect healing to take place.

Today so many people are looking for a certain kind of therapy or a certain kind of doctor to make them well. Many people have never realized that spiritual truth is therapy. They spend a lot of time, a lot of money, just trying to find out how they can get well. They search far and wide, never thinking the solution might be just under their noses. Peace and harmony are such simple things. Perhaps only a few of us have come to understand that finding peace and harmony on the inside has a profound effect on the outside, the physical side of the person.

Let us begin to spiritualize our thinking. Let us learn how to reach deeply inside ourselves to bring a godlike expression to our living. Everybody needs love. Every *body* responds wonderfully to love. And we can only get the kind of love we need, the kind of love our bodies need, by seeking spiritual uplifting.

There are unseen things that can come to us through God, from God through nature, from God through people. We regard these things as mysteries. Man has yet to understand them, but we know they are very real.

We find that in each of us the physical, the mental and the spiritual are so closely related they appear as one. We find that in his essential nature man is one — one with God. We are able to reach a pinnacle of health through doing that which is right and that which has the approval of God more surely than when we try to depend on man's limited ideas.

There are many aspects to the art of healing. You have to take up not only the physical, mental and spiritual sides but the nutritional, mechanical, chiropractic, osteopathic, naturopathic, medical and surgical sides as well. We live in an age of specialization, as we all know. How do we put this all together?

When you think of all the arts and all the techniques that we have today, you realize there isn't any one art that serves man completely. You can't go through life just eating well and expect that to take care of everything. You can't be just spiritual and still expect to have a good body if you don't take time to eat and enjoy some of God's own foods, properly prepared.

The Spiritual Side of Healing

I am going to share with you some of the ideas and experiences that have come across my path in the last fifty years. Most doctors refer to what they do as a "practice." By now, I should know fairly well what ought to be done! I wish I had known what I know now fifty years ago. I could have helped people more.

Yet, God takes care of those things. Those people who were meant to see me at the start of my practice received what I could give them then and probably came only to get what I had at that time. But those who come to me now need to draw deeper from the well of healing than those who came to me at first. Of course, I still have patients who continue to come to me after all these years!

We can look at health from the perspective of a divine purpose so that we don't toil without direction in this life, so that we can get the best there is in this life and know that God will never let us down. Sometimes we have to take a little time out just to be aware of God.

A Look in the Mirror

Where do we get our inspiration? Where do we get our goals? Where do we go with our imaginations? What image do you hold of yourself in your mind's eye? Is it just Mr. America? Or, Miss America? Is it just muscles? Just physical beauty? Of course, I am exaggerating, but you know what I'm getting at. If we are caught up in only the physical level then we're going to have to dig a little deeper.

Imagine yourself outside the door of a great warehouse in which all that you could possibly want is being kept for you. All you have to do is knock, and that door will be opened to you. When it is opened, what will you seek? We have all come through the door to be in the room we are in now. What are we seeking? Christ said, "In my Father's house are many mansions." There are many rooms. As we go from one room to another, we should expect to find wonderful things.

What is beyond the river?

Sometimes we may get a little tense thinking about this life and its problems. I will try to loosen up some of the tightness. I will try to bring more relaxation. I *could* do it through massage. I *could* do it through adjustments. I *could* even do it through telling you to eat certain foods that bring relaxation to the body. But then you would be missing something.

You would be missing the greatest relaxation therapy there is, the spiritual side of life. The greatest relaxation we have is when we have peace and harmony with God, with our fellow man — with our family, our neighbors, our fellow workers, our employers. This peace and harmony always brings relaxation.

Tension Within Shows Without

Let's examine tension from a physical standpoint. First, realize that even as we talk we can have tension in our throat. We can have tension in our voice. You can tell when a person is tense through his voice. When a person is very tense, you can even tell it from his eyes.

Emotional strain produces physical tension. When we have tensions, all of the muscle structure of the body wears out more quickly. The cells of a tight muscle have to be repaired and rebuilt often. If we do not know how to wear this old world like a loose coat, we'll end up with no time to repair and rebuild.

Fatigue is found in all who are sick and ailing. Now, to get rid of tension is not an easy thing. We teach tension-relaxation exercises. You can take up yoga if you wish and you can take up meditation. But it would be good to know what to meditate on and in which direction to tune your mind. That person who has trained himself to let go, and to let the rest of the world take care of itself for a little while, takes care of himself through being still, through being quiet. And at this time his muscles and nervous system will begin to relax and to recuperate.

Every muscle tension first begins in the mind. Your hands and your arms have more to do with your head than you think. This may sound strange to you, but I mean exactly what

I say. You walk with your brain! You grab and you reach with your brain. You act from your brain and your muscles follow that which is in your brain.

If you are vindictive or malicious, you produce tension in the body. When you feel rejected, there is tension in the body. When hate and fear develop, they begin in the head first and then seep into the body like poisons.

There is an old saying that goes, "To hate a person means the same as to strike him." You only strike a person in hate, don't you? For your own good, you can't afford to strike people because you are doing it in tension. You are wearing yourself out. Even to give someone a piece of your mind, you have to give up your peace of mind. You are not going the harmony way; you are going the chaotic way. You're going the "fight" way. You are trying to get to your destination, but you are going the wrong direction. You have to change directions.

Looking At The Map Of Life

There is a right direction to go. I think if we can begin to see this, we really have something. For instance, kindness is a way to go. Courtesy is a way to go. Manners are a way to go. I have heard it said that having manners is like adding color to life. Manners set others at ease around you.

A man who is going the harmonious way knows that he cannot go through life and "get even" with people because to get even with people is to bring on tension and to create acids in the body, which can produce arthritis, rheumatism and joint troubles. I don't say that these things can only be produced with inharmonious thinking. I don't say that all our physical ailments come from fear acids. But I am convinced that our spiritual attitude can add to our physical good, the health of the whole person.

I don't care what church you go to. I don't care what books you read or what your personal faith is. There is a spiritual approach to this physical side of life which is good for us. It makes no difference whether you are Catholic, Jew, Protestant or Buddhist. If it is truth, any church would accept it. If it is truth, any church would like it. Your mind will like it. It is for this reason that you must have a spiritual approach to health in order to be well. Yes, I said *must*.

This is why I feel that the spiritual side of our physical healing must be examined. Maybe for the moment, you don't see it. You will. Maybe for the moment you don't have enough understanding or training. Maybe you haven't awakened to it. If I could be the one to awaken you to it, awaken it in you, or bring you a new thought, a new perspective, it would be a blessing to you, and you would be in better health. Then I would be doing the job I want to do. This is the only point I am trying to bring out — that is, I'm trying to bring a more relaxed life to you from this religious aspect.

What's On Your Mind?

When we have sickness in our lives, we need to look in other directions besides the physical. There is an attitude toward our work, an attitude toward our families, an attitude toward the ups and downs of life — and these attitudes can build or destroy. There is an attitude in the way we handle sickness. Here at the Ranch we have had so many who were despondent, blue, dejected; who feel left out, lonely, fearful; who even live in resentment, hate, anger and rejection. In all of these cases, when we moved them a little bit and eased them into better attitudes, their physical bodies changed for the better. As we change our consciousness and our level of thinking, the physical body comes along.

The change works both ways, of course. I notice that as the physical body improves, the mental attitude improves. The two are intimately related. We work not only from the spiritual side but also the physical. Each is only one aspect of the total healing of man.

You can't meditate with a toothache. You can't think sweet thoughts with a sour stomach. We must take care of the body physically as well. I feel there is a divineness in this creation as a physical body. It has been called the "Temple of the Living Soul." Many of us are making a mess out of this temple. Many of us don't know how to repair it. We don't even know what color bricks to use to repair this temple. We don't know what size the bricks should be. We don't know what we can digest. We don't know how much to eat. These are the bricks of life. These are bricks for building and rebuilding the temple.

That is what I'm trying to show you, to teach you.

I only see a temple beautiful for your physical body and I'm working for that. You must have a radiant temple. It was made spiritually and wonderfully. I want you to see that. I know the potential beauty there, and I know it can be brought out. Our attitudes affect not only ourselves but those around us. If you'd like to have some of my attitude rub off on you, be my guest! Let it do that. You are the receptacle for this because while it is the temple of the living soul, the living soul is in constant growth, reaching and searching for the finer things.

Your Body Uses What You Feed It

I don't think the cells in your body care whether you eat donuts and drink coffee. The body uses whatever you put in it to repair and maintain the body as well as it can. I believe it is only through soul growth, through your attitude, your religious view, your psychological view, your philosophy in life that you're going to make a better hand, the kind of hand that will reach for the better things in life. And if you don't reach for the better things in life, that hand will never be better. The physical life will never improve.

That is why it is necessary so often to come to the mind and start at the source of your troubles, the source of the problems. I am convinced that most of the glandular conditions start with our thinking. It is said that twenty percent of the women who are sterile in this country today have developed this condition from emotional strain. It is time that we begin to think about the emotions that we go through in our daily lives. Fear can cause physical trouble. I learned that years ago, and I also learned this: It feels good to feel good.

There are passages in the *Bible* that describe the countenance of certain men as being so bright that the people could not look upon their faces. For example, when Moses came down from Mount Sinai with the stone tablets containing the ten commandments, his face was so radiant that the people had to turn their eyes from him. We hear people being described as having a beautiful countenance, a soft countenance, a hard countenance, a poor countenance. Don't ever let anyone point at you and say, "There goes a poor soul." Our countenances reveal to a great extent the state of our physical and spiritual well-being. Our countenance reveals what is going on inside us.

The inside is the most important. We express from the inside to the outside. I am convinced beyond a shadow of a doubt that we live on what we give forth. What you have on the inside is going to make your body repair itself or destroy itself, regenerate or break down, whichever you choose. You have the choice. What happens on the inside of your body is your responsibility and yours alone. This day you will choose. This moment is the beginning of the rest of your life. Not what happened yesterday. Yesterday is dead. Don't try to revive it. Not what is going to happen tomorrow. Tomorrow has not yet been born. We can't do anything about what is not yet in existence. Let's not try to live our yesterdays and our tomorrows so that we spoil today. There are so many walking through life letting their yesterdays and their tomorrows destroy their bodies. They are not living fully *now* and they cannot be harmonious, loving people. You have to love people. You don't have to love what they do, but you have to love people.

One day a very great man was praying to God. He had been unjustly attacked by certain people in a very unpleasant sort of way, and in his prayer he said, "God, I'm finding it impossible to love these people. I just can't do it. I just can't feel any love in my heart for them." Then he thought for a moment and said, "But, maybe, God, you could love them through me."

Manners Are Like Colors

As we mentioned before, our manners are like colors. Colors of certain hues either pick you up or let you down. They can make you feel elated or depressed. I have heard it said that we should never eat in a blue room. Blue depresses the appetite. A yellow room will bring joy to us and our friends. Children have favorite colors. Adults have a special fondness for a sportcoat or dress of a certain color. Wearing these clothes makes you feel a certain way, a way you like to feel. Color is very important. In the same way, manners flavor and color life.

There is a club for men in Los Angeles that requires its new members to complete a course

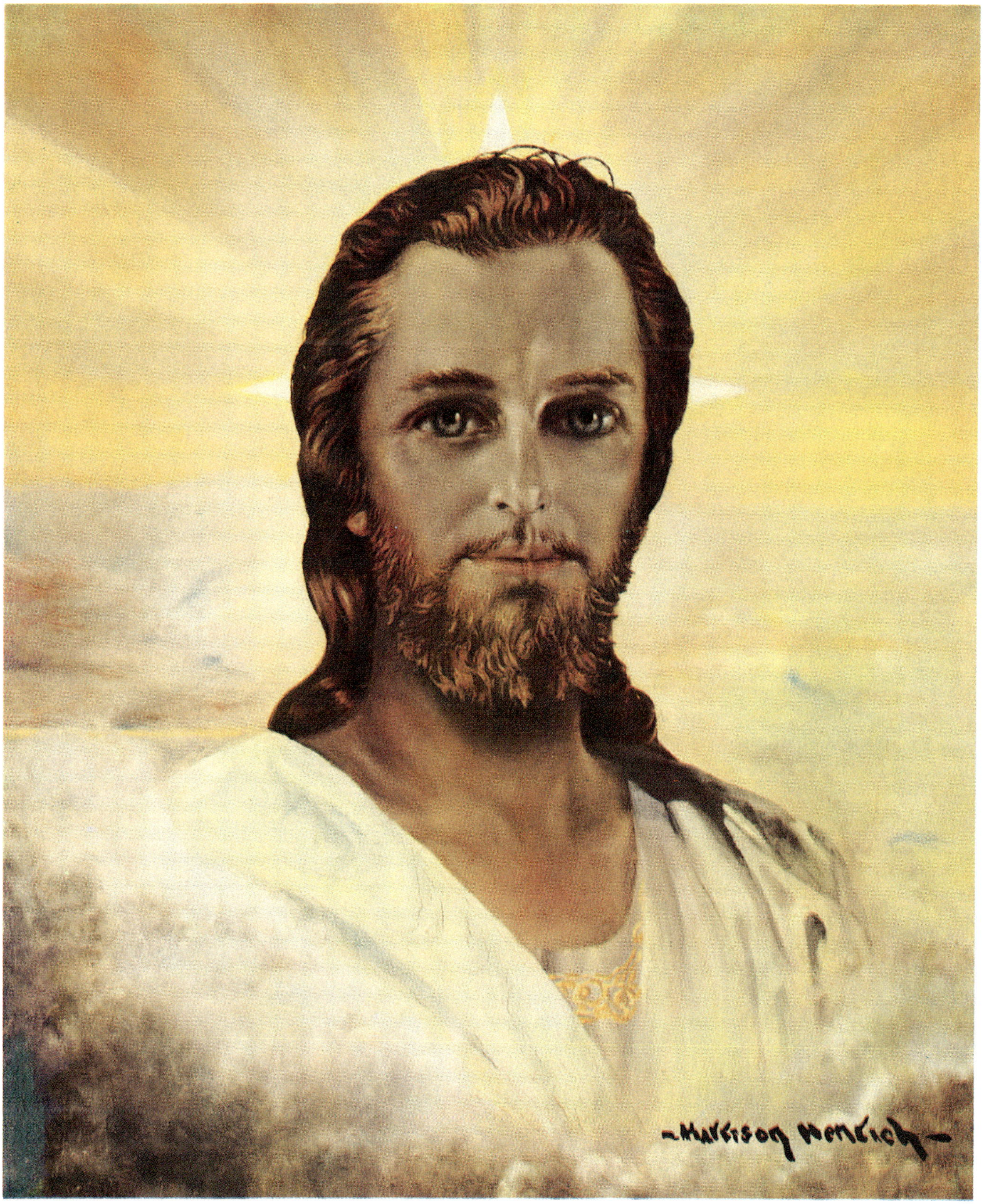

Artist Harrison Henrich titled this painting ***The Great Healer—Christ, the Man.*** *While in Europe studying under several great art masters, the American-born painter was inspired to do this great picture of the Christ. Henrich, who died in 1944, left behind paintings of many prominent people including William Jennings Bryan, John D. Rockefeller, Pope Pius IX, Porfirio Diaz and others. This original hangs in Dr. Jensen's library.*

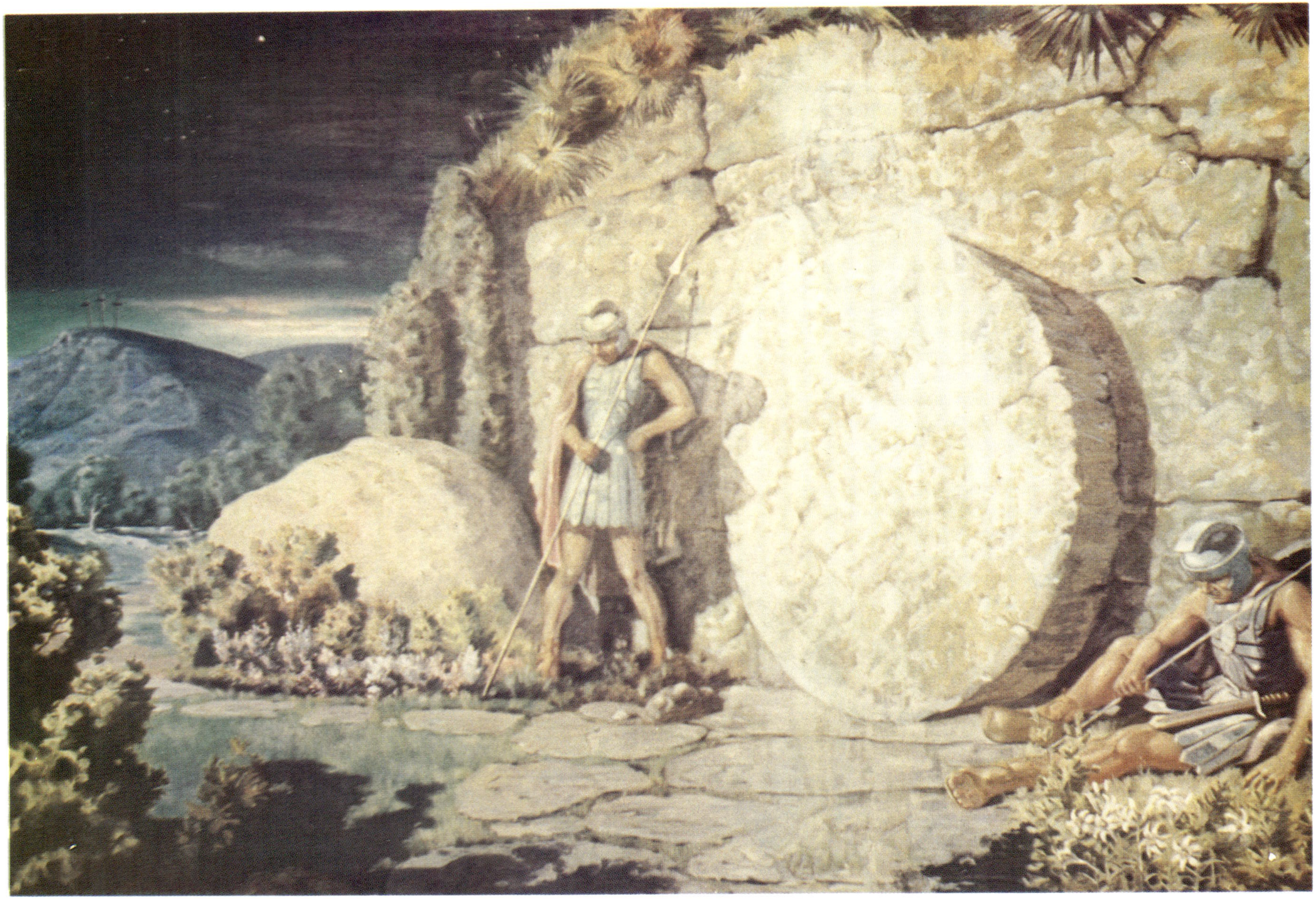

I want you to look at this picture . . .here is my tomb . . .I was locked inside. I was buried... because I have ways "Ye know not of . . .and I go to prepare a place for you. I came forth unto my Father through all circumstances of life, death and hell, and . . ."

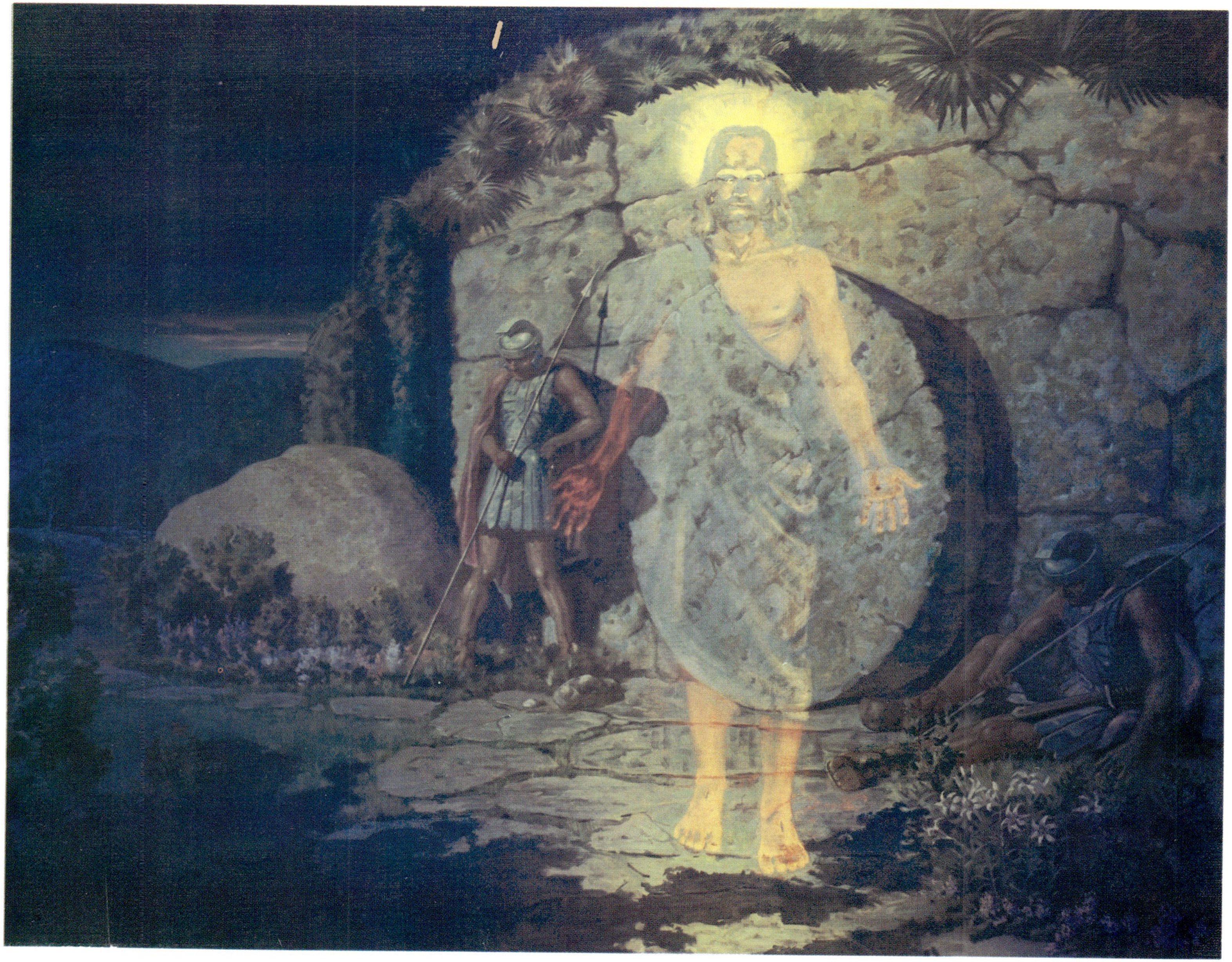

On the third day I arose again as I promised you I would do. Though you doubted me showing myself to you, I nevertheless did this for those who would like to follow and arise again and go to Father Consciousness and realize that I go continually unto my Father. My resurrection was accomplished before you that you may do likewise and know that at any moment, any place, all is well as long as you realize my teachings that when we become one with the Father, "All is well...."

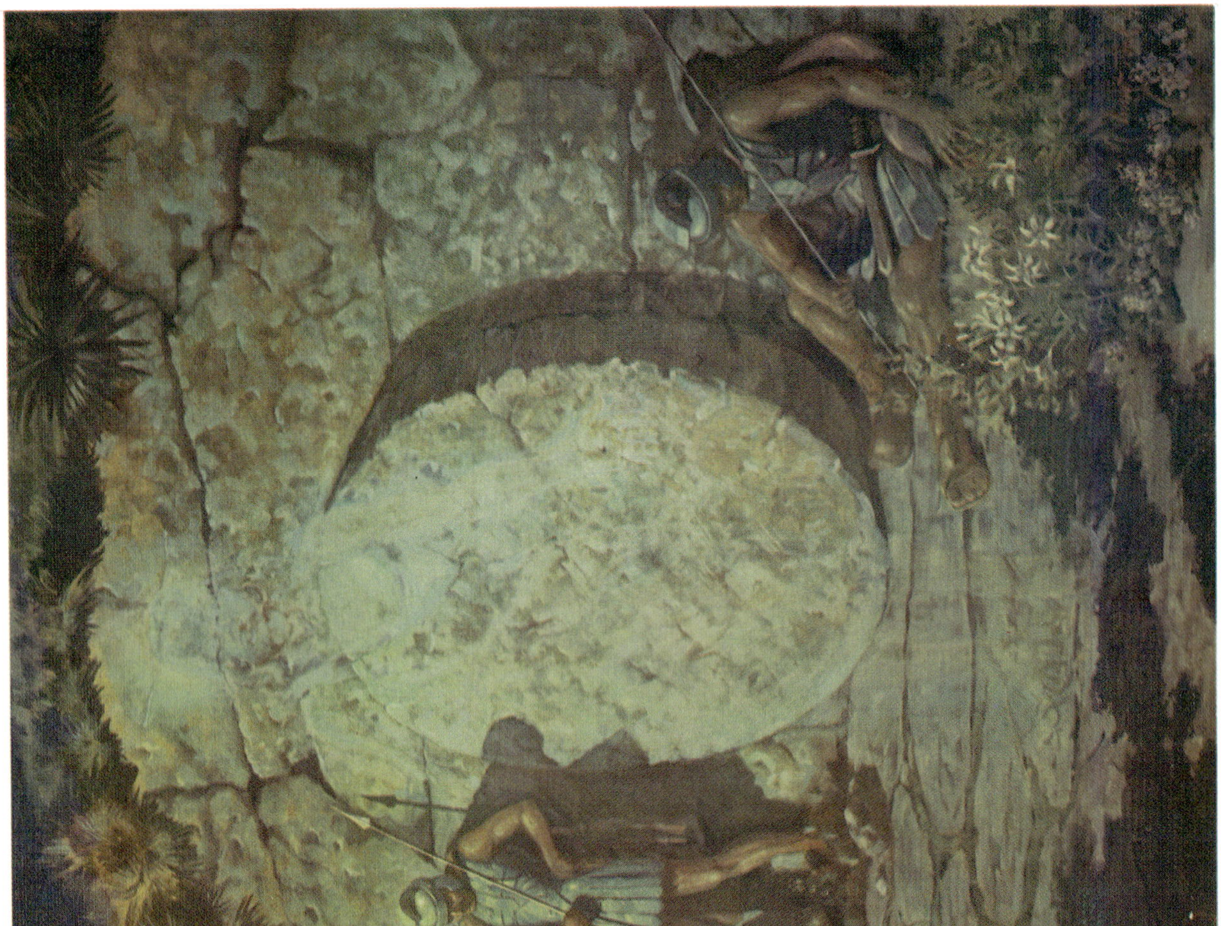

of instruction in table etiquette before they are allowed to eat with the other members. Your manners have to be just so. You have to know how to pull the artichoke leaves apart and fold them around the plate in a neat circle. You have to eat spaghetti a certain way, hold the knife a certain way, use the napkin just so. These men enjoy etiquette, and gobblers and slurpers are not allowed. One sloppy eater would break the harmony in this room, like a splash of gray or brown on a rainbow.

So we color our lives with our manners. We color our lives with our attitudes. Mother taught me — and this is so true — that our *attitude* is our *altitude* in life. If you want to get out of your physical troubles, you will have to raise your mind to a higher level of thinking, because the mind and the body, as I have been pointing out, work together.

This lowering of spirit or attitude adds another complication to the physical problem. It compounds the trouble. A person who lets this happen will have two problems, the initial problem itself and the new one brought on by the mental attitude. A vicious circle begins. Above all, we must never allow the will or the imagination to become negative. If the imagination alone becomes negative, it will drag the will down with it, for in my experience the imagination is much more powerful than the will. That which you imagine in life will come forth.

That's why we hear and read so much about "outpicturing" from spiritual teachers. When we picture certain things in our minds, we can hold to that picture and express it more effectively than we can by using sheer willpower. If you have a picture clearly fixed in your mind, all the will in the world will never move you. You find out that what you have uppermost in your imagination, the image, that is the most important thing.

Don't Accept Less Than Perfection

You are created in the image of God. So don't allow your will or imagination to take you to any lesser place. I want you to understand this. God is perfect. You've got to see yourself in that perfection or you'll never get out of where you are.

Repeat to yourself, "I must be getting better. I certainly *am* better." With this attitude you can gain altitude. You can go up. Aren't you thinking better thoughts? Aren't you striving for better things? Aren't you doing better today than you were yesterday?

I learned early in life that it isn't trying to make things happen that works. The secret is letting the good life flow through you so the body has a good time. Give your body a good time. Give it a chance to heal. This is where the healing will come from, through spiritual truth as well as through foods and through the physical things.

It is only in the past few years that the Church of England has been formally allowing healing. We should be able to go to our churches for healing. Why should the churches just be interested in our souls from eleven a.m. to noon on Sundays? That's like the lady who said, "I had a salad last week, and it didn't do me a bit of good." Living our religion only one hour a week is not the answer. What do you do on Monday from eleven a.m. to noon? On Tuesday? What about the rest of the hours in your day?

It isn't what you do once in a while that counts. It's what you do most of the time. So spiritual truth is a matter of daily living. It's a flowing thing, a pouring forth, a matter of your attitude coming through your hands so that the hands have a good time, renewing themselves faster than they are breaking down.

I heard a story one time about faith. A ship struck a submerged obstacle and was sinking rapidly. The captain herded the passengers together and asked, "Is there a minister here, or someone with a lot of faith?" One man replied, "I have a lot of faith." The captain said, "Good. We're short one life raft, and you'll have to get along on your faith."

I like that little story about faith and the sinking ship, because faith really can function as a life raft in an emergency. It is more than that, of course, but it can save our lives in times of crisis. What is faith? It is said that faith is a substance. A substance? Now, the cloth of my suit is a substance. The wood of my chair is a substance. The flesh of my body is a substance. Do you believe that faith is a substance? The *Bible* says, "Faith is the substance of things hoped for, the evidence of things not seen." That is faith. I can feel cloth, wood, the physical body; but I can also feel joy, love and satisfaction. These have substance to me. So does faith.

Faith is getting hold of something—*something*. It is said, "Faith is the substance." You can get hold of a substance. You can get hold of faith. And if you can do that, it will carry you through crises, through troubles and problems, even through "the valley of the shadow of death." You will have something because faith is substantial, it can be grasped, felt. Following the words of the Bible quotation, "Faith is the substance of things," are the words "hoped for," meaning *yet to come*. Faith is the substance of the future, our future in the making. To me, that is a wonderful thing.

We need have no fear for what is yet to come when we live by faith. So we are going to live in this wonderful moment. The future can't even come yet. It is unborn—but we know when we arrive there, and we will live in good substance.

Strive For Mental Maturity

When premature babies are born, they must have oxygen. They must have certain formulas and they must have extra care. I don't want a premature moment. I want a mature moment. I want a moment that is good and clean and I want to be ready for it. You're never going to get a mature moment if you go through life too hastily. That's what gives birth to premature moments. If you prepare yourself, you are going to be ready for everything that comes. If you bring it up too much ahead of time, you won't be ready for it.

"Faith is the substance of things hoped for, the evidence of things not seen." It's difficult when you come to the phrase, "the evidence of things not seen." It's hard when you realize you've got to believe in something you're not going to see yet. But everything is going to be seen in its time. Faith starts at the mental level, reaches into the spiritual level and seeks out the truth. There isn't a thing that we won't be able to see in time.

Let good conquer evil. Give blessings, not curses. That is how we prepare ourselves to meet the future moment. We have to have an equal regard for one another. Don't be too ambitious. This is a health rule! Don't blow this moment to pieces! The person who is too ambitious kills himself.

Living The Higher Law

Be at peace with all men. That is something to think about, isn't it? We don't seek vengeance by our own hands. The Good Book says, " 'Vengeance is mine; I will repay,' saith the Lord." Vengeance belongs to the Lord or the Law. Don't you know that judgment comes to the person who doesn't do the right thing? Let the Law take care of it. Now, we are talking about Law with a capital "L" in this case. According to God's Law, we get back what we give forth from our lives. Those who live by the sword shall die by the sword.

The Law will take care of all things. We are not to take justice into our own hands. We are not even to judge others, according to the Good Book. God does that through the Law. Don't you try to be a law of retribution, a law of harm and disaster, unto yourself. Live within the Law, but don't go around inflicting your interpretation of the Law on others *You live the Law,* and realize that the Law knows better than you what others need and how they are to receive it. Often people have to hit bottom before they realize there is such a thing as "up."

The person who kills will suffer more than the one killed. He will have the real suffering. Have you ever felt sorry about what you've done? I am sure you have! There is sorrow, there is regret, there is despair — and these are terrible forms of suffering. I mention these only as examples of the kinds of retribution that Divine Law may inflict on those who walk the path of violence on the lower plane, until they learn to look up. I mention them so that we may know that vengeance and judgmentalism are not for us. They, too, are of the lower plane. It may be hard to break old habits of anger, fear, distress, sorrow, regret and despair, but we must realize they are unhealthy for us. They have no place in us as we seek the higher things. When they come, we must let them go quickly.

When we go the uplifted way, are we vindictive? No. Are we malicious? No. Are we destructive? Are we chaotic? Do we have a fighting manner? No. We choose to have good manners, lovely bright-colored manners. We choose to work hard toward the better things with the finer substances of life.

Let the justice of God take its own toll in its own way. We are going to have peace with our bodies when we have peace with our minds. If we are going to have peace with our neighbors, we must have peace within our own minds. If we are going to have peace with our arms, legs or any of the parts of our bodies, peace first has to come into our minds. The mind is the bridge between the spiritual and the physical.

Let's Be Good To Ourselves

I am convinced that our minds often get in our way. If your mind is not uplifted and inspired, it can be your worst enemy. It can be an enemy to your own health and your own world. Why shouldn't we let it be our friend? Be good to yourselves today. Be good to everybody, and when you are good to everybody, you are good to yourself as well. When you're good to yourself, you'll be better to your family — better to your husband, better to your wife, better to your children and better for the work that is yet to come.

Be good to yourself through your mind. Let it go to the spiritual things that tell you all is well, all is good, that "I am with you always, even unto the end of the world."

We realize that the spiritual aspect is only one therapy which we use, only one part of what is necessary for the body. Let us realize that we cannot do without it. May each and every one of you go your way blessed. This is my wish for you.

Just one more thought: A retired business executive was once asked the secret of his success. He replied that it could be summed up in three words: *And then some*. "I discovered at an early age," he said, "that most of the differences between average people and top people can be explained by these words. The top people did what was expected of them — and then some. They were considerate and kind — and then some. They met their obligations and responsibilities — and then some. They were good friends to their friends — and then some. They could be counted on in an emergency — and then some."

His philosophy for success in life certainly comes close to what Jesus was saying when He talked about going the second mile and giving your cloak also to a man who asks for your shirt.

It is God's way. He always blesses us with as much as we need—and then some!

TRY IT!

From the Doctor's Study . . .

MIND OVER BODY

Queen Elizabeth, during a trip to the United States, came into the Pediatrics Cardiac ward of a hospital to visit the children. A number of these children were wired to electronic vital sign monitors, and one little fellow's heart, beating at 70 beats per minute, jumped to 130 beats when he saw the Queen. What is it that brings a blush to a girl's cheeks when she receives an unexpected compliment? What brings the sudden chill and trembling to a jungle traveler when a tiger leaps on the path in front of him? Emotions clearly have their effects on the chemistry, tissues and organs of the body. Stress or anxiety can cause the skin to perspire. The pupil of the human eye dilates when it sees something pleasant and contracts when it sees something unpleasant. During a long period of stress, some people develop a skin rash. Chronic worry can cause ulcers. Soothing music can act as a sedative. Because the mind exercises such strong influence over the body, we have to take care that what we put into our eyes, ears and minds brings positive benefits both to mind and to body.

Chapter 4

The Joy World

Strength without a joyful heart
does not exist...
You only have strength with
joy in your heart.

Many years ago I started out with my physical work — working with the spine and working with the physical body's need for nutritious foods and so forth. Then, failures came along to rock my boat, to disturb me, to awaken me. Some of my patients failed to respond to treatment the way I expected. Now many times, things which come along to disturb us bring important lessons in life. So, in those days I sometimes wondered whether there was something wrong with me and my training or whether there was something wrong with my patients' responses.

What Can You Feed A Malnourished Mind?

I began a search, trying to find out what the problem was. I probed within myself to try to understand what was wrong in other people. I began to discover that there were many problems that had to be taken care of besides physical adjustments and improper diets. I discovered there was food for the mind and food for the soul as well as food for the body. People sometimes have malnourished minds or overweight attitudes. People sometimes have malnourished souls — even to the verge of starvation. I finally realized that people needed something besides just the food on the table.

I learned that it is not so much the kind of food that goes into a person that matters, but the kind of person the food goes into. I found that it wasn't always a matter of physical things but sometimes the unseen things, the intangible things, the unexpected things that bothered a person to the extent of producing a distraught condition and acute indigestion. I realized that I would have to search for ways to deal with several levels of the person.

Through the help and suggestions of teachers and others, I decided to approach this from the spiritual standpoint.

As I began to explore the spiritual level of life I found new levels of meaning in some of the old truths. For many people seeing is believing. But I found something further — that believing is, or can be, seeing. Many people want a demonstration before they will believe. If we believed first, we wouldn't need a demonstration. We would be satisfied. I have found that many of the beliefs we have, we live on. Our beliefs determine our reality to a very great extent. People who believe in a lie, live a lie. You have to believe in something that is very, very good to be able to reach the good life and the good of life. That is why we must be very careful about our beliefs — full of care about choosing them and living them. If you want to live in peace and harmony, you have to believe in something that can give you peace and harmony.

All Truth Comes From The Same Fountain

Now, the truths of life come from many different sources, many different religions, many different churches. I want you to go to your own church. I want you to go into your own beliefs and I want you to go into the truth that you carry in your life and believe in. It will help you be well.

Bringing out the spiritual values helps us in our healing work. I feel that truth makes us free. So do as your freedom dictates to you. And above all, don't believe that I am the one to follow. I don't want anyone following me. We must follow the truth. The spiritual values are so impersonal that it makes no difference which church you belong to. I just want you to be a better person in your own church.

People in our society need an awakening. If it came to them, if it was broad enough, then this whole nation would be uplifted. People everywhere would be stimulated to live a better life. The churches would be filled to overflowing.

Where Is Our Church?

I feel that church is within us. If it isn't, what could you get inside a church? It is within yourself that you are going to make the final growth — that you are going to do something for yourself. We go into a church on Sunday because inside the church we go inside ourselves. We may forget to do that most days of the week. As we awaken to the truth we are shown, we will go inside more and more. This is what I feel we should realize from a health standpoint and a healing standpoint. There is a "withinness" we have to care for. It is this "withinness" that will lead us to the higher levels, to new worlds.

My teacher used to say, "What we are deepest, we really are." Have you ever been deep inside yourself? Have you ever gone really deep? Have you closed your eyes and gone back into your own being?

Many people are looking for a joy world "out there." "If I were only married, I'd be happy." "If only I had money, I'd be happy." Well, look at the people who are married and unhappy. Look at the people who have money and are unhappy. No, that is not the way.

While I was in Switzerland many years ago, I spoke to a Communist, an officer in the Russian army. I asked him what his goal was. He said, "If everyone could have a radio in Russia, we'd be happy. If everyone could have an automobile, we'd be happy. It's this happiness we want." And then I began to think. In the United States we have all this. At least the majority do. Yet, are we happy? Well, where does happiness come from? Is the happiness in the thing, or is it in the appreciation? Do you buy appreciation? Does it come in bottles? Is it a thing you develop? Is it always just over the next hill, or on the other side of the fence? Appreciation is something that you practice and work with until you finally put a praise on things. Then you have an appreciation for them.

Appreciation is an attitude and it comes from values within. The soul seeks the good and seeks to express its own good. It does this by working through the mental and the physical, relating its values to the mental attitudes, the mental values. Appreciation is one of those values which, when applied to the right things, is both food for the soul and an outward expression of the soul. Joy is another of these qualities.

Beyond the Power of Words

I think that joy is one of the highest, most precious expressions of life. It lies beyond the power of words to describe or explain. We can live in joy from the contemplation of what is yet to come, yet, unless we are grounded in truth, joy can be spoiled through expecting too much or the wrong thing, and then reaching a disappointment. Joy which awaits its time, its place, its true objects, is never spoiled.

If I could take negative expectations away from my patients, I would also take many disappointments away from them. With fewer disappointments, they would experience more joy.

There are also too many false expectations. There are people expecting something great to happen on July the 2nd at two o'clock, and it never happens. They remind me of the little girl who prayed every day for a horse for Christmas. When Christmas arrived, there was no horse. Her brother said, "Well, you see, God didn't hear your prayers." She replied, "Maybe He did. Maybe He just didn't want me to have a horse." To make joy depend on the external world, on external objects, is mistaken.

What do you expect? Something for yourself? Is it for your physical pleasure or for something within? Do you really want the material thing on the outside? Is that the only way you can express or receive your joy?

Some people must be flooded with gold before they can believe they are happy. But they find as the gold goes their happiness goes with it. Any potential threat to their gold makes them miserable. Remember the story of King Midas and his golden touch? He believed that gold could bring him joy but it became a curse on his life.

We should seek treasure of the eternal kind not the temporal kind. Joy that is spiritual is permanent because it comes from the inside out not the outside in. This kind of joy will carry you through thick and thin, through troubles and problems, even through those walls you say you can't break through. If you have a joy within, you can take care of any problem! Who doesn't have problems? Children have problems with their parents. Parents have problems with their children. These problems have to be faced—and sometimes facing our problems is an even bigger problem. But with the light of joy shining in us, we can find our way through the darkest valleys of our lives.

Take Care Of Your Problems Today

If the problem is ahead of you, it is the unborn thing. Some people become so concerned about this unborn thing that they develop physical ailments. Most of the people who come to me have people problems. They come into my office to say, "My mother did this, my father did that, my children won't do so-and-so, my landlord does such-and-such, my wife gives me a pain in the neck, my husband makes me sick to my stomach." They are all people problems. If they would take better care of themselves and leave worrying about other people behind, they would be in better health.

We make a problem out of facing problems. You must meet problems. You can't run away from a problem, because unless you have learned the lesson it has come to bring, it will find you again where ever you run. My mother used to say, "If you don't take care of your problems now, you'll have to wake up tomorrow to take care of them again." A problem is going to get to you sooner or later. The best thing is to face it and then put it behind you.

How do we do this? It takes practice. You don't love well unless you practice love. You don't overcome things unless you practice overcoming. You don't face problems well until you move yourself in front of them and confront them. You don't learn to overcome your fear of water and learn to swim unless you start overcoming and swimming. The more you practice swimming, the more you overcome your fear of the water. Once you overcome something, you let go of it — and it lets go of you.

When you once overcome your fear, whether it is swimming or people or problems — it doesn't matter what it is — once you have let go of it, you have reached that point where joy is possible. This is the most wonderful point in the world for your well-being. You will be well when you are joyful.

If we could only see this marvelous body wearing away and renewing itself we would be inspired. You are building new skin on the palms of your hands every twenty-four hours. Just think of that. But if you want *better* skin, you will have to provide better nutrients, better care, for the inside from within and develop outward, just as happiness and joy must come from within and work their way out.

Let's Face Tomorrow With Joy

In order for me to help nature heal you, I have to help you find a way to change the kind of person you are within. The kind of person you are within must go forth in joy. You must learn to meet problems with joy. You must learn to face tomorrow with joy. I mean you have to go forth with a joyful attitude. We have to learn to express peace and joy even throughout the changing chaos and tumult of civilization. We have to make our peace with change.

I remember the time when there were no radios. I was working with the first radios ever built. I took a *Quaker Oats* box, wrapped copper wire around it, got a little cat whisker and put on some silica. I'd slip into my pair of earphones and listen for hours, trying to pick up some music coming out of the air. It brought me joy to finally hear that music. The invention of radio meant change, and change will always be in the air. We must learn to live with it.

When the first airplane flew over our home I ran outside to see it. It was a joy to watch it make its way across the sky and to listen to that motor growl and purr. Something about it seemed alive! Something had to be actually holding that plane up in the air! I felt real suspense for a moment. Would it fall? How was it possible that it could stay up there in the sky? What a marvelous thing! What marvelous things man has accomplished to be able to keep airplanes in the air, not to mention sending men to the moon in rockets!

Today we turn the radio or TV off when we tire of it. We frown and go inside the house when a noisy airplane — usually a jet — approaches overhead. I am exaggerating a little bit. But I think you can see the point. We grow used to those earthly wonders that once gave us joy. There was a day when we used to ride in Model-T Fords at twenty miles an hour, and that was very fast for those days. Recently I drove to Santa Ana, California to give an evening lecture, and when I started from the Ranch I only had an hour to get there. I had to almost fly down that freeway to make it on time — but I made it. When I arrived I started to remove my hands from the steering wheel, and do you know, my fingers seemed glued to it! I couldn't move my hands! They were actually stuck to that steering wheel by the tension, the strain and stress of freeway driving.

I remember a time when we went riding, and the car would go so slowly that we would sing along the way. You can't sing today when you drive. You have to concentrate every minute. You have to watch what you're doing. Today there is humming on the freeways, but it comes from tires, not people.

There is a definite tension, strain and stress in the atmosphere today. But we must try to find peace in it. I can't say that the day of freeways and high-speed auto travel is coming to an end. There may still be more to come. But if you don't learn to relax and accept change, there is every possibility that there won't be enough doctors to take care of all the sick people.

Will You Be Among The Survivors?

Sometimes I wonder where all the problems are coming from — but then again, I think I know. Our civilization hasn't gone along with a song in its heart. People are so rushed they haven't the time to recuperate, to develop a better life, to discover the joy world that longs to be awakened inside them.

The moment some aspect of civilization starts crowding people, they start a resentment program or a resistance program. One of the first casualties is joy, and close behind it is peace. And who suffers the most because of the resistance and resentment? Those who resist and resent. You can't afford to join their program or you will be killing yourself like they are.

I can tell you sincerely that joy will never kill anyone. Instead, joy will save you. You have to find this joy within yourself. In fact, joy, in its own special way, is something like a broom. Once you open your mind and your heart to it, it begins sweeping troubles and problems away — from the inside out. What comes to replace them? More joy!

Who enjoys being miserable? Who enjoys being dejected? Who enjoys being depressed or blue? There is a story about a minister, one of whose parishioners, Mrs. Jones, would visit him regularly and carry on for hours about her troubles, aches, pains and her latest illness. One day as he was hurrying along a downtown street, he rounded a corner and bumped into Mrs. Jones and several of her friends. Caught by surprise, he blurted out, "How nice to see you, Mrs. Jones! Are you still enjoying ill health?"

Of course, we come to realize that people don't like to be around us when we're miserable. Be honest, now. Do you actually like to be that way? No, you don't. We must understand that whatever you have within yourself goes into the lives of others, so when you are around others, you owe them the very best you have in you.

Let's Be The Best We Can Be

When a young fellow is courting his girl, he tries to look his best. She puts on her prettiest dress when he comes over. He brings her candy or flowers. They both want to look and behave their very best. Why shouldn't we be at our very best all the time? I see people invite their friends over and put out the nicest silverware and their prettiest things. Then when the company is gone — it's back to the old things again.

We have a chance to be rich, to live richly, and we should live that way all the time. Find the joyful path. Those who are not seeking joy in their lives are not opening themselves to the richest and best in life. They have closed and locked the door, so to speak. Joy is still outside. If you are a joy seeker, then you will leave these people alone, you will let them learn their lessons until they decide for themselves to unlock their door and let joy enter. You have to let a person search for the place where he or she can find joy.

Joy is essential to health. It has a vibratory effect on the inside. But it evades us when we aren't open to it. A wife may say, "Darling, you're killing yourself with the things you're doing." A husband may say, "Those friends you're running around with are tearing you to pieces." Haven't you heard such things before? Some activities keep us from joy, and we must let go of these.

"My, you look beautiful this morning!" A friend says. "Oh, I just had a wonderful talk with a friend of mine!" Someone tells you. These things are joy-spreaders. Why shouldn't your friends do something nice for you? And, what are you doing for your friends? Friendship and the activities it involves can be a wonderful door-opener for joy. You can't give joy away without it bouncing back to you!

You've got to remember that the communication we are talking about is a neglected art. We have to practice it. We have to be in a place ourselves where we can say kind and loving things and mean them sincerely. We don't go through our life meditating. We don't sit down to be quiet with ourselves for a few moments and say, "Well, now, I'd like to talk to you for a bit. What is it that you really want? Do you want peace and contentment?" We have to ask ourselves these things so that our communications with others come out of the best in ourselves.

Is there anyone who wants to resist peace and contentment? Is there anyone who doesn't like gratitude? Is there anyone who doesn't like the contemplation of something beautiful yet to come? These are inside faculties. You work with them on the inside.

Peace Within Or A Wreck Without

I am only bringing this out because if you can't be peaceful and kind to yourself on the inside, you're going to be a wreck on the outside. If you are living in the outer part of your body only, it will decay quickly. But the person who has a joyful spirit within has a healthy body.

"I feel wonderful this morning!" How is it possible to feel wonderful? Where do you think it started? Would you try to tell me that I feel wonderful just because my joints are healthy and active? Well, possibly there are people whose joints feel wonderful to them. Possibly there are people who breathe sixteen wonderful breaths each minute. But then you find that they have a mean husband or a nagging wife. Is everything physical? No, it is not.

If the spiritual part of your life is drab and doesn't bring you joy, I advise you to change it for the sake of your health. If you don't have contentment within you, then something is lacking, and you need to find it. If you can't find God or haven't looked, then you're missing the great joy and peace that comes from knowing Him. The reason I'm telling you to do this is that the kind of good that we find only in God and through God works from the inside out in each of us to help us get well and stay well.

I offer knowledge, and from this comes wisdom. But I can't force you to accept the good. I can't force you to be healthy. I can't force you to be happy and joyful. Nobody can. I can awaken you to this. That is what we have to see.

We once had a man at the Ranch with what is called a hiatus hernia. In other words, he had a pocket down inside his esophagus that sometimes trapped the food he tried to swallow. When this happened he had to regurgitate. He found that when he and his wife were not getting along with each other, or when she was nagging him, this contraction would come in the esophagus, which would hold the food, and he would have troubles. Do you know what advice I gave him? I told him to "get lost" from his wife. I told him to get lost from his family for a while.

What do you do in a case like this, where the wife or the husband is working against the one who has the problem? Do you advise divorce? No. But you must advise reasoning together. You tell the person to lay his whole inner self right out on the table and say, "This is what my problem is, and this is what my doctor advises me to do. Now, we must get together on these things." We must cope with whatever aggravates the condition. We have really, just gradually, built up a bodily tension, a threatening feeling, so that physical conditions are worsened by the foods we eat and the air we breathe.

Without a spiritual and mental philosophy there is no use trying to treat the physical problem today.

Back in 1900 people spent most of their money on food. Today we spend ten to twelve percent of our income on food. We are spending more money on our environment — automobiles, houses, appliances, clothes, shoes and many other things. We are fortunate to have all of this — in a way. In a way we are not. If we become caught up in the spiral of never getting enough, of always wanting more, more, more, then we are in hot water.

People have increased their consumption of alcohol. There are more alcoholics than there used to be. There is an increasing problem with drug abuse. Many nursery school supervisors say that the three- and four-year-old children sent there by working parents have been given tranquilizers to keep them quiet all day. The children are a side-line, a business to these people. They are not part of the family. The rearing of children in our society is poor, and most of us just escaped the type of treatment of children we see going on today.

Accept Joy Whenever It Appears

The world of troubles and illness is the same world in which we find and express joy — the joy world. There are lessons to learn; we are learning them. There are things to work out; we are working them out. We are in this world — but we don't need to be of this world. We can arise to a new level, and from there we experience the joy world. We accept joy whenever it appears.

Can you understand what I'm trying to bring out here? I'm not talking about going on a spiritual search for holiness so that we forget the physical body. The physical body is a counterpart of the spiritual. We are on this earth for a purpose. This body is the temple of the living joy I have been talking about. We should be able to express this living joy in a good healthy attitude at the physical level. We should be ready to accept all the joyful things that come to us.

Why should we try to be joyful with sore knees? Why should we try to be joyful when we have an ulcer? It becomes a physical, a mental and a spiritual process. This is what I have learned over the years. There are people with lung trouble, with heart trouble, who bring on these ills with stress and strain. One of every seven people is taking tranquilizers. Is this living with joy? No. If we hold on to our anxieties they will kill us, but pills are not the answer. The *Bible* says, "Resist not evil." It says, "If a wise man contendeth with a foolish man, whether he rage or laugh, there is no rest." In the resisting of evil, the contending with the foolish, we set up tension and stress. Christ did not war with the devil. He just peacefully said, "Get thee behind me."

Now, can you see this thing? Why should I have to take care of people who are resisting, contending, fighting, to the point that the negative things of the world have dragged them to the level of disease? Go peacefully and leave fear behind. You may be worn out. You may be weary from the struggle. Stop it. Stop struggling. I am treating tired people. You can get your energy back. You can have it by just being joyful.

The Secret Of Finding Joy

Joy is a substance. It is a mental quality. What is this quality called joy? "He went forth with joy." What did he have? What did it look like? How big is it? Is it yellow? Green? Does it come in a bottle? Where can you buy it?

Joy is nothing more or less than an extension of your own understanding. When you really understand, you will have joy. Understanding is found within. And when you expand this understanding, you begin to do what? The nicest way I can think of to put it, although a bit difficult, is that you *appropriate* joy. You claim joy. You accept joy. You take joy because it is already yours. There is enough joy for everyone to appropriate. Joy is not just limited to this person or that person. There is so much joy that, to use a physical example, it is like pouring a little oil in water, for it will cover the entire surface. As you appropriate joy and express joy, it multiplies and expands. You can feed the 5000 and have 12 baskets left over, to use a biblical comparison.

Spiritual joy is for everybody. Nobody owns it. You can't buy it. It isn't like a material thing.

The joy I have is the joy I want you to have. My joy is for each one of you to use, but it must be shared to hold its value. It doesn't belong to me. There is a fleeting moment when it comes through my mind, a fleeting moment — just imagine it, like a flying saucer flashing through my mind at some incredible speed — it is called joy.

What a crime it would be if this beautiful thing called joy passed through your mind and you missed it because you were thinking about some problem or about what happened yesterday!

You know, you can't think of joy and depression at the same time. It's one or the other. So the joy road is one that you have to train yourself to travel. You have to be ready to accept it when it comes. And here it is. Do you see? That is joy, but you have to practice appropriating it.

Joy is a form of praise. It is found in contentment. It is found in peace. You have to practice these things. That is what we mean when we talk about "conducting" our life. It is your conduct. How do you conduct your life? Joy is part of our conduct. So, don't mis-conduct!

There are times in my office when it is difficult to like a person, but I change it around and I practice joy. I have found that the moment I feel joy toward the other person, he or she is joyful. It's catching. I want you to be happy and joyful. When you are happy and joyful, I am happy and joyful.

I want you to feel good. That is the reason we are exploring the joy world. The more joy you have, the happier those around you will be. The more joy that's spread around, the happier the whole world will be.

One of the great secrets of healing was revealed by Christ when he said, "What you have done unto the least of these, ye have done unto me also." When you are unhappy, I feel that unhappiness and respond to it. But if you come to me with a happy thought, it builds me up. If a person comes to you with a happy thought, take it. It will bless both of you. It is joy that has come to you: Accept it; appropriate it. We find joy in pleasantness. We find it in optimism. There are many people who are not pleasant and happy, who are always looking for something wrong. Wouldn't it be nice to suggest to a person like that, "Something good will happen to you today, because I am looking for something good to happen for you"?

I used to know a Dr. Tucker who would look his patients in the eye and say, "I'm afraid you're going to get well." This humorous touch of reverse psychology was based on the strange fact that what you fear will come upon you. Don't be afraid. Everybody is going to have some problems and troubles. I fear something wonderful is going to happen. Why don't you appropriate that thought? Why don't you take on the joyful way of being?

Take The Joy Path

The path we take is formed by the carpet of our thoughts. Keep this in mind while you are walking and thinking. If you are thinking a depressing thought, what are you walking on? You are walking on thoughts. You talk in words and you walk on a carpet of words. In the Old Testament of the *Bible*, King David in one of his Psalms of praise to God wrote, "My mouth shall praise thee with joyful lips." These are the words from the Good Book, ". . . with joyful lips." This is the only kind of thing worth hearing. This is the kind of carpet I want to walk on.

I want pleasantness to come from your lips. I want something that makes me feel good. Does that sound selfish? No. Because when I love my neighbor, according to the Good Book, I am to love him as I love myself. If I want lovely things to come to me, I am also to want those lovely things for my neighbor. It can't all be just for me. I want to know what this spiritual joy is and I want to see that it is passed on. Joy expands as far as you want it to go. Our brightest hopes can be dashed to the ground by fears. That's why we have to go to optimism the joy way.

There was a grandmother who only had two front teeth. Someone approached her and said, "Isn't it terrible that you only have two front teeth?" She replied, "Yes, but they both bite!" We choose the way we want to look at things. We can choose the bright side.

We have a joy in seeing all of this come together on the higher way. So I bring this out — it really is something to think about. Why don't you adopt a pattern in your life? Adopt a pattern so that you can see these wonderful things.

Be Happy In Your Work

Joy comes, not always in doing the things you love to do, but in loving the things you have to do.

One of the best things we can do for ourselves is to find joy in our occupations. This may be difficult for you at the moment. But I will say this: If you are having problems and you have any idleness around you, get busy. Do something. You can do it physically, mentally or spiritually. But never, never get into idleness. And don't wait for the "right feeling" to get you started; feelings can be misleading. Sometimes we have to separate our thinking from our feelings in order to have control over our feelings. Don't let negative feelings tell your thinking what to do. If you just start doing something constructive and positive, even the smallest and most humble thing, I know you'll get through.

It's the idleness that doesn't allow good things to happen. It's so easy to get into a rut with idleness — a negative rut. Many people are so negative in this world, even when they appear to be trying to get with and learn love, that on their present level the negative thinking overcomes them. We all know there are lots of burglars, lots of thieves, lots of people who lie and cheat. They haven't learned yet. They let idleness and negative thinking overcome them.

Of course, we've all done our share of negative thinking. But aren't we glad we've finished with it now? I'm so glad I'm all through with that. There is joy even in this thing — knowing that I am finished with negative thinking. I can look in your eyes and say, "My friend, it's a wonderful feeling!" I have a lot to feel wonderful about.

Grab hold of some of the things you can start feeling wonderful about, and you are going to have fewer problems with health. After all, you are your own best spiritual and mental doctor. Exert yourself. Employ yourself to do good. You will find that being busy with an occupation will really help you to go forward and will do good things for you. Be better. Be happy. You will find that when you purchase a thing in life, you bring something good to yourself. But you don't purchase the spirit. You appropriate it. It is similar to purchasing something nice. But you *appropriate* it. Don't forget this word because it is a very, very wonderful word.

Contemplate the good things. Reflect on the good things. The power is within you. The kingdom of God is within you, and if you don't think that is where all power is, then you had better start thinking about it. There is no power on the outside that can operate on you, and when you operate on anything that is good, you must have the most powerful thing in the world, and it is within you.

The power of God is within you. Ignorance is responsible for your illness. And we can do something about ignorance. We fear darkness. Darkness is just the absence of light. Put light there. Put joy there. Joy brings enlightenment into our lives.

I say again, you have to search for what it is that you need to put into your life, then take up your life and your health and concentrate on molding them "nearer to the heart's desire."

Don't work against evil, as I have emphasized before. We must open to and acknowledge the God within us, the good within us.

I'm bringing this out because you want to learn to let your old ailment decay on the outside. Your body needs a good direction. Go in this positive direction as if you have bought a ticket on a Joy Coach, and you will go through life leaving your troubles behind. If you are riding the Joy Coach, you are not looking for trouble.

Jesus knew joy. He went forth in joy. There was joy on His lips. There is joy in our hearts. Let us rejoice! Let us rekindle our joy! Keep that joy going! Everybody wants joy, everybody loves joy, and there is plenty of joy for everybody. Remember that joy and sorrow often come together and work together—but we turn sorrow into joy. We don't turn joy into sorrow. We always turn the negative into the positive, the lower into the higher.

The counselors of peace bring joy to people. The wise child will have joy. First come knowledge and wisdom, then comes joy. The people shall increase in joy, and we shall go forth together in joy!

Let us remember always to carry two very special words with us: JOY and APPROPRIATING. Let's keep it just that simple.

The Good Book tells us, "Consider it all joy, my brethren, when you encounter various trials, knowing that the testing of your faith produces endurance. And let endurance have its perfect result, that you may be perfect and complete, lacking in nothing."

So what do we do? We consider it *all* joy. We greet our trials with joy. Why? Because in trials, through trials, we may become "perfect and complete, lacking in nothing." That means all of us! I don't want to be the only happy person in the crowd! So why can't we go as one?

We Are All One With God

We are one in spirit. There is only one God, one Father. And that makes us all brothers and sisters. We are one family. This is what we have together. Spirit is one. If we could find a way to bring this into our lives, we could all go together in joy.

Joy is an attitude. It is an attitude that we have toward all things, including our trials. Since we must always be expressing an attitude of some kind, why not let it be joy?

When we have joy we are capable of our best thinking. We make good sound decisions. When we are sick, blue and dejected we shouldn't make decisions, because any decision we make will be a bad decision, poor in judgment. I have to smile at this, because many people come to me in their suffering and say, "Oh, doctor, I'll buy you a new car if you if you cure my sinus trouble." But when the sinus trouble is cured, amnesia seems to set in. They forget about the new car.

Don't make an important decision when you are sick because you will make a sick decision. You will make a poor decision. But if you can greet your problems with joy, you will make a good decision. Then you will have contemplative, reflective joyousness. Always work for joy and make your decisions fit the joy. Then you will attract more joy.

When you follow this way you can expect joy because you are working on that level. You have changed the vibration of your life. Your physical body will change. The physical body just follows. It doesn't know what to do, so let it follow you in this joyful way.

Put A Song In Your Heart

If we are going to have peace and truth and good will, we must have joy. Joy will improve your breathing. When you have joy in your heart, the heart will beat better, more rhythmically. When you have joy in the stomach, the digestion will work better. When you have joy, you will always have good friends around you.

I am not going to worry about your physical condition if you accept joy in your life. You have a responsibility, and now is the time to take care of it, because no doctor is going to take responsibility for the way you live your life. The only responsibility the doctor has is to share his knowledge, to show you the way and to encourage you to take it. But he can't eat for you. He can't drink for you. He can't breathe for you. He can't think for you. You have to *appropriate* joy. Then you will eat, drink, breathe and think in joy!

In our meditation and in our quiet moments, let us just go back into ourselves and say, "I have, Father, a place in this world, I am your child." *We belong here.* We were placed here. But you must know this one thing — that you were created for joy.

All God's creatures begin life with joy. Just imagine for a moment the romping puppies, the playful kittens, the frolicking little colts and their wobbly legs, the newly born sweet-faced calves, the lambs. All God's creatures begin life joyfully — until they are taught something else. That puts a damper on their joy and starts them on the road to sickness. Then they are moving deathward instead of lifeward. Has that "something else" taken the joy from you? Maybe you have one of those devoted mothers who never tires of discussing your first year or two of life and showing baby pictures where you're laughing with joy. When was the last time you laughed like that? From deep down inside? Think about it.

Why not let your original inheritance shine forth? Hasn't the Father said, "All that I have is thine"? Didn't the Christ say, "It is your Father's good pleasure to give you the kingdom"? Remember that God's kingdom is joy and light and love and wisdom. With this inheritance you have the strength to accomplish every good thing. Appropriate this with joy. Give thanks for it. Peace will come to you when you have joy in your heart. Time doesn't exist for the person who is happy and joyful. Time only drags for a person who is disliking his moment, living in resentment, wanting to get rid of it and not wanting to face the new day.

Time sheds the burdens of those who have joy in their hearts. So today we have really and truly been blessed because we have come face to face with the joy world. We realize that joy is the only thing we will allow to rule our body, rule our heart, rule our life.

Go forth with joy in your heart!

Youth

Youth is not a time of life
Measured by the years,
The young are often aged
By sorrow and tears.

Youth is but a state of mind,
Measured by ideals;
Those old in years are often young,
The game of life reveals.

Wrinkles in the face appear,
Painted by the years,
But wrinkles etched upon the soul
Are put there by our fears.

Faith and hope will keep us young,
Courage kills despair,
Time cannot take the toll of years
If enthusiasm's there.

So hold fast to your ideals,
Fill your life with worthwhile things
So that in the end we marvel
At the joy such living brings.

— Ida M. Forrest

Chapter 5

Mother's Day

"Mother is the name for God."
— Thackeray

I would like to dedicate this chapter to my mother, who has done so much for me, and to mothers everywhere, who have done and are doing so much for their children. When we think about it, mother is more than a person. Mother is an idea. We speak of motherhood and the mother principle. These concepts, in turn, bring to mind the notions of the bringing forth of life, of nurturing, of caring, of loving or protecting. These are vitally important aspects of health, and we will be looking at these things from a health standpoint as we pay our respects to motherhood today.

What can we say about mother? Mother is the childbearer, the nurturing being in whose womb the seed grows into the babe, who then comes forth into the world as life. It is the mother who, with tender loving care, feeds, bathes, clothes, watches over and protects the newborn infant as it grows first into a toddler, then a child, a teenager and finally a grown young man or woman. Motherhood involves suffering and pain. Motherhood involves wonder and joy. As the mother watches the child grow and mature, she herself grows and matures. There are many lessons in motherhood, as every mother knows.

Now, we also have the mother principle, the female principle in nature. We have the positive and the negative polarities in nature which correspond to the male and the female principles, the father and mother principles. We have an attracting principle and a repelling principle, and the interplay between these principles, so to speak, is what makes the world go around. We might say these things are complementary opposites; they go together, they work together, they belong together. Without mothers, there would be no fathers; without fathers, there would be no mothers. Each of us should have the positive and negative principles in balance in our life, because this, as we will see, has an effect on our health.

This interplay between positive and negative forces is going on constantly throughout the universe. We have negative and positive planets. We have negative and positive electricity. We have the negative and the positive in ions, in molecules and in the atom. We are not just looking at these things from the scientific standpoint, we are looking at them from the standpoint of life itself. You see, I believe the female principle carries the healing. The mothering aspect is the healing aspect, and we will expand on this as we go along.

Life Begins With Mother

Mother is the beginning. The Good Book says, "And Adam called his wife's name Eve, because she was the mother of all living." Mother is the one who really gives us our start and our beginning in this earthly life.

We honor our mothers on Mother's Day, and as we do this we remember the unique things about her and we think about her with love. Mother doesn't ask for much. She doesn't necessarily want to have a day off or a leave of absence or a Mother's Day card. But she does want to be remembered and loved. I think this is really all any mother ever wants from her children — to be remembered and loved. Our mothers are the embodiment of *givingness*, and it is from this standpoint that I say the mothers are the healers. The mother principle is the healing principle.

There are times when I have been hurt, there are times when I have fallen and have gone home crying. My mother would just touch me and say that everything was all right. I believed in her so much that it *was* all right. This is a healing principle. Any mother can do that. The mother principle does that. That spirit of givingness in which we were raised has a healing power that we recognize from deep within ourselves, and we reach out for that when we are hurt or sick. Now I don't want you to personalize this just to your mother or mine. We all have the same principle operating in us.

The mother principle expresses its healing power in many ways.

Look at the mother songs we have today, the lullabies. Look at the mothers who sing to their children in the rocking chair or by the bedside. The mother principle is entirely different from the father principle. They sing in higher voice, a sweeter voice. They live in and express a different vibration. They are usually more finely tuned to their children. They are closer to them. Many of them, in fact, have never severed that birth cord of the child.

The story is told of an elderly lady at her son's funeral. She was some eighty years old, and her son had just passed away in his sixties. She said, "I just knew I'd never get that boy raised." She was always tied to that boy. We can see there is a very closely knit relationship between mothers and their sons and daughters. Sometimes the mother takes on more responsibility for her children than she should.

A mother came to visit her son in San Quentin prison, and upon coming to the visitor's window with tears in her eyes she said to him, "Where have I failed you, son?" She felt she hadn't properly reared this boy.

In my work I treat a good number of children. The mothers of these children are often so close to them that it creates problems. For example, if I want to put a child on a fast, I have to take it up with the mother. She is the one who will have a hard time with the fast. She will want to give food to that child because she doesn't want him to miss a single meal. If she does, that will ruin the whole purpose of the fast. It may be right for the child, but in her over concern she doesn't always see it. You see, the mother is sometimes so close to the child that she doesn't recognize the physical needs of the child.

Mothers Have Lessons To Learn

Abraham Lincoln once said, "All that I have ever been, all that I hope to be, and all that I am now, I owe to my mother." Great men frequently pay tribute to their mothers. And it is right and proper for this to be done. But we must recognize that mothers have lessons to learn, too. Mothers grow mentally as their children grow physically.

I have heard one mother say, "When my children were born I didn't know anything about raising children, and here I am fifty-two years old, and my children have left me. Now I know all about them."

It doesn't seem like we have the knowledge to work with our children in the beginning. But perhaps that's how it should be — because I think children are born to teach parents lessons. I think they come to help the parents grow. They make you think, don't they? Oh, the things they can get the parents to think about! Where is my child tonight? What is he doing now? He needs a good spanking. Shall I spank him while I am angry and upset, or should I wait until I calm down? Many a child has been hurt — physically and emotionally — by enraged parents. We should never spank a child at such a time. At the same time, we must remember that anger and rage are just as destructive to us as they are to the child. The negative emotions are always more destructive than instructive. That is a lesson we must learn. The negative emotions always block the healing power of the mother principle. A misbehaving child is as much in need of healing as one who is physically ill.

Never discipline a child at mealtime. A good mother never does this, and it is likely that more fathers are at fault in this than mothers. But I have seen many children sitting at the table being disciplined and having their digestion ruined. Some parents don't know that they can't discipline children at the table without a serious risk of causing digestive problems for the children — and for themselves.

There are backward children, mentally retarded children, children with tumors and other serious problems. What is the purpose of this? Is it to destroy the parents' lives? Is it to drive them into pity for the children and self-guilt for themselves? No. It is to develop strength, compassion, patience, perseverance and hope. It is to lead the parents on a search for the higher things. As they try to find what is best for the child, they uncover what is best in themselves. We should never express pity toward a child — or anyone. Compassion, yes. Pity, never.

Detours Have Lessons To Teach

We are all on a journey. As we go through life we have to realize that our children are forcing us on detours. But a detour will always show us something new. The more detours we go on, the more we appreciate the beauty, the wisdom, that life's journey has in store for us in the days to come. It is out of what we give forth to our children that this comes to us. So you see that the mother principle not only gives out blessings, but returns blessings to the giver.

Mothers give a good deal of thought to what they can do for their children, what they can give to them. Consider the wealthy mother, for example, the mother who has given her child an inheritance of money. On the physical level, this means that the son or daughter can satisfy many needs and wants. Now, we must ask, is that the best aspect of the mother principle, the best gift for that child? Will money help that child take satisfaction in doing good for others or in being an honest, upright, sincere and spiritual person? Which is more important, an inheritance of money or an inheritance of solid, decent values? Which would make the child richer? We must think about these things.

There is an old story that says the wealthy man misses something worthwhile by not being poor. He will never realize the satisfaction and delight that comes from making the last installment payment on his house or car! Of course, there is more to it than that. Wealth tends to give people a false sense of security that can distract them from the search for spiritual values. Then when the bottom falls out, or they lose their health, they are lost. There are things money can't buy, things like courage, faith, happiness, patience, hope and joy.

The Essenes gave their children a wonderful inheritance. When a child was born, they planted a tree for him. They considered the tree as the one thing in nature free of all sin. Each year on the child's birthday they planted another tree. At the age of eighteen the young man was given his inheritance, the trees and the land they were on. Land to live on, trees to provide nourishment and shade. These would nurture him and take care of him the rest of his life. This is the mother principle at work.

The Earth Is Our Mother

Do you know why so many of the sages in history have called this planet "Mother Earth"? Because it gives us a home, it feeds and sustains us. Mother Earth is a good example of the mother principle. It is God's creation along with all else in the universe, and there are certain natural laws at work by which Mother Earth maintains a balance among the living things nourished by her generosity.

People often ignore the lessons that Mother Earth tries to show us through natural law and the balance of nature. We have mothers who are out of balance. We have mothers who smother their children and we have mothers who spoil them by permissiveness. We have mothers who interfere too much and mothers who don't care enough to interfere when they should. But these children grow up, and many of them are healed by the work of the mother principle within themselves. Each generation sees the dawn of a new hope amidst the troublesome clouds on the horizon left by the previous generation. Life goes on here on Mother Earth. When I think of the work that is yet to be done, I hope for a generation of good mothers, mothers who will bear and rear children who are strong enough and courageous enough to do the work that needs to be done.

The Responsibilities of Motherhood

Today forty percent of all the female alcoholics in this country are mothers. Nicotine is in the smoking mother's breast milk thirty seconds after she lights up a cigarette. Can you understand this from a health perspective?

One time a lady came to one of my former professors and said, "I am five months pregnant and I would like to start living so that I can have a healthy child." He said, "Little lady, you should have come here twenty years ago." It all starts way back. It would be wonderful to see a generation of mothers who have the proper idea of health.

Mothers must learn these things. That is why we talk to those in the field about kitchen planning. We talk about foods. Usually the mother takes care of the food, the food shopping and preparation. We talk about food buying, how to select the right foods. We talk about how to make soups, how to take care of fruits, dry the fruit, revive the fruit. Mothers need to know this. Nutrition is a vital aspect of health, and this is the job of the mother.

All healing in this world should come through the mother. The maternal relationship is very important. In biology we talk about the mother cell from which all life begins. We talk about the mother tongue, or native language that we grew up in. To mother means to bring forward or toward. It means what you are akin to, your family. What you are akin to is always traced back to the mother, the one who gave birth. The country that gave birth to all the veins and arteries of gold and silver in El Dorado and Amador Counties in California is called the "Mother Lode Country." The mother principle gives birth to everything.

What The Bible Says Of Mothers

The Good Book speaks very highly of mothers in many places, and it boldly warns, "The foolish man despiseth his mother." But the most wonderful description of a good mother is found in Proverbs, and it goes like this: "Strength and honor are her clothing, and she shall rejoice in time to come. She openeth her mouth with wisdom, and in her tongue is the law of kindness. She looketh well to the ways of her household and eateth not the bread of idleness. Her children rise up and call her blessed." Now this is the mother principle, and its healing power is made evident where the prophet Isaiah tells how God rewards those who keep faith: "As one whom his mother comforteth, so will I comfort you . . . and when ye see this, your heart shall rejoice, and your bones shall flourish like an herb." This is the givingness of the mother principle, and through it "your heart shall rejoice." In joy there is no sickness; there is only health.

When we think of how healing can come about, we have to approach it as children from a spiritual standpoint. We have to open ourselves to receive the healing as children open themselves to their mothers. What can you accept? I think back to my mother. My mother was a very wonderful person, a healer in our family. She used to say to me, "Sit down, son. I want to talk to you a moment. You know, you can have anything you want in life. I want you to think about that a while." So I would sit there and think about all the things I could have. Then she would say, "Oh, I forgot to tell you — you can have anything you want in life, but you have to take everything that goes with it, too." You have to take the consequences that go along with what you ask for, what you decide to receive into your life. I am very careful now about taking coffee and donuts into my body because I have to take everything that goes with them.

Seek And You Shall Find

Another principle my mother taught was, "You can go through life and you can seek things on many levels, on many streets, but I want you to remember that whatever you are seeking in life is also seeking you." This is a very wonderful principle. This is a healing principle. If you are seeking the higher and better things, they are also seeking you. If you are seeking health, it is also seeking you. If you are seeking joy, joy is also seeking you!

My mother taught me from a kind of healing wisdom that she had. She said, "Son, you could lose all of your money one of these days and you'd lose a lot. You could lose your health and you'd have lost still more. But if you ever lose your peace of mind, you have lost everything." She taught me peace of mind. She taught me what it was to be quiet and still. She taught me what it was to go to church, to listen. She taught me to realize that there is healing in being still and quiet. This is one of the important healing principles.

The following poem brings out afresh what we were saying earlier about how the children that come forth from the mother help the mother develop and grow:

I know a busy mother
With a thousand daily cares,
Who will say each time I meet her,
"I have just found more gray hairs.
It is the housework and the children
That are turning my hair so gray.
All these problems and this pressure
Are just wearing me away!"

I wonder as I listen
While she frets about her curls,
If she has ever looked at diamonds
Or admired the glow of pearls.
If an oyster has a problem
When some sand gets in its shell
Then it covers it with beauty
And it makes a pearl as well.

And a worthless lump of carbon
Hidden deep beneath the earth,
Changes form because of pressure
And the diamond is given birth.

Without problems, without pressure,
They'd both have been sand or coal.
Let us be thankful that our problems
Help to make a lovely soul.

— From a Collection of Poems for Charlotte Greenwood by D.H. Johnson

Among the travails of life we will encounter problems and troubles and we have to accept them. Mothers especially will face problems whether they wish to or not, because problems are a natural part of child rearing, and the growth and learning of the mother accompanies the growth and learning of the children. They have to take that broken leg. They have to take the fight on the baseball field. They have to know what it is to soothe, to stimulate, to get a person to go on. They have to know what it is to slow a person down, to stop him sometimes. Mothers learn a great deal in life because there is so much for them to look after. Because of that, they develop many wonderful qualities.

So as we remember that the Good Book tells us to "honor thy mother," let us realize that this godly principle, the mother principle of givingness, of reaching out to make a better person, a person who will be able to carry to the unfinished job ahead, will always be with us.

In God the complementary opposites are One, and it is from God that we have the Mother-Father Principle in highest form. When we work with and through the Mother Principle, when the Mother Principle works in and through us, we are life givers, we are healers, and God will never let us down. We will always be able to carry on.

Let us be thankful for what is yet to come. Let us love what comes to us. My mother taught me that we must not just love this friend and that one — or even just this enemy and that one — but we must love everyone we meet on the path of life, for our own good.

Father-Mother God, bless each and every one — and it is so.

Mothers have the power not only to rock the cradle, but to rock the world.

Chapter 6

All Power Is Yours

You have to go inward to come outward.

We're all striving for the finer things in life, and I believe the finer things are the spiritual things. We are all striving toward beauty, and I believe the real beauty emerges from the spiritual perspective. I also believe that the natural world and the spiritual world are closely interrelated. Being nature students, we no doubt are in contact with or have a feeling that a magnificent creative power underlies the awesome beauty and variety that we find in nature.

I don't think we can completely rely on the physical work. I think we have to know something about the effects of love on and in a physical body. Is love physical? Can you buy it and drink it? I don't think we can go through life and just be interested in how many breaths we breathe each minute. I think we have to be interested in how healing takes place, which is not just all physical. I know, too, that many times things need to be adjusted in life and I don't think it is always a chiropractic adjustment we need. Sometimes we need our head adjusted! And I don't believe that only a doctor, only a physical adjustment, only what comes from a prescription or vitamin bottle, is going to give you what you need to change and become a better person, a healthier person. You are going to have to do some doctoring, some adjusting for yourself — on the inside.

It is possible for us to realize there are things we can do psychologically, mentally and spiritually that help this physical body. We are not considering these spiritual things from a church standpoint but from a healing standpoint. You have to look at healing from many different directions.

Balance Your Life

If you are just going to look at life from a nutritional side, you are going to miss living. You are going to miss living, and if you aren't living, you're dead. There are many people living on vegetarian diets — and they are vegetating! Vegetables alone are not enough. You can't go through life as a vegetable! You have to live! And there is more to life, more to health, than the mouth, the digestive tract and what we put into them. You have to realize that it isn't just nutrition that adds zip and vitality to our lives. We have to get going. We are vibrant beings. We have to meet life with that quick and confident stride that takes us surely along the path to the higher and better things.

Often we become tired when our health is not the best. When this happens we seem to be powerless to do things. I want to spend time here talking about power, how we get it and what we can do with it.

You may think that an elephant is the strongest and most powerful living creature, but I believe that we are the most powerful of all the Lord's creations. Certainly, an elephant can't build a house or fly a jet plane. An elephant can't build a future. Look at all the things we have the power to do!

But many people use their power in a negative way. They are using their power to destroy instead of to create. Many of you are using your power to kill yourselves, and if I can persuade you to turn this power around and build with it, it will be the most wonderful thing I can do for you

Remember:

Inferior conversation is gossip and
detrimentally speaking of others;
Mediocre conversation is about
places and things;
Superior conversation is about
ideas and ideals.

To tell you to stop using this power negatively, to tell you to forget that, is not enough. People just don't forget. You have to train yourself out of it, you practice your way out of it. It takes constant practice to change life-long habits that bring on problems and troubles. I tell each one of my patients that if he wants to get well, he must grow out of sickness and into health. You grew into the problems you have now, whether physical, mental or spiritual; and if you want to leave them behind, you must outgrow them, just as a child outgrows a coat or dress or pair of shoes. It is just like growing up from childhood all over again. When we are in the scribbling stage of kindergarten, what do we understand when the wise man tells us a parable?

Grow Up And Live

Too many of us are still scribbling. Too many of us are still in kindergarten. We just don't understand because we haven't expanded our understanding. We haven't come to the place where we can be aware of the actual power that can come and lift us and save us. What can save us? I think love can save more people than anything else. Many of us are anemic for love. We are lonely and starved for love. Many of us are starving for kindness. Many of us are hungry for something, but physical food doesn't meet that need. The hunger is for something else. That's something to think about, isn't it?

It is the constant little drop of water on the knee that can cause a disturbance there over a period of a year. A drop of water coming every few seconds on that knee. Your body can't take it. You have heard about the proverbial water drops that wear the stone away, haven't you? As you walk up to the end of our Hidden Valley Health Ranch, you come to a place where there used to be a thriving Indian settlement. They took their baths in large hollows in the rocks, hollows that had all been worn away by water. Water will wear a rock away — and that is power!

In India where people don't believe in killing animals or insects, the townspeople had to decide what to do when they captured bandits or looters. This was many years ago. What they would do is to let drops of water fall on the bandits' heads for many months — until they went crazy from it. Then the people would untie them and take care of them. Now that may sound strange to us, but they didn't have prisons in those days, and they didn't dare let the bandits go or they would return to kill and loot again, and the villagers didn't believe in killing them. So they would let the bandits go crazy from the water drops.

Words are as powerful as drops of water. The point is worth making, because, like those constant little drops of water, negative words can wear us away over a period of time. They can drive us crazy or make us sick. Water—and words—can work in beneficial ways, too. As water carries nutrients to the roots of plants, words can nourish our minds and spirits. Words carry power. We must remember that.

Build The Power You Need

We can talk about power in many ways. These days people are in a hurry, and most of us have seen how a huge crane can lift a heavy steel girder hundreds of feet in constructing a skyscraper. In ancient times people didn't have cranes. But they had something else that was very powerful. They had time.

People will look at a large piece of granite, and they will say, "I can't possibly lift that!" But you can lift anything with enough people and enough time. That's how the Egyptians built the huge Sphynx and their magnificent pyramids. That's how the Great Wall of China was built. Thousands of people working patiently for many years built these impressive wonders. Think of the power we have when we work harmoniously. Think of the power we have when we take the time. Now, look at the power we could build up by thinking good thoughts from now on. This is a power we can use to build good health.

If you have this power working, you can be well in a hurry. Personally, I believe that a good deal of the power that works through faith in a religious person's life comes because that person has broken out of his old negative ways of thinking and believing. He believes in something new. He is no longer hindered and burdened by negative thought. I believe there is a great power in working with love.

The Good Book tells us, "God hath not given us the spirit of fear." He has not given us fear. We give that to ourselves. It goes on to say that we are given power. If we go out and use this power in fear, we use it negatively. We use it backward, and it destroys. When we do that we are not using power in faith and love toward a good purpose. We must use it in faith and love to be using it constructively, to build good health.

Without Power We Can Do Nothing

You will agree with me that we should all be healthy. We should be wise. We should be capable. Would we consider an impotent man as powerless? Yes, he has no power. He doesn't have the power to rejuvenate. He doesn't have the power to produce, to activate. Here again, I would like to tell you that when Christ said, "All power is given unto me," He meant this power to be invested in you likewise.

Do you realize that all of the power that works in Christ can work in you, too? It makes no difference whether it was Christ or Buddha or a Hindu master. It doesn't make any difference. The power is there. Their power can be invested in us today, right now.

Your heart beats seventy-two times per minute, year after year, your whole life. What a motor! What a powerhouse you are! The blood in your veins and arteries travels 30 feet per second in your body. What a powerful body you have! Look what powerhouses we all are! We can easily use this power to destroy, to harm, to kill — but what a waste! We can just as easily take this great power, turn it around the other way, and use it to rejuvenate and rebuild ourselves, then to reach out and help others. But we are only going to have the power to do this when we work in joy, in love, in happiness, in good feelings — blessing other people, being thankful for today and for what is yet to come, being unafraid of tomorrow. If you use this approach, this concept, your health will return to you automatically.

When I say automatically it is because I am thinking of the great power of this universe. The earth is traveling though space faster than a bullet, and that is power. Do you realize the power that is in sunlight alone? Do you know how many flowers each day receive the power to bud from sunlight? That's flower power. Do you realize how much chlorophyll is developed each day in the plants of the earth because of sunlight? Scientists say that without chlorophyll, there would be no life on this planet as we know it. The power of the sun is working around us constantly. Think about seeds pushing their first tiny roots into the soil, pushing their little cotyledons up toward the earth's crust, seeking the sun. The same sunlight power working in the garden makes top vegetables and root vegetables grow. We find that the same energy of sunlight that gives us light and warmth is also found in the consuming flames of fire. This power is everywhere around us.

We Live By Our Words

Like sunlight, our language is in such constant use everywhere around us that we tend to overlook its power. In fact, the words we live by are so powerful that we need to take great care in selecting and using them. We may need to change them. Because people think in words, we must change our vocabulary to be sure that we are using words that are good for us.

When I speak of eggs, you think of e-g-g-s, don't you? If I want to tell you about ham, I tell you h-a-m. This is how we communicate. This is how we give out, how we receive. We use words. If we say "damn" it is a different feeling in comparison to when we say "joy," isn't it? Every word has its own feeling—its special vibration.

We find we have to live in the world of feelings these words create in us. Words can be harsh. Call a person a name, and what do you get back? Words can be golden. Express a compliment, or bring joyful news to a person, and what do you get back? That's obvious, isn't it? Yet, there are some people who seem to remain unaffected by harsh words, and there are others who respond with little feeling to compliments. This can mean they have something of a problem, or it can mean that they have simply learned to control their feeling responses to words. Doctors must learn not to get trapped into responding to the negative language used by a very sick or hysterical patient, or they may find themselves so disturbed that they are unable to think properly about what needs to be done. You don't have to let words hurt or destroy you. The power of a person's words cannot harm you unless you give your consent. Did you know that? It may take practice, but you can accomplish that; you can control your responses to peoples' words. In the meantime, you can practice upgrading your own vocabulary.

Most of us have not in the past taken the trouble either to examine the vocabulary we use in our own thoughts or the vocabulary we use with others. Nor have most of us learned to control our responses to words. Under these conditions, words have had a strong effect upon us. Words have a power akin to that of tree roots, and in time they can inflict great damage. Some of you may have seen pictures of the tree roots found in some of the ancient stone temples in India. The roots came up from the ground, into the temple walls and just cracked and split those stone temples apart! Growing roots have broken them up.

The Forces Of Nature

Nature, of course, is impersonal and doesn't intentionally look for ways to destroy the works of man. But we must take nature's ways and nature's laws into consideration when we build. We must learn to work in harmony with nature and with each other, for there is almost unbelievable power in us, through us and around us all of the time. We must learn to be good to one another and to be good to nature. Then we will be taken care of. You can't fight nature or nature's laws; nature always wins. We must do our work in faith — in good faith.

We say, "If we only had the faith of the tiny mustard seed, it would grow in time to great strength and power." And, believe me, there is power in the mustard seed! It takes time. It takes time for the seed to grow into the plant and to send its roots deep. It takes time to develop its size and strength and power through the action of the sunlight and water and soil nutrients. We have the time. And if we take that time and use it wisely we can have that power.

We talk about the power of the arms, the power of the legs, the power of the chest, the power of the breath — the power that is in our physical body. The power that is found there has to be developed. It is the power of droplets of water to wear away stone that we put to work for ourselves, until finally the body is changed. The arms, legs, chest and stomach are changed. It takes constant practice to make a new arm, to make a better arm, to make a better muscle. And the same is true of our minds, our attitudes. We have to practice and constantly grow with our minds and attitudes.

I speak of this because if we wash and bathe ourselves daily in better attitudes and better thoughts, we can expect better health. The power is there. Health is cumulative. It doesn't come overnight. You have to make it, little by little. Disease comes little by little. Disease comes when we have brought bad habits into our lives and then our health gradually breaks down. To invite a bad habit into our lives is like asking a thief to spend the night on our living room sofa. The room will not be the same in the morning. Some good things will be gone. Good health comes as an accumulation of doing the right things each day. This is important to realize.

Now we find that in the godly things we have a great deal of power. God is all powerful. He is everywhere. He is all powerful, all seeing, all knowing and all intelligent. He is also all good. Do you think God could be a destructive influence in your life? No. God-less-ness is the killing thing in life.

Choose Your Environment

I believe that the spiritual aspect of life gives us access to great power. It can tear you to pieces if you use it wrongly. Many of us have experienced this power being used wrongly. We hear people say, "You give me a pain in the neck. She makes me sick to my stomach. I just heard the most revolting thing!" Don't you feel revulsion when you are in the "wrong" company? The wrong place? We must choose our environment.

We have to pick out pleasant companions, good friends. It is essential. It is healing to be in an environment in which you can feel good. It is destructive to be in an environment in which you can't. Unless you go where you are wanted, unless you go where you are loved, you will not feel right. And you will not be well. You can't constantly spend time in places where you are not wanted. That is destructive. You have to be where you are loved. How do you do that? You love — you love those around you — and they will want you to be around them. You create this atmosphere yourself; you create your own environment.

It is good to have ambition, to want to do things. But don't overdo. Ambition will kill you if you don't know when to quit, if you don't know when the game is over. The hard driving, hard striving environment is hard on health. Overambition can create envy, strife. It can create jealousy and vengeful feelings. They can wound, slash, kill. We hear people say, "I'll get him." What is that? Christ said, "Not that which goeth into the mouth defileth a man, but that which cometh out of the mouth."

We Live On What Comes Forth From Us

There are certain spiritual laws at work in our lives, whether we want them to be there or not. We have to recognize that what comes forth from us has great power. We live by what we are giving forth in life. That's the way life works.

The power that goes forth from you will affect every cell in your body. Why do you think people become mentally disturbed? Why does a person have a nervous breakdown? The reason is that we are powerhouses, and we can use this power to tear ourselves to pieces. We can break our bodies down faster than they can repair themselves.

I want to show you how you can rejuvenate and revitalize your body. You have the power to do this. All this power is within you. How many times have I heard, "The spirit was willing, but the flesh was weak"? I can't count the times. Now, when I buy a horse, I buy it for the spirit it shows. I've seen horses that are so high-spirited that unless they are properly ridden, they can't run a hundred feet before they are all sweaty. Uncontrolled spirit can kill a horse.

The same thing happens with people. I see people who sweat on the slightest provocation. I see people who sweat in fear or hatred. This is a misuse of power, of spirit. Many times these people have to use all the power they can muster to make their bodies move. They are almost immobilized. If only we could learn to use this power for our own good, we'd have something.

Most people haven't been educated to understand the power we have as human beings. We have much more than most people realize.

I once saw in the newspaper where a man who can normally lift 150 pounds was able to lift 400 pounds after being hypnotised. Now, hypnotism isn't magic; it can't give you power. It can only help you use what you already have. Is it possible that we have this much? Yes, it is. A mother and her young son were driving along in a Ford station wagon when suddenly the car swerved out of control and overturned on the bank of the road. When the mother climbed out, she found that her little son was pinned underneath the car. This little mother, only five feet tall, lifted that station wagon off her boy! She threw her back out of place but she did it. In the hospital she was asked, "What on earth gave you the strength to do that?" She replied, "I had to do it."

This is the kind of power we have in the body. We can tear ourselves to pieces — and often we use it that way. Doctors make a good living on the effects of people misusing this power.

The Power Is Yours

I can't help but think of the words given to me years ago by one of my teachers. Every time I met him, he would say, "All power is yours." We have this power — but how do we use it? Do we use it thoughtlessly? A little story might make this clear.

A man was once given three wishes, so with the first one he said, "I wish I could have a big plate of sauerkraut and weiners." And, poof! There it was, right in front of him. What a powerful thing that wish was! Just then his wife came in, and he told her about the three wishes, and what his first wish had been. His wife scolded him. "Why did you wish for that silly thing? You could have wished for something much better!" The man's face grew red, and he retorted, "I just wish the sauerkraut and weiners were on your nose!" And you know, the wish was granted. There was his wife with the sauerkraut and weiners stuck to her nose, feeling foolish, embarassed and hurt. He felt sorry for her and said, "Oh, I wish they would just go up the chimney." And they did. In a sense, his three wonderful wishes had also gone up the chimney, completely wasted.

Thoughts, hopes and wishes are powerful. Because of this power of producing results, we say the *thoughts are things.* I know that prayers are thoughts, and there is power in prayer. I know that you have to be careful how you think of other people because you may bring harm upon yourself by thinking negative thoughts about them. From a health standpoint you have to think good thoughts. I'm telling you this as a doctor, from my perspective. If you don't want to be doctored, you don't have to be. I can't really order you to love other people. You have to see the value in what I'm saying and do that on your own. For the sake of our health we need to be good to one another, to uplift one another.

A person who chooses to go the uplifted way is placing himself in the right environment. When you put yourself in the right environment, the right thoughts, the right feelings, you find that the power flows in your life to bring health to the body automatically. Your body naturally gets well. This is what I want to see you do.

Power means the ability to act. It gives the potency in any activity we perform. It is the ability, the capacity, the energy that is working in you. This power works best when we use it with love.

We find, too, that there is a great deal of force working through our attitudes of life. Of course, we know there is an enormous amount of power in nature. But have you heard of the power of the pen? Have you heard "the pen is mightier than the sword"? Many powerful things have come from the pen. But you see, it has no power of itself. The only power my pen has is what I give it. That is how powerful you are. You have the power to change nations, the power to change the whole world.

Ours is a powerful nation. We have power in our legislation. We have power in our leadership in government. We say, "That man is powerful. He has a great deal of influence. He can get things done." Power can be compared to electricity. Electrical power has the capacity to destroy or do good. That is why we need the spiritual values, because like electricity our power can be used for harm. Mechanically, we can be compared to steam engines. If the steam power isn't put to work properly, it will build up in the engine until it blows a valve.

I have heard of people "flipping their lids." I have heard of people "sounding off" and "getting all steamed up" over some event. I have heard of anger "getting the best of a person." This is like steam, out of control. What powerhouses we are!

Power To Change

Power gives us the ability to use the body normally, mentally or physically. Now we have the right, the ability and the capacity to exercise control. We have legal authority when we have the power of attorney. But you have the power to actually change things. There is word power. There is the power of the vote. There is military power. If we could only realize how much power there is in such things!

Power is the energy we have available for doing a job, for getting work done. Do you want good health? You have the power to get it. We have access to the kind of energy developed by mechanical or electrical means, and it must be used with wisdom. It has to have spiritual values directing it. That is why I think spiritual power is more important than physical power.

There is no morality inherent in power.

Power is just there. Acid has the power to corrode metal or to corrode our bodies. There is the power of a lens to focus light, the power of a mirror to reflect light. Power can be a very positive and active force, but when it is out of control, we have to return to the spiritual truth, don't we? The spiritual intent is very important. Spiritual power is the greatest power we have to overcome resistance.

When we have this power working through good words, good thoughts, we find there is a powerful effect on mind and body. There is power in seeds—the power to rejuvenate, to bring forth life. There is power in the growing plants. There is power in the egg yolk, power in vitamin E, power in foods. We can transmit the power of the foods to the body, but what a wonderful thing it is that we have this power with God!

We cannot take pride over this power, we cannot put our pride in it. It isn't our power. Yes, we have access to it, it flows through us, and we can use it. But it isn't ours. It is God who has the power; "For Thine is the power and the glory." God is the power. We find that in His hand is power. And we can do powerful things with our own hands because of it. We can plant gardens. We can build and create with our hands. Do you know how the handshake first started? Men used to carry swords and daggers in times long past. When two men met, they would extend the right hand—the hand that usually held the weapon. The empty right hand signified peaceful intentions. This is how handshaking began. Consider the power that can go with the handshake. When we do this, we are powerfully giving forth all the good we can. Great meaning can go with that extended hand!

God gave us the power to change. God gave us power to eat. God gave us power not to eat. We have the power to refuse. There is power in wind, in nature. I want you to realize what this power is: what word-power is and what God-power is. I want you to realize what David used when he overcame the power of the giant Goliath. David was a small man, but he was powerful. He was "taller" than the giant, more powerful than the giant — because he had God power.

Mind Is Power

What a wonderful thing it is to have this power! The power we have in love can change this whole world. The kingdom of God comes to us with power. The kingdom is loaded with power—and we can use it to rejuvenate, to bring our bodies to health. We cannot get well in the kingdom of hate or in the kingdoms of fear, jealousy or resentment. There we become powerless, impotent, sick.

The power of God is the kind of power that destroys those who use it wrongfully; it is removed from those who use it negatively. We have talked about the power of hate and the other negative attitudes and emotions, but we must realize that over a period of time the negative use of power wreaks havoc on the instrument through which it is used — the body. Then the power is lost.

I want you to have all the power for good that you're looking for. This process starts with the mind — with mind power. Remember, the mind is the intermediary between the spirit and the body. Spiritual power flows through the mind to the body. There's no limit to the power that is available to us. When we carefully channel this power, we gain control over it. We have to be careful of the man who has become berserk with power. If he isn't using it in accordance with spiritual principles, he can do a great deal of damage with it for a while.

We speak of the power of darkness. But there is no power in darkness unless you give it power. There is power in light. We find that all the power we need is found at the spiritual level.

You are all-powerful and you must use that power wisely. An automobile speeding down the street without a driver has become a dangerous weapon. Stay in the driver's seat. Follow the spiritual rules of the road. A driver without love can be a menace.

The next step in the consciousness of man is to learn to avoid any activity or occupation that would be harmful to people. If you want to have a powerful, healthy body, you will have to live right and do right , because only in that way will you retain the power to do what you want to do. If you take the higher road, the good road, the godly road, you will have health.

Because God is all-powerful, He works through nature. He works through foods; He works through companions; He works through kindness; He works through love. These are the godly things.

So today, know that as a child of God you have all this power invested in you. It gives the Father great pleasure to give you His kingdom. His kingdom is filled with glorious and powerful things to use for your good health. I want you to be healthy. When you are healthy, I am happy. When I am happy, I am healthier. Let's spread this around. Let's use our health, our happiness, to make others happier and healthier. Let's widen the circle of happy, healthy people. Then the world will be a better place. So get healthy. Get happy. Go the good road, the higher road.

I have to live the good life to be able to show you what it is. Then you can show others. This is being good to one another. I need you very much. You need me very much. We need each other! When we recognize that our need for others comes out of spiritual principles, we find that God approves. Let us live so that whatever we do, whatever power we express, has the approval of the Wise one — the approval of God.

Avoid being like the little seed that was —

Too Critical

A little seed lay in the ground,
And soon began to sprout.
"Now which of all the flowers around,"
It mused, "shall I come out?
The lily's face is fair and proud
But just a trifle cold;
The rose, I think, is rather loud,
And then its fashion's old.
The violet is very well,
But not a flower I'd choose,
Nor yet the Canterbury bell —
I never cared for blues."
And so it criticized each flower,
This supercilious seed,
Until it woke one summer hour —
And found itself a weed.

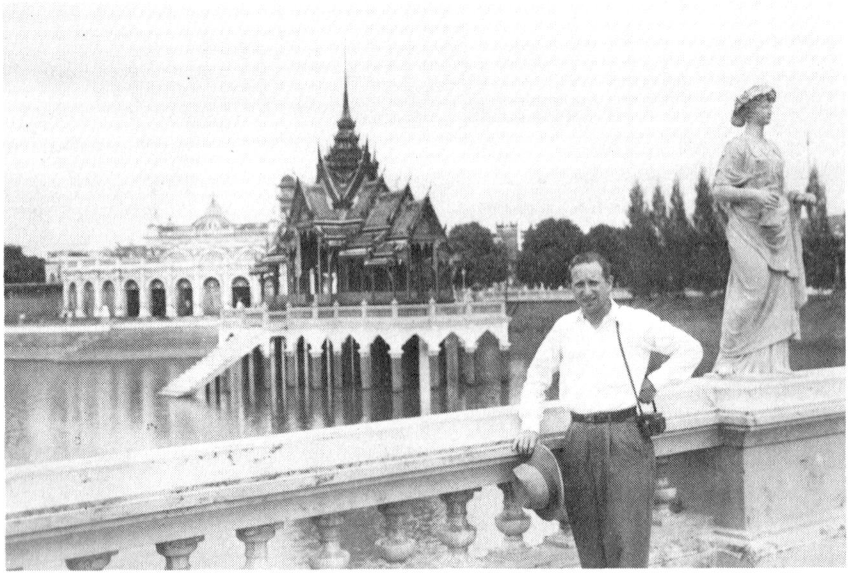

During a visit to India, I came to this beautiful shrine in the midst of the waters.

Chapter 7

Selflessness In The Enlightened One

Harmony creates...
Chaos destroys.

We would all like to have a little more enlightenment from an inner standpoint, from an upliftment standpoint, from the standpoint of what we could do for ourselves.

How much *do* we do for ourselves? How much do you do for yourself? Selfishness, I believe, is one of the hardest things to overcome in life. Selfishness is something we have to carefully look at, think about and take care of in life. Does selfishness really work to our benefit? We will have to explore this question with some care, for we are constantly finding selfishness wherever we go.

We know that happiness helps us to be healthier. We know that joy helps us to be healthier. Is it selfish to seek happiness and joy? No. These things must be shared to become real in our lives. It isn't selfish to seek happiness and joy in order to share them with others. We have to find happiness and joy in order to be well.

I have been teaching about the need for happiness and joy for many years, often to people who have lost theirs. It isn't easy for me to be joyful when everybody around me has problems. When a problem comes along we get serious and we move away from joy and happiness. Somehow when a problem comes along we have the idea that we have to be so serious that we can't be joyful. Problems and joy don't seem to mix well together.

Most people have the idea that when problems come along, we have to get harsh, we have to get tough, to solve those problems. But by being harsh and tough we make further problems for our bodies and minds. We must learn how to take on problems and not fall into those attitudes. I am treating people for nerve depletion. I am treating people for nerve tension. We doctors are making a living on your stress and strain.

I believe that ninety percent of stress and strain today is self-made. I think it would be helpful if we looked at this together from a spiritual standpoint. I want to show you that the enlightened way gives us an opportunity to choose for ourselves how to create a new and better life.

It is only through enlightenment that we are going to become better people. So with regard to those problems and troubles that you encounter each day, don't pray for fewer problems and troubles, pray for more enlightenment. Pray for more strength and more power, because, after all, having problems doesn't automatically increase your personal growth. You can grow through problems, but you will not graduate from life's first grade, eighth grade, high school or college until you learn to work out those problems.

Life flows along like a river. You bump into problems and you know you must take care of those problems as they come. Take care of them now. Otherwise, you'll wake up tomorrow morning and find yourself staring them in the face again. It's very frustrating to work hard to get through the eighth grade only to find out at the end of the term that you didn't pass, and you have to go through the same problems over again.

Let's solve those problems now so we can graduate. We want to grow and we want to graduate from the eighth grade. It's all right to be thirteen years old and be in the eighth grade, but we don't want to be there when we are sixteen. Some of us are still in the eighth grade at the age of thirty-two. The same patterns of job problems, the same patterns of marriage problems, the same patterns of health problems, come to us again and again. Some of us haven't grown up yet. We just haven't grown an inch — on the inside. We haven't gone beyond.

Now, I think the one thing that hinders growth the most is selfishness. I'm not certain how to approach the subject of selfishness. I sometimes think I've had a lot of selfish attitudes in my life, a lot of selfishness that I've tried to overcome. But I'm not alone in this. You've helped me to be selfish. Maybe I've helped you to be selfish.

This is one of the things that we have to see, that selfishness is a matter of how we govern our lives. We often govern our lives through selfishness. I am wondering if we can't use the spiritual connection to help us here, since selfishness has to do with material things. You can't be selfish with spiritual things. You may hoard money but you can't hoard truth. I can have truth as well as you can. You can have more money than I have but you can't have more truth than I have, if I'm willing to accept it.

Selfishness Means Misery

Does selfishness really work toward our own benefit as some people believe it does? Does the "what's-in-it-for-me" approach really bring happiness? I'm going to be very blunt about this.

If I treat you spiritually, I treat you with love, because love is of spirit. Then I can never hurt you. When we act from selfish motives, we always hurt other people — and ourselves.

Selfishness is of the material world. Many times, psychologically, we think we have to skin the other fellow before he skins us. Some call that "smart." That's based on the dog-eat-dog philosophy of life, and it is rooted in fear, fear that we will not get our share, that we will not get what we want, that we will not get enough. Some brands of psychology say that is how people are. There is magic in psychology, there is good in psychology, but there is also some "black magic" there, some spiritual blindness.

Let's Try Looking Up

If we seek the spiritual things, we have the opportunity of making our bodies well. When we raise our eyes from the material level, when we have the spiritual aspect worked out, we are present with the Law, with God, and our needs are taken care of — abundantly. So many people think that the Christ came to us as a man, but He also came to us as Truth. The Lord brought us the Truth and wanted to be known by the Truth He expressed. He said, "Ye shall know the truth, and the truth shall make you free." That is real selflessness. As a man He could not make us free. But the Spirit of God, the Spirit of Truth, can make us free. Christ dismissed from Himself all personal attachment, all selfishness. And He taught that lesson everywhere He went. The Truth flowed through Him, to us.

We go through life saying, "Look at me!" This is the pride that comes before the fall. Christ never said, "Look at me!" He was always busy sharing, teaching, healing, ministering to the needs of others.

When I tell you I feel wonderful, I feel happy, I feel good, that has to come from the inside out. Those things don't come from the outside in. Selfishness has to do with things you could take from me, the outside things, the material things. There is something that you can't take from me, and that is what I have on the inside.

This inner part of the person can never be harmed — unless you give your consent. Where is your consent? It is within, isn't it? It's not in the fingers. It's not in the material thing. Your consent is deep within you.

It is from within that we give our consent to be unselfish, to live in a world that is not of this world. I am in this world but not of this world. Can you see the difference? That which is real, that which is permanent is the unselfish thing. The material thing, the material pleasure, is the short-term thing, the selfish thing. You are going to be unselfish one of these days. You are going to be unselfish, happy and healthy.

There is a line in James Russell Lowell's poem, *The Vision of Sir Launfal,* that says, "For the gift without the giver is bare." Giving of oneself is unselfish giving. Giving of oneself is selfless giving. Self-less giving. There is less self in this giving. We could go on looking into the inside meanings of these words and phrases, but I think you understand. You understand that true happiness lies in unselfishness, in giving up loving material things.

The Unselfish Person Is Rich

True wealth is measured by how much selfishness you have given up and by how much selflessness you have grown into. The selfless person is truly rich.

Grow into selflessness. Selflessness is the gate to happiness. It is continuous joy, and the person who has grown into selflessness has risen above the body. There is no joy in sickness, is there? But there is no sickness in joy, in spirit. Our happiness lies in spirit.

You can't go around saying, "I'm a spiritual person." The person who does that is obviously not spiritual, is he? This is something you work toward. You can't even go around saying, "I'm a healthy person." I have never seen a healthy person. We all have something to work on, something to strive for. We all have a certain amount of selfishness. Of course, we all have a certain amount of unselfishness, too. It seems that some of us were born into this world with a great deal of selfishness to overcome. This is a difficult thing to understand, that we are born selfish.

Harmony Is A Breath Of Fresh Air

Wouldn't it bring a fresh breath of air into our lives if we hungered for the spiritual things? Some people want the spiritual things. Wouldn't it be nice if people would set their minds so they wanted harmony more than anything else?

There are people who want to have music, people who have to have music. They want this music not for the inner self but the outer self. Sometimes you have to wonder how far we can go with our wants. This is a form of selfishness.

Some people help others only in order to fulfill their own wants. This is also a form of selfishness. I feel that when we are helping another person we should avoid doing it for our own personal gain. If we work this way, we'll be avoiding the selfish life.

Perhaps the greatest form of selfishness today is making a living by taking advantage of other human beings. Too many people are doing this. In nature we would call this parasitism. However, civilization itself seems to emphasize and encourage selfishness. We are selfish when we live as Americans, Frenchmen, Germans or Chinese. I think that the pride of nationalism, the pride of racism, are forms of selfishness.

We must get away from this. We must learn to live as human beings. If all you are going to do is to preserve yourself on the material level at the expense of other people, you have picked the greatest form of selfishness to live in. We need to get away from that level. If we would let go of selfishness at the physical level and find the real self, the governing self, at the spiritual level, the body would be better off.

From a health standpoint, we must realize that our needs on the physical level are well taken care of when we live on the spiritual level. It isn't a question of accepting voluntary poverty, of leading deprived lives, when we decide to take the spiritual path. I believe that health and wealth are more spiritual and mental than we know. I am convinced that they are more inner than outer. I am convinced that they are rather higher than lower, if you follow me.

Be Unselfish — Be Healthy

The selfless person gives. My mother used to say, "If you keep holding on to what you already have, you will never have more than that. Always keep your hands empty, and more will be put into them!" Give everything you have, keep your hands open, and you will receive more. You will be filled again and again.

There is a great lesson in the Good Book. When the Samaritan woman came to the well to fill her water vessel, the Christ was sitting there, and he said to her, "Whosoever drinketh of the water that I shall give him shall never thirst again." He offered her the living water, the water that quenches the spiritual thirst. You know, many of us are so filled with the water of selfishness that we don't have room inside for that living water. If we would just empty our vessels of selfishness and take in unselfishness, we would find ourselves filled with something wonderful. We have read, "He is filled with the Spirit. He is filled with joy. He is filled with happiness." Do you want to be filled? Then you must empty yourself first. When you have done that, you'll be filled with the water of life — and with health as well.

You won't need to fill yourself with vitamins. You won't have to keep "chasing" good health. You won't have to chase anything. You will have it all if you become one with the Great Within.

What Is Real Security?

The search for security, so common these days, is one of the most misleading aspects of our civilization. We have to have life insurance, health insurance, home insurance, car insurance and many other forms of security. But the only real security we have is in opportunity, constantly letting that which is good flow through us. We don't have to become the most powerful and important person in this world. It is only that which we allow to flow through us which is really important. This is spiritual power.

When Scripture tells you that "All these things will be added unto you," how much more do you want? You can work hard and make seven dollars an hour, but I'll tell you how you can have seven times seven. You do it from within. A lot of people wish to themselves, "If only I had a business that would support me." That isn't the way it works. You support the business. When you open your business on Monday morning, whatever you are is what that business is going to be that day. You can chase customers away by being rude and uncaring. Or you can draw them to you.

You don't have to try to give. You can wear yourself out through trying; you can wear yourself out emotionally. You just give. I give you everything I have. I can't give you any more. This is me, and it's done nicely. It's all I have. All I have is yours, and that's it. It's not a matter of squeezing a quart out of a pint. Don't worry whether you have given enough; you've given all you have. You give according to what you have, according to the capacity of your mind, the capacity of your body, the capacity of your vision. We see as we think and we think as we see. If you can see this, you can start going the enlightened way — and wonderful things are in store for you.

Do You Want To Be Liked?

Nobody really likes a selfish person. Nobody really likes a materialist minded person. Such people may have a gang of cronies or pals around, but they are all out to get what they can from each other, and there is no true friendship involved. We can even make the spiritual way of life obnoxious — by boasting about how spiritual we are. That is why Christ would say, "Go, and tell no one," after He had performed a miraculous healing. He never boasted about His miracles.

Sometimes it is best not to speak of spiritual matters. In Italy I saw a wonderful sign that read, "Your prayer is your work." Think about that for a moment. "Your prayer is your work." You may feel a compelling urge to persuade others to believe in your particular faith, to believe as you do. I don't want you to do that with me. Let me see how you live, how you work — then I will *know* what your faith is. Then I will know whether it is something I would want to find out about. I will believe in your faith because of what I see you doing, not because of what I hear you claiming about it.

If a person goes around talking about doing good, do you care what church he belongs to? On the other hand, if he goes about doing good, you would certainly like to know what church he belongs to. We should teach people by example, by being the kind of person we should be. What we are shows in what we do.

All we want right now is to let go of the self and let the love of God come forth. We should be asking for more and more spiritual help, not material help. We should ask for Inner Help.

Lao Tse, a great sage of the past, once said, "By being the most unselfish, he is the most secure." I never realized this until I heard the story about the man who wanted all the king's jewels and all the king's gold. He was given that wish. When he got it, all he could do was to sit in the king's treasure chamber and count it all. He handled all of this gold every day. He lifted up the sparkling diamonds, rubies and emeralds and feasted his eyes on them. He was just like a banker — thousands and thousands of dollars touch his hands every day, but none of it is his. The treasure was only cold and hard. Can you see the lesson in the selfish, material thing?

In selfish living, you'll find that you must lose the inner values to gain the outer material values. When you seek selfish ends, happiness will elude you. Happiness is from the Inner Self; selfishness is from the outer self. James Allen said, "When seeking in selfishness, happiness will elude you and sow seeds of wretchedness." This, I think, is right. Wretchedness is not found in the spiritual realm. One of the truest things ever spoken is, "Whatsoever a man soweth, that shall he also reap."

If you sow selfishness, you'll reap selfishness. What you sow on that level will come back on that level. If you insist in living on the material level, it is the only harvest you can expect.

Get Out Of Your Own Way

Do you understand what your self will do to you? You've got to get rid of the self and go the self-less way. Have you ever heard of a person being self-destructive? Or self-disciplined? There is self-help and self-regard. There is self-satisfaction. There is self-pity — lots of it, and what a waste it is. Then we have the self-starter, the self-made man, the self-styled person. Can you see, can you feel, what this self is, what it does to us?

We have to get out of our own way. We have to grow out of the self, from the spiritual standpoint. We have to say "goodbye" to the self and give joyful "welcome" to selflessness. We have to let our spiritual nature overcome our human nature.

Mark Twain once said, "The only thing wrong with human nature is human nature. It's the nature of the beast." To overcome your self is to overcome your own worst enemy.

When people become unselfish, you know they have put something good in its place. You can tell. You can see it in their faces. You feel good around them. The unselfish way is the enlightened way.

When you have enlightenment then you choose your own destiny. You choose your own success. You choose health. The person who lives in selfishness harms other persons by expressing unhealthy misery. We have to beware of the selfish person. You don't have to beware of the spiritual person, the unselfish person. These are the people to pick as friends, people that you are glad to know, people that you never lose faith in.

These are the kinds of people in whose hands you can trust your life itself. These are the people you give your all to because you know it will be used for a good purpose. I've had money come to me as a gift, a gift given with only one thought behind it: "We want you to use this for the Ranch, for beautifying the Ranch. We want you to use this for something good and we know you will use it that way."

Even in India while taking photographs of an enlightened Master, it was lovely to hear him say, "I know you will use these pictures for good." And, you know, I couldn't use them for anything else but good because I felt I couldn't do a selfish thing with them. It is a very wonderful feeling when things are given to you to use unselfishly.

If we go about unselfishly, we are going to give of ourselves. I can't help but think of the crucifixion when the Christ said, "My God, my God, why hast Thou forsaken me?" It was as though he said, "Well, here is my self. What have you done? Where is my God?" After all the things I believed in through Christ, I thought, "My goodness, if you're going to lose His philosophy and all of His goodness the last minute . . ." But then Christ turned to the thief crucified on the cross next to Him and said, "To-day shalt thou be with me in paradise." Now, to-day! So another thing has turned!

If we could turn ourselves into that unselfish person, we would realize that, no matter what we have done or been, we can have paradise with unselfishness. We have to go through life and make a success out of this body, but you can only do it through harmony, peace, joy and happiness. These are, together, the way to health, the way to make the body run smoothly. Any other kind of body will be running to the doctor, and the doctor makes a living on bodies that do not run on the spiritual path.

I hope we go the enlightened way. If we go the enlightened way and know that we are raising ourselves above selfishness, leaving behind all our misery, we will turn and see the other side of this picture. We'll be able to rise above our selves.

A SPECIAL OCCASION—MY KNIGHTING

On September 7, 1984, I had the honor of being elevated to Knight Commander in the Sovereign Order of St. John of Jerusalem, the Knights of Malta, at the Basilica of Xaghra on the Island of Malta. It was, at the same time, a great and humbling experience.

As the Grand Prior explained, "The virtues of a knight are courage, good faith, courtesy, piety and respect for women. No details of such a life can be unimportant. It originates in natural dignity. The loftiness of demeanor is part of the true knightly character, distinguished from pride as clearly as admiration is distinguished from envy."

We are all knights in our own right. We carry a "righthood" as well as a knighthood, and there is no true knighthood unless it carries righthood along with it. We carry this according to our own level of consciousness.

Knighthood originally developed as an ideal way of life to follow. The leadership qualities of a knight begin to emerge only as he has learned to overcome the problems and obstacles in his own life, and it is only then that he becomes qualified to lead others.

Many people are looking to others to help them through their problems and troubles. Sometimes the wisdom of knighthood requires that we leave people alone to learn for themselves. At other times, this same wisdom requires the knight to hold a person's hand, to work with a person so they may awaken to a higher state of consciousness.

Knighthood is an ideal of service to mankind, embodying an attitude of helpfulness toward those around us—our children, friends, colleagues and humanity in general. Knighthood is associated with strength of heart, valor in word and deed. We have all heard the expression "lionhearted" and have a sense of what it means. People look up to strength. Our strength should not only be an asset to ourselves, but to others in meeting needs they are unable to supply on their own.

Those who are strong in love, mercy, kindness, justice and righteousness are often strong in body and purpose as well. While it is true that we may inherit a strong body, we can also develop strength by following what is right.

Just as the knights of old were adorned in suits of armor, each of us carries a kind of "armor" by which we can resist temptation, corruption, selfishness, greed and threats to our well-being. Nothing can disturb us unless we give it our consent. As we become stronger within ourselves, we put on the "armor of knighthood" so we can live our lives undaunted by obstacles or disturbances, prepared to accept the best there is in this life.

During my knighting ceremony on Malta, the Marquis don K. Vella Haber, Grand Prior International of the Knights of Malta, described the meaning of the distinctive white eight-pointed cross on the capes we wore, as follows:

"We wear this White Cross as a sign of purity. Wear it also within your hearts as well as outwardly, and keep it without soil or stain. As you know, the Cross has eight points and four arms, not without reason. Remember that the four arms represent the four cardinal virtues: Prudence, Justice, Fortitude and Temperance, while the eight points are the eight signs of the eight beatitudes which ye must ever preserve, that is: Spiritual joy; to love without malice; to weep over your sins; to humble yourself to those who injure ye; to love justice; to be merciful; to be sincere and pure in heart; to suffer persecution."

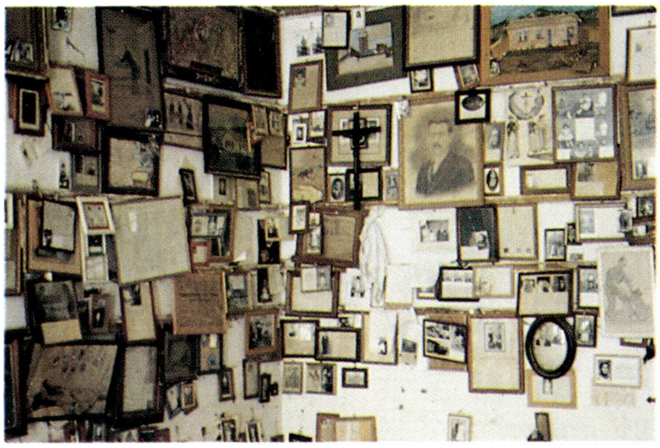

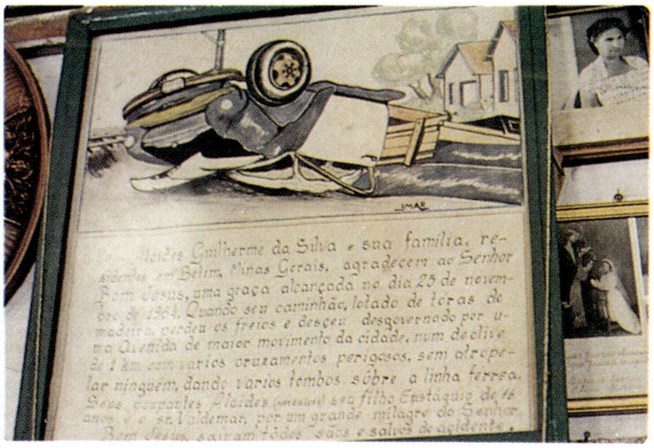

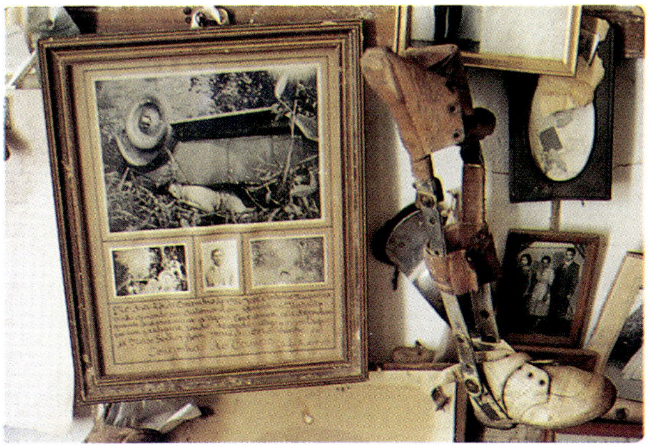

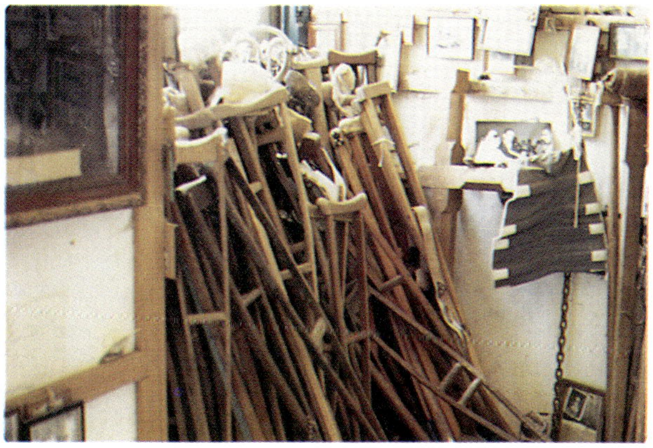

In many churches we visited, we have seen the power of faith working where people would arise and walk. They would take their beds and carry them, after they had been in them for years. We have seen crippled people leave their wheelchairs. There are many wonderful things that can be done through faith. Even in this little church, one room was set aside for crutches that were thrown away when people walked away healed and well.

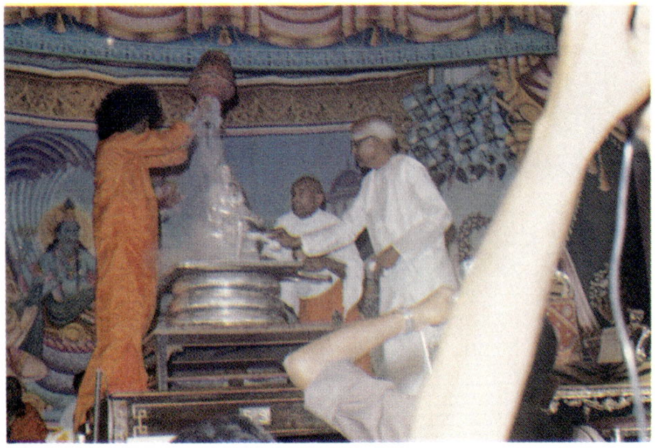

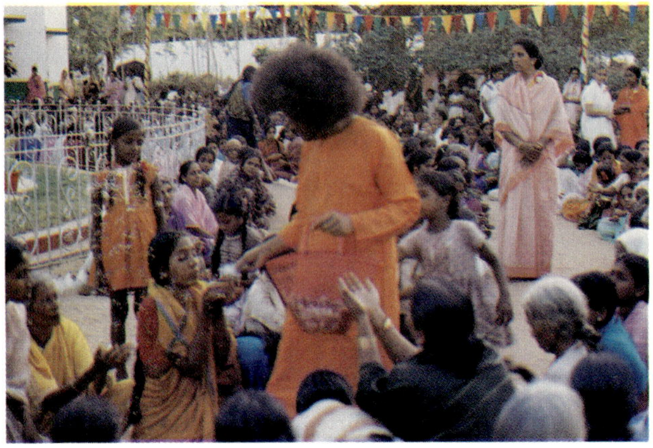

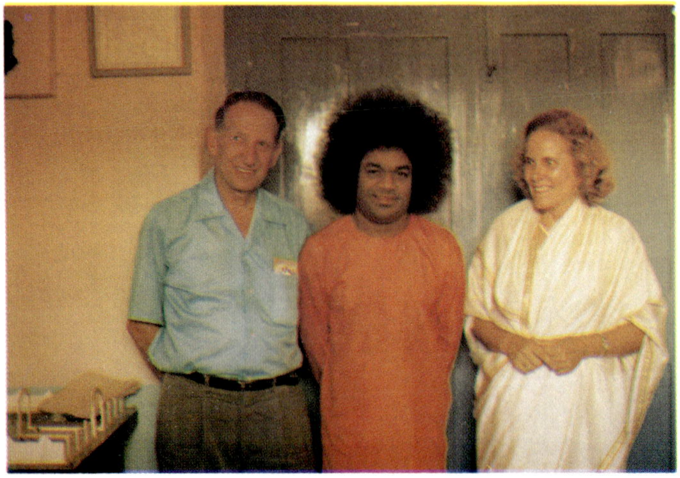

Sai Baba, one of those avatars of India, with more than two million followers who adore him for his philosophy. He has done many miracles, work that people consider some of the greatest of all demonstrations in the world today. It was our great pleasure to have a visit with him and to sit with 20,000 others and hear his teachings.

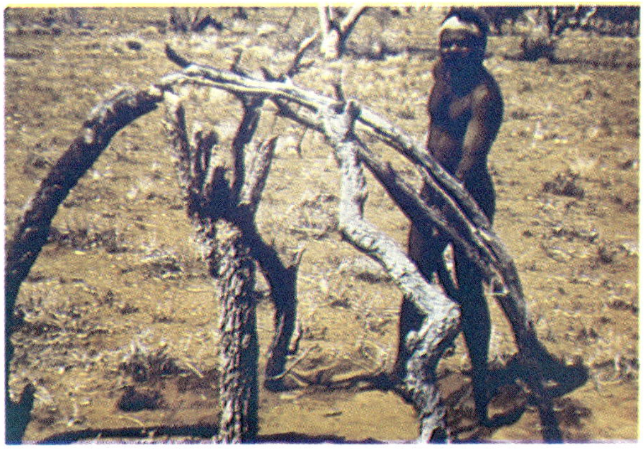

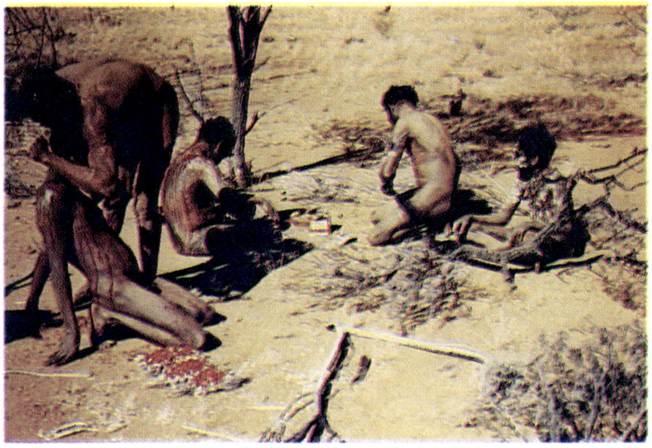

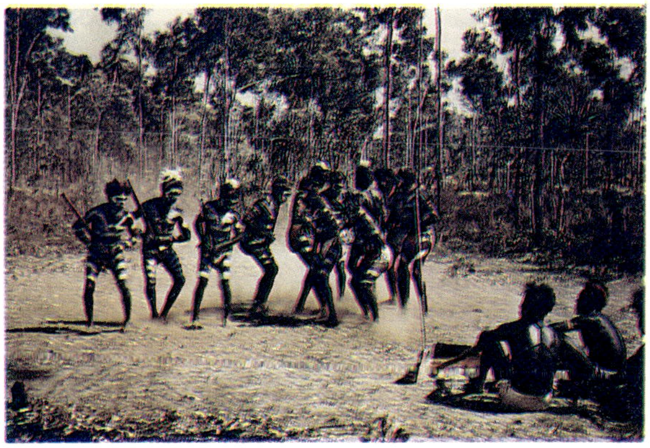

Aborigines, native to Australia, still live in the old way in remote areas of the country. Top: This man is making a home of what little nature has to offer. Middle: The Aborigines are becoming blood brothers by this ceremony communicating that they must share with each other. Bottom: Aborigines here are stomping the ground to awaken the gods to their needs, so they may have a good harvest, something coming that is good for their families so the next generation will have all the health possible.

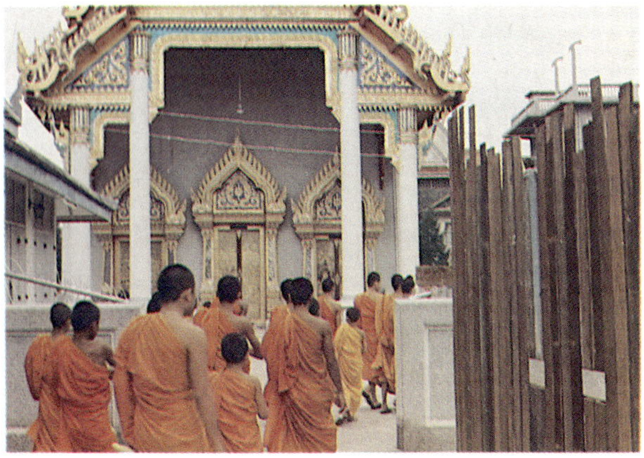

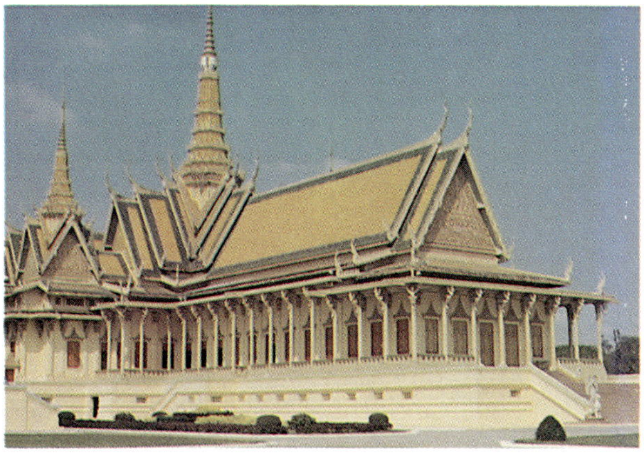

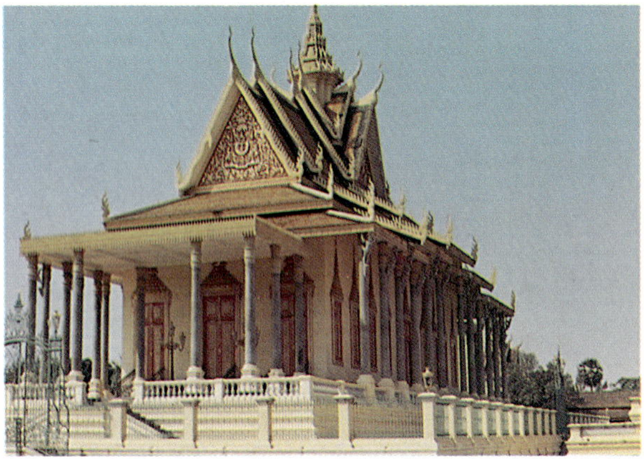

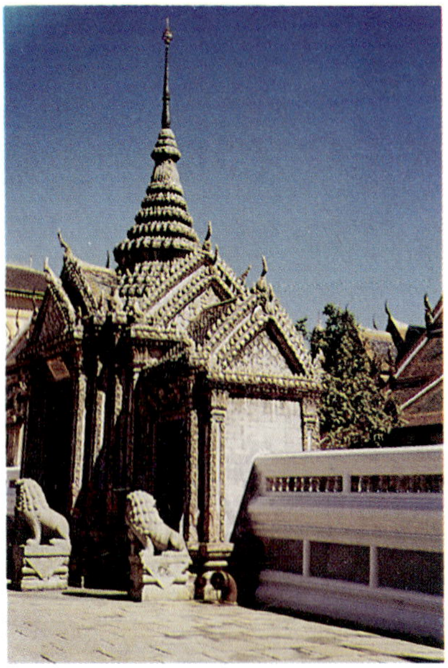

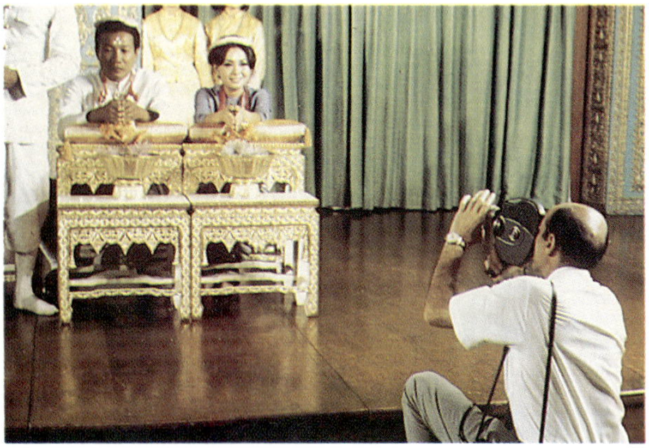

Upper Left: The young men from 15 to 19 are taken in for spiritual work in the temples of Thailand. They must practice spiritual ethics for one year. They must live on what people give them, usually just a bowl of rice left out on the porch for them as they pass by each day. Discipline is what they teach these young men in these temples. Lower Left: Beautiful temples in Thailand. Lower Right: A marriage ceremony taking place in Thailand.

Chapter 8

From Poverty To Riches

It is easy enough to be pleasant,
When life flows along like a
song,
But the man worthwhile
Is the one who will smile
When everything goes dead wrong.

How do you meet each new day? Do you meet it gladly, believing that it will reward you richly? Or do you meet it with uneasiness, believing that it will impoverish you, take you down another notch? Do you see each new day as full of new opportunities or do you see it as full of potential troubles and woes? Think about it. Look back at what was on your mind when you got up this morning. How do you meet the day?

One night I was having a good talk with friends about all sorts of things and I said, "What do you think is the real cause of poverty?" So we got into the subject of poverty and came up with some fascinating observations. Maybe poverty isn't what we think it is. Maybe there's a state of mind, an attitude, a mental thing going on. And certainly there's a spiritual aspect of poverty as well. You hear people say, "That poor dog!" What does that mean? It means that whatever kind of problem came to the person, he met it with a poor spirit. We hear people say of the man who has no money, "The poor fellow!" Why is that person poor? What is poverty?

My dictionary defines poverty as, "The quality or state of being indigent or poor; need; destitution." Concerning the word "poor," the dictionary gives one of its definitions as "spiritless." A poor person, in this sense, is one who lives in a spiritless manner. From the spiritual standpoint, a poor person is one who has not risen to the spiritual level at all. He is spiritless.

A person who is poor doesn't have the means to form good substance. The poor lack certain qualities, they are scanty, they have no sustaining values. Now, we have to be careful about who we define as poor. As we will see, some people who are very wealthy in material things are very poor in other ways, while some who are materially lacking are rich from the spiritual standpoint.

The man who is really poor today is the one who is poor in spirit. If you are going to buy a horse, you look for one that is full of spirit. If someone sells you a horse without any spirit at all, you have bought yourself a dead horse.

The poor are deficient in vigor. To accumulate vigor, we have to accumulate it in good health. You can't expect to have strength and power of mind unless you also have strength and power in the physical body. From a health standpoint, the person who is ailing is poor.

The Person Who Is Never Satisfied Is Poor

Now the person who lives constantly in physical want lives in depression because he can't get what he wants, and the person who is greedy is just as poor because no matter how much he has, he is never satisfied.

When you are fed physically, after a while you are hungry again. But the person who eats the spiritual food can always be full. When you have that spiritual fullness, you have stopped being poor. You have ended your poverty. Suddenly, you are rich. Suddenly, you have something, something of value. When this happens, life changes for you.

We know that it is not possible to grow healthy foods — healthy fruits and vegetables and nuts — in poor soil. Poor soil is soil that is lacking in proper nutrients. If you try to raise a garden in poor soil, you will get poor plants, unhealthy plants. Because they are poor and unhealthy, disease comes easily to them — disease and insects. If you have some healthy plants near the poor ones, the insects will attack the poor ones first, then move on to the healthy plants. If you enrich the soil, if you fertilize it well, before you plant the garden, you will get strong, healthy vegetables. In the same way, if you enrich the mental environment with the spiritual values, the attitudes will rise, and the body will quickly follow.

What Is The Good Life?

Most people believe that the good life is to have lots of material possessions, things you can see. Many people who are physically impoverished believe that if they can just get started on the road to having more material possessions, their problems will be solved. I believe this attitude is mistaken. I believe it is upside-down.

The way out of poverty is to start with peace on the inside, to start with harmony on the inside, to start with joy on the inside. Then happiness will come. Then satisfaction will come. Then everything that is right for us will come. Would you like to have happiness? Would you like to have good friendships? Would you like to have good health? These are riches, but where do we find them? Can you borrow these things from someone who has more than you do? No. Can you get them by demanding that Congress pass a law ordering these things to be distributed among those who lack them? No. You can't get such things by organizing a march on Washington, D.C., or on your state capitol. They aren't there or anywhere else on the face of this earth.

The *Bible* tells us that the poor will always be with us. This would be true even if everyone on the face of this earth had plenty to eat, a nice house, two cars in the garage and money in the bank. Those who choose the path of material possessions, those who shake their heads "no" when you suggest that they look within, will always be poor. When a person lies, he is poor. When a person cheats, he is poor. When a person steals, he is poor. The federal government tells us that "white collar" crime is seriously on the increase. These people are among the affluent poor. They are poor because they are hungry to get more, so hungry they are willing to take from others.

There is an end to poverty. We choose the higher path; we leave poverty behind us. We take the Joy Coach; we leave poverty behind us. Perhaps you were poor once, but now you seek the truth, and the truth will make you free.

Come Up To Riches

The idea is this: When you get away from this perpetual gnawing hunger for material things, you will find that you are truly a rich person. Then you will stop saying, "I am poor." Then you will stop saying, "If only I could have this or that." You will have a new consciousness. You will be taken care of.

I believe that poverty, like sickness and disease, is deeply affected by the mental attitude. I believe that when a wretchedly poor person says, "I need bread," he is saying something very similar to what the sick man states when he says, "I need medicine to get over this thing." Neither person is dealing with the real cause of his condition. Both need an education. Both need uplifting. And this must start from the inside, not the outside.

When I was in India a great realization came to me. The Communists are taking over part of that country. Do you know how they are doing it? They are putting hoes in peoples' hands. The

Communists are putting tools in the hands of the rural poor people there, tools that will help them grow their own food. Those people are beginning to say, "We can feed ourselves." This is a new attitude. This is a new start for them, a new hope to replace the old hopelessness. There's a saying that goes, "Give a man a fish, and you feed him for a day. Teach him how to fish, and you feed him for a lifetime." There is a mental concept behind this. The person begins to say, "I really *can* do it!" Now, what has the United States been sending to India? We sent them five million dollars worth of vitamins. We sent them a "fish." Do you see what I mean?

Poverty Is An Inside Job

Every now and then a bank or corporation is robbed of a great deal of money, and the robbers know just exactly where to find it and what day the most money will be in a certain vault. The police will say, "It was an inside job." To a considerable extent, poverty is an inside job, a kind of robbery where someone or something on the inside is assisting the situation. Something on the inside of the person keeps that person poor. What is it that does that?

We have previously talked about how people live their beliefs. You can live by a positive belief, and it will do you good. You can live by a negative belief, and it will reap a negative harvest, a harvest of harm. You can live believing you are poor, and you will reap a harvest of lack, of want, of need. This is a law: As you believe, so will it be done unto you. Christ said, "For unto everyone that hath shall be given, and he shall have abundance; but from him that hath not shall be taken away even that which he hath." Is Christ saying here that the poor are doomed to perpetual poverty? No. He is saying that those who refuse to look at and be thankful for the richness of life itself have not yet learned to be receptive. They have not yet learned to have faith in the abundance the Father has promised them. Their hands are clutched tight around the little they have, and even that will be taken from them — so they can learn to reach out with empty hands to receive their inheritance, their birthright. There are some very hard lessons in life, and poverty is one of them. Poverty is an inside job, an attitude, a belief. As long as we continue in that belief, we allow it to rob us blind.

You can't pray and expect God to do all the work. You can't make God work. You can't ask Him to pedal a bicycle up a steep hill for you; but you can ask Him to give you the strength to pedal it up that hill yourself. We are the ones who have to get to work. We are the ones who have to get going.

We must also realize that wretchedness and poverty, as states of mind, have an effect on the physical body. As I have said before, our thoughts affect each cell of the body. When people get too nervous, they begin to lose their hair. Improper thought can cause the skin to dry out. When we dwell on thoughts of poverty and lack, our bodies begin to reflect this, and other people notice. There may be a dejected appearance, a forlorn appearance, a "poor me" appearance; the body lacks vitality and vigor. Such a person seldom draws or attracts happy, healthy friends and companions. Instead, he is usually surrounded with people like himself. Like attracts like, as they say. Have you ever heard someone say, "He is caught in a vicious circle"? Poverty is a vicious circle. And it must be broken from the inside. You can't break it from the outside by giving food, material things or money to the poor. The circle only closes up again because it is a mental thing, an attitude thing.

I am not saying that we should not give to the poor and needy. All the world religions teach that we should give to the poor. But none that I know of teaches that poverty will be cured by giving to the poor. The cure lies elsewhere. It is within.

We have talked about the "vicious circle" of poverty. There is an interesting aspect to the idea of the vicious circle. We have certain lessons to learn in life before we can go on to the higher things. But if we are in the eighth grade and we don't learn our lessons, we have to repeat the eighth grade, don't we? This is the vicious circle we are talking about. It continues until we learn the lesson. Sometimes we have to go all the way to the bottom before we realize there is such a thing as "up." Sometimes we have to get to the place where we are sick of being poor before we realize it is time to seek a cure. Then we go within. We find hope there. We find peace there. We find love there. We find there is a state of well-being inside ourselves and we find the keys to the kingdom.

Build A Better Kingdom

When we unlock the door of the inner kingdom, we begin to discover some wonderful thoughts, ideas and attitudes that we can use to build a better outer kingdom. We must raise our sights so that we can build a kingdom worth living in. God's kingdom is the only one that will not pass away. When we begin dwelling in it, we find that the mental kingdom, the physical kingdom, begin to take on some marvelous changes.

We can look upon these kingdoms as gardens. We get our seeds from God's garden, we plant them in the mental garden and water them with the living water of God's truth, then we find that we reap good fruit at both the mental level and the physical level. When we are learning our lessons, we are planting the seeds of knowledge. Over a period of time when we have gained enough experience, our knowledge begins to mature into wisdom. And wisdom is one of the most important things we can have in life. We find that experience gives us the wisdom to handle the experiences that are yet to come. We grow in wisdom. It takes wisdom to build a better kingdom.

When I hire a person, I always ask, "What experience have you had?" Often I find that the one with the most difficult experiences, the worst experiences, can do the job best. But only if that person has learned from his experience, only if he has gained wisdom from his experience. Too many people let their experiences batter them around. The experiences have grabbed ahold of them instead of the other way around.

Now I want you to be rich. I want you to be able to meet the experiences that life brings you and still keep your health. It isn't hard to get knowledge these days because you can read good books and you can associate with people who know. You can become rich in knowledge and wisdom. You can use that wisdom to build a rich and wonderful kingdom.

I Am A Millionaire

I've got my name on the river,
I've got my name on the sea;
I've got my name on the summer skies —
They all belong to me.

I've got my name on the violets
That grow in their corner fair,
And wherever nature has planted peace,
My name is written there.

As far as my eye can travel
From where I stand to the sun,
I've got my name on the things I see
And I own them, every one.

I've got my name on the singing birds
That mate when the spring is new;
But I won't be selfish with all these things —
I'll share them, friend, with you.

There is no deed to the river,
There is no lock on the sea;
Not all the power in all the world
Can take their joy from me.

There is no fence in the heavens, No vaults
hold the sunset's gold,
And the earth is mine, and the heaven's mine
Till all the suns grow cold.

And though I may be a pauper
And stand in my rags apart,
I'm richer than all the kings there are
If peace is in my heart.

The stars are my thousand jewels,
And life is my bread and wine;
And all that I see was made for me,
And all that I love is mine.

There Is Plenty For Everyone On This Planet

I believe there is enough on this good earth to provide abundantly for every human being alive. Why shouldn't we simply give the poor a substantial amount of money and let them buy what they want? Well, by now we should realize the answer to that one. God, in His wisdom, has put each one of us on this earth to learn certain lessons in truth. When we turn away from that truth, when we refuse to lift our eyes to that truth, when we deny that truth, we suffer the consequences. The consequences are at the same time pointing us back toward the truth.

People who consider themselves poor are poor in mind, poor in spirit and poor in purse. There is only one thing we can do for them that will have lasting value, and that is to show them something to grow toward. To become rich is to know that in consciousness you can have everything you want.

But people who focus only on their physical wants get caught up in the lower values, the temporal values. Food can be given to them, but they will get hungry again. Money can be given to them, but they will spend it and be broke again. A temporary patchwork solution isn't really what we want, is it? We want to get out of that rat race! We want to get out of that wretched way of thinking! We want to leave all that behind and go on to a new life!

Today Must Be Better

You can shed the old like a butterfly sheds its cocoon. You can start shedding that cocoon of old troubles by realizing that you are doing better today than you did yesterday. If you aren't doing better, you're still caught up in "I haven't got all I want," and by now you should realize that approach simply doesn't work. When you have reached the place where you realize that every day you are getting better and better, where you are thankful that you are getting better and better, where you are blessing each moment because you are getting better and better, then that attitude will bring you a better life, a healthier body.

Often poverty and sickness breed fear. "God hath not given us the spirit of fear," it is written. Where did you get fear? You made it. You invented it yourself. Scripture tells us, "The fear of man bringeth a snare." You bring fear into existence, and it snares you. If you were walking down a jungle path, and a tiger walked out of the bushes, what would you do? You would run and climb a tree. There is a smart thing to do, and you do it. You don't have time to be afraid while you are running and climbing that tree. But if you walk down that path thinking a tiger might jump out from behind any bush, you will be afraid. You will get the cold sweats. Fear will drain your energy. Then if a tiger jumps out, it might possibly get you. What have you done? Through fear you will have wasted the energy you needed to meet the situation and do the right thing.

You know, the world is full of tigers. The world is full of troubles and problems. And if we fear them, they will come upon us. Some people are busy still fearing yesterday's tigers. Others are busy fearing tomorrow's tigers.

Seek right thoughts. Replace ugly fear thoughts with lovely thoughts. We need to change, and we are already changing. We look to the desert and we see the rose in bloom. We make it bloom by the way we see, by the way we think. Do you understand?

What Is It You Need?

What do we really need? What are we really hungry for? I see hungry people. You see hungry people. Maybe you are hungry. The *Bible* says, "What man is there of you whom, if his son ask bread, will he give him a stone?" God has not put that stone on anyone's plate. We put the stone there ourselves. We are starving and we give ourselves a stone! We need to balance our lives. We need to arrive at a spiritual-mental-physical balance. Being out of balance is what makes us sick. Being out of balance is what makes us poor. We have to deal with whatever it is that keeps us off balance.

There is something about wanting, the thought of wanting something, that makes it very difficult to get what we want. The more desperate our want becomes, the more elusive its object becomes. I'd like to show you a way to break through this frustrating situation. It is a fact of life that those who already "have" tend to get more. You have to have something in order to receive. When I was just starting out with the Ranch, there were so many things that needed to be done that I could hardly count them all. I wanted someone with money to come along and help out. I needed people to help with the work. But when I didn't have anything, nobody wanted to help me.

Now that everything is going well, everybody wants to help. You have to have something of value for your fellow man before you can progress and grow. Now I have all the help I want, but it didn't come until I learned to stop wanting. Logically, I realize, this would be called a contradiction. The ancient philosophers would call it a paradox. But life doesn't take place by human rules of logic. There are many paradoxes in life.

There's only one thing you can do. Let go of wanting and be thankful for what you have. Realize that you already have much that is good in your life. Focus your thoughts on what you have, not what you don't have. Reach for the inner values, the higher values, and put them to work in your life. Get the foundation built and build it on rock, not on sand. Build it on the rock of the higher values, the eternal values. Then people will come to you. Then you will get help.

Laziness Travels Slowly

Many years ago Benjamin Franklin wrote *Poor Richard's Almanac*, and his thoughts are still good stepping stones out of poverty. Ben Franklin, in the guise of Poor Richard, wrote, "A lazy fox never catches any poultry," and "Early to bed, early to rise, makes a man healthy, wealthy and wise." Poor Richard was an enthusiastic spirit; he tells us to get moving in life. "He that riseth late must trot all day." So, it's better to get up early because, "It's the early bird that catches the worm." We can do quite a lot for ourselves, can't we?

"Laziness travels slowly," wrote Poor Richard, "Poverty soon overtakes him." These sayings really have "bite" in them, don't they? You have to overtake problems and deal with them. A person who handles each day as it comes is much better off than the one who always lets his problems wait until tomorrow. He will be a richer person.

"Be ashamed," Richard said, "to catch yourself idle." There is always something to do, to learn, to discover.

Now what is the key to all this? What is the most important idea? We must realize that we have access to the infinite power of God. With that Infinite Resource within, working from the inside out, we can have that spiritual-mental-physical balance we need. With the power of the Spirit working in us, we are equal to any task — we have a quality that we can go within and draw on.

We have to draw on this power. People look for God in many places. People look for power in many places. Where is He? Where is the power? We will find both in the quiet place inside ourselves.

God doesn't make a lot of noise while He is at work in our lives. We sit on an earth that is speeding like a bullet through space and we accept this very calmly, don't we? Godly things take place very smoothly, according to law, with no confusion whatsoever. The power is there. It is up to us to use it. What is the first step? Unclutch those hands of yours. Let go of what you've been holding onto so tightly. Let God see that your hands are empty — and He will fill them up!

If you want to get away from the poverty side of life, you'll have to get on the giving side. If you aren't giving to others, it doesn't matter how much money you have in the bank or how little — you are poor. If you are always feeling sorry about that splinter in the eye of the poor, it is time to take the log out of your own eye. You have been down there with them, mentally. Rise up and get on the giving side. A person who is giving is one who is lifting people. I'm not just talking about giving money. Money really doesn't count for much, you understand. We can only help uplift people by those things that come from the heart — kindness, peace, harmony, joy. This is what we are looking for.

Who Is Rich?

One time when my accountant was going over my books, he said, "You know, doctor, when I look at these figures I see you have a wonderful business, but I would like to ask how much cash you have in your pocket, right now?" I took all my money out, and it came to $1.30. Then he said, "Look, I want to show you something." He reached into his watch pocket and took out eight $100 bills. "How would you like to have that?" he asked.

"Oh, yes," I thought to myself at first, "It would be nice to have that in my pocket."

"Doctor," he said, "you walk around like a poor man all the time." Still looking at those eight $100 bills of his I thought, "Gee, is he rich!" So I asked, "What do you do?" When he replied that he was an accountant, I said, "I know that, but what do you do in your spare time? What do you do with your home life?"

"Well," he said, "when I go home I take off my shoes, fix a bite to eat, then go into the living room to sit and read the newspaper. After that I watch television for an hour or two before going to bed."

"What do you do the next morning?" I asked.

"I get up, shower, shave, eat breakfast and go to work," he replied.

"How long have you been living like that?"

"Oh, for about fifteen years," he said. I began to grow curious then about that $800 he carried around, so I asked him how long he'd had that in his watch pocket. "I've carried that with me for twelve years!" he said proudly.

My accountant, I began to see, was not a rich man, because he lived a poor life. That $800 he carried around wasn't money to him, it was just paper! He didn't even use it! He didn't get any good out of it whatsoever. He hadn't discovered the joy of giving or receiving. In fact, for a man with $800 in his pocket, he was the poorest man I'd ever seen. I put my $1.30 back in my pocket and thought about the lovely trip I'd taken just a few months before. Would this man have gone with me? Would he have taken the time to enjoy himself? I spend my money. Why put it away where it doesn't do any good for anybody? It seems as though I'm always too busy to watch television, and when I'm learning something new or talking to interesting people or on a trip, I miss a lot of meals. I spend my time and money on things that I often value more highly than my meals, but what I receive in return is wonderful. I don't feel sorry for the man who is dying, I feel sorry for the man who has never lived. Such a person is truly poor.

What Are The Best Gifts?

Who is rich? Is it the person with the big bank account, the expensive home, the big new car? Or is it the person who lives a full life surrounded by friends, the person who is needed and wanted? You can't buy the joy life. You have to live it. The joy life is one of those rich gifts that we simply appropriate as we go the uplifted way.

In the *Bible* Paul urges us to "Covet earnestly the best gifts, and yet I show unto you a more excellent way." He is talking about the uplifted way, the higher path. As we go through life, changing and growing, there are always ways for us to do good. I'd like to present a poem here called "The Legend of the Raindrop," a poem that has meant a lot to me because it serves as a wonderful reminder that you can have much more than you think you have in any given moment.

The legend of the raindrop,
Has a lesson for us all
As it trembled in the heavens
Questioning whether it should fall.
For the glistening raindrop argued
To the genie of the sky,
"I am beautiful and lovely
As I sparkle here on high,
And hanging here I will become
Part of the Rainbow's hue
And I'll shimmer like a diamond
For all the world to view . . . "
But the genie told the raindrop,
"Do not hesitate to go,
For you will be more beautiful
If you fall to earth below.
For you will sink into the soil
And be lost awhile from sight,
But when you reappear on earth,
You'll be looked on with delight;
For you will be the raindrop
That quenched the thirsty ground
And helped the lovely flowers
To blossom all around,
And in your resurrection
You'll appear in queenly clothes
With the beauty of the lily
And the fragrance of the rose;
Then, when you wilt and wither,
You'll become part of the earth
And make the soil more fertile
And give new flowers birth . . . "
For there is nothing ever lost
Or eternally neglected,
For everything God ever made
Is always resurrected;
So trust God's all-wise wisdom
And doubt the Father never,
For in His Heavenly Kingdom
There is nothing lost forever.

We must remember that we are eternally rich, for as the *Bible* tells us, "It is your Father's good pleasure to give you His Kingdom."

You Can Make The Sun Rise

If you are in a poor kingdom today, you can change. You can look again and see a brighter side to life. There was never a sunset without a bright new sunrise the next morning. The sunrise always follows. So if you are one of those who think of themselves as poor, one of those who feel down and out, think of this time as the sunset. You can make the sun rise tomorrow.

This lesson is brought out nicely in the parable of the Prodigal Son. This fellow asked his father for his inheritance ahead of time, so he could go out and see the world. His father agreed, and the son went off to the nearest city where he quickly spent his fortune in riotous living. Broke, destitute, the young fellow searched for work, but all he could find was a job slopping pigs for a farmer. Hungry and miserable, he recalled how even his father's servants ate better food than he was getting, so he decided to return home and to ask his father for a job as a servant.

With his head hanging in shame, he approached his father's house. Instead of being angry when he saw his son approaching in rags, the father rejoiced at his return! He ran out and kissed him, calling for his servants to bring a fine robe, new shoes and a beautiful ring to put on his son's finger. He ordered that a fatted calf be killed for a feast in celebration of his son's return.

For the Prodigal Son, a new day dawned, a new sun rose, when he came back to his father's house. He had thought of himself as poor, and he had approached his father's house ashamed of his poverty, ashamed of wasting his inheritance. But his father received him with joy!

One of my teachers always left me with this reminder when we parted company: "It is your Father's good pleasure to give you the kingdom."

We can make the sun rise on the new day by accepting the Father's gift. Look outside. See that beautiful sky, that wonderful earth? All the earth and all the lovely things on and in it have been given to us! Man has been given all this to use and enjoy! So be thankful. We have been given life so that we may rejoice and be glad in the day. Recognize that you cannot go through life without being touched by Divinity. Recognize that you belong to God. You will never lack because your Father has given you the kingdom, and everything you could want or need is there.

There is much richness to recognize in life. We are the highest of all created living things. We were made in the image of God. How can we ask for more than that? As we live in that image, the image of God, we are given every good thing.

God Created You To Be Rich

If we live in God's kingdom, if we realize we have been created for joy, we are truly rich. So many people look to the earth for its riches — its gold, its diamonds, its pearls. It is true that the earth can give us these things, but there is one thing the earth can never give. You can, but the earth cannot. You can love.

You are part of the divine creation, and the divine creation has given you the gift of love to pass on to other people. The person who loves his fellow man is a rich person. The person who has risen above hate and fear and jealousy is free — free to love, free to give. That person has left bondage behind. That person is rich.

Don't be an earth-clinger. Let it go. Let loose of it and be free. When you help free other people, you free yourself. When you let go of the earthly things, you let go of your stress, strain and worry. Leave that prison and learn to take care of yourself. Lift your eyes to the stars. Recognize that it is your purpose on this earth to take the higher path because you have the earth and more.

When you think of yourself as free to be filled with love, you begin to see love in others. Eyes purified with love see more love, because good finds itself in others, brings itself out in others. When you see only love, only good, you have become one with love and good. You have come into harmony with all life. You have peace, happiness and joy.

All this is yours if you seek it. Above all, let's not just think giving these things lip service is enough. Don't let them fall into platitudes. Live these things.

Say to yourself, "I am rich. I have left poverty behind because I have chosen to return to my Father's house, my Father's kingdom." You may not see it. You may not hear it. You may not feel it. But it is there, greater and deeper than man can penetrate with earthly senses.

You have been blessed!

LETTER WRITTEN BY HERMES TO HIS SON TITIAN

Thou wouldst contemplate
the Great Spirit, the Creator,
even in perishable things,
in things that are of the Earth,
or in the deep.
Reflect, oh my son,
on the formation of man in his mother's
  womb.
Contemplate the skill of the workman.
Learn to know Him
according to the divine beauty of the work.
Who formed the orb of the eye?
Who pierced the openings of the nostrils and
  of the ears?
Who made the bones hard?
Who covered the flesh with skin?
Who separated the fingers and the toes?
Who made the feet broad?
Who hollowed out the pores?
Who spread out the spleen?
Who made the heart like a pyramid?
Who made the side wide?
Who formed the caverns of the lungs?
Who made the animal parts of the body
  conspicuous
and concealed the others?
Who made all these things?
Who was the mother?
Who was the father,
if it is not the only Invisible God
Who has created all things by His will?

Chapter 9

Then There Were Two

Nothing just happens . . .
Everything happens just.

There was a time when I didn't realize that thoughts and feelings were so important. At that time I believed that the physical side of life was everything. I believed that everything was mechanical. Adjustments of the spine, so I thought, could cure almost anything. A change to a better diet, so I thought, would improve a marriage. I believed that if you drank enough carrot juice, you'd never have to worry about diseases any more.

In those days I believed I was treating only one thing — the physical body, the outer self.

But I've learned over the years that the deeply satisfying things of life, such as harmony and peace, don't come just from food and physical pleasure. I began to see that there was such a thing as the inner self.

My gradual discovery of this inner self began when I became interested in the power of thinking. People always talk about how the grass seems greener on the other side of the fence. While I was still involved in the physical side of health I thought I'd do some investigating, and I found that there *are* some lush green pastures on the other side of the fence! I met Napoleon Hill and read his book *Think and Grow Rich*. I was fascinated. There were many things in that book that I hadn't known before. For a while, Napoleon Hill and I lectured together before the same audiences. Then I decided that thinking was everything, that you could, in fact, grow rich just by thinking.

Of course, getting rich seemed to be the most important thing in the world. Hill's book was selling very well, and many great men have copies of that book on their bookshelves. Napoleon Hill had interviewed a number of the richest, better-known men of his time, and in his book he described what each of them felt had brought him his great wealth. Then I realized that I had lived long enough to see all of them die.

Are Rich Men Happy?

In previous chapters we've talked about the effects of selfishness and greed, mostly on a philosophical level. Now we are going to get down to actual case histories.

Five of the seventeen men who were the subjects of Hill's book, men we were taught to look up to and think of as leaders, committed suicide.

They thought so little of their lives that they decided to end it all. Is that happiness?

Livermore, with all of his riches, ended up in prison in Leavenworth. Apparently he couldn't get enough money by legal means to satisfy himself. He wanted more — but he was caught at it. Needless to say, Leavenworth is not noted for its joy and merriment.

Two of the men in Hill's book fled this country to hide what was left of their wealth in secret Swiss bank accounts. Many of the original seventeen men died broke! Yet many people still believe that growing rich is great, and among them are many who are still trying to think themselves rich.

So I began to wonder, "Is happiness perhaps more than a matter of gathering wealth and accumulating material possessions? Could there be something more powerful than thinking? I began to see that there was a life more abundant, a life that money couldn't buy. I began to hear a voice inside myself saying, "What is that to thee? Follow thou Me."

The Good Book tells us that it is easier for a camel to pass through the eye of a needle than for a rich man to enter the kingdom of heaven. The rich man has the hardest time getting into heaven! Well, I wanted into that wonderful kingdom and I thought to myself, "The poor man has a better chance." Perhaps I shouldn't tell you this, but I prayed that I would have all my money taken from me. And God heard me.

I reached the point where I'd tell somebody, "You need it worse than I do." Then I'd reach for my wallet. Before long, I'd given most of my money and a considerable amount of my possessions away. I wore the same suit for nearly two years! I was taking care of it — I won't tell you all the nice things I was doing for that suit — but I really wasn't taking care of myself. Here I was, telling everybody, "Take care of yourself, now — you need this more than I do," until I reached the place where I didn't have a thing. There were times when I went without food just to be sure others had enough.

Then I began to wonder, "Is this really the right way to live? Is this really the way to work things out?" I thought again about the life more abundant that is so often spoken of: "I am come that they might have life, and that they might have it more abundantly." I began to ask myself, "What is this abundance of life?" I had just lost my wife and had to start life all over again with a one-year-old boy. I was living in depression. The world wasn't good. What was wrong with me? Why should these things happen to me? I had so many questions. But where was I going to get the answers?

Before my wife passed away we had planned to take a voyage with seventeen others on a cruise ship to the South Seas. I wanted to get rid of everything. I couldn't even seem to move my arms anymore. I couldn't drive my car. All I wanted to do was to run away from everything. I thought I would go to an island in the South Seas, live under a coconut tree and let coconuts fall in my lap. I am exaggerating a little bit, but you know, you get to wondering, "Where am I going? What do I want in life?"

The ship left without me, because after my wife passed away I couldn't stand the thought of going alone. When that ship arrived off the coast of Acapulco, fire broke out and it burned! A couple of the people were seriously injured. I couldn't help but think, "Maybe I wasn't supposed to be there."

For a while I let myself get wrapped up in earthly things. I used the principles in Napoleon Hill's book, and they worked. I was wrapped up in money. I was wrapped up in a human foolishness. Can I put it that way? So often, man has such foolish ideas. I could see they were foolish after they happened but not while they were happening. Wisdom comes from hindsight, they say. While they were happening it seemed wonderful, and I was part of it. I think many people are doing that today, enjoying themselves in ways they will later come to regret.

For me, the riches I obtained through positive thinking were simply not satisfying. They lost their value. Something was missing. I began to see how we bring these problems and troubles on ourselves. I was just like the atheist Ingersoll — he didn't believe in God at all. He felt there was nothing in this life outside of physical things. But on his deathbed, he told his wife, "There's nothing more that I seem to be able to get from this world. There is only one thing left for me in life, and that is to pray to God." At the end, he reached a turning point.

I asked myself, "How could a man like that, an atheist all his life, come to such a conclusion just before he died?" Wouldn't it have been wonderful if he had come to that conclusion long before? So many of us have hindsight. Why can't we have foresight? Perhaps that's why the Good Book tells us that without vision we perish. If we are unable to take that step of faith that leads to truth, we are in trouble.

What Is It You Want?

I started on my search. I think we are all on a search of some kind. What are you seeking? Have you thought about it?

Lots of people only find out how to live correctly when they reach their sixties or seventies. That's a bit late considering the amount of damage that has often been done in the earlier years. Scars are produced — internal scars as well as damage to the health. Psychologists call some of the internal scars "blocks." People develop fixed ideas, fixed beliefs, fixed patterns of living. It's difficult to change into a right way of living as you get older, but some have the wisdom to do it.

If we could only recognize it, by changing our lives at the right time we can release ourselves from the need for doctors. We can release ourselves and really enjoy life without sickness.

There is an answer. I've been searching for this answer for years and although I don't think I've found all of it, I'll share what I've found. It has to do with physical health. It has to do with brain rejuvenation, with keenness of mind, alertness. It has to do with the bowel, the stomach, the kidneys, the heart. I know these well from a doctor's standpoint.

For many years I treated only the outer person — the physical body. Then I discovered the inner person and its effects upon health — the thoughts, the feelings, the beliefs, the spiritual thing. First there was only one thing for me to treat. Then there were two.

Stop and think for a moment. Do you just want financial success? Do you want it badly enough to have people hate you if you get it? Or would you rather have people bless you? Would you rather have time to enjoy life?

In a previous chapter we mentioned a man who wished to have all the king's treasure. When his wish was granted he spent thirty days counting it, thirty days admiring it, thirty days locking it up all the time, thirty days worrying whether thieves were going to get it; and by then he was so tired of taking care of the king's treasure that he didn't want anything more to do with it. He wanted to mingle with people, to share love, kindness, courtesy and good feelings.

You don't acquire these from gold or money. One of the hardest lessons to learn in life is that wealth gives so little inner satisfaction. The psychologists and the psychiatrists say that money is very important, that money is at the heart of many mental problems. I believe that. But, money doesn't give us all we need. I certainly found that to be true in my own life, and that is why I began my personal spiritual search.

I was just a novice at these spiritual things and one day while I was giving a physical treatment, I heard, "I will find thee, even unto the marrow of your bones." What will find me? Who will find me? What's this voice I'm hearing inside myself? I knew that the marrow of the bones was the hardest part to rejuvenate, to rebuild, to take care of. In the marrow of our bones the new red blood cells are formed, and the Bible says the life of the body is in the blood.

So when I heard, "I will find thee, even unto the marrow of your bones," I knew that message referred to the most valuable physical process in the body. When the marrow of the bone goes, the physical body goes with it. I was seeking something — and something was seeking me — at the deepest level.

The Inner Food

I knew all about nutrition for the physical body. I knew that to affect the marrow of the bones, I would have to think of certain specific foods for a person's diet. But was there such a thing as food for the mind? Food for the spirit?

So I began investigating these questions, these other foods. When a person is dying and someone says, "Here's a cup of herbal tea that's good for the heart," that's not the right food to offer that person. He needs spiritual food. And I'm telling you — how I needed that spiritual food! I consumed it like a starving man who had just found his way out of the wilderness.

Love is such a food. Another is patience. A lady once told me, "All I need is patience, doctor. If I could get a bottle of patience from you, I'd pay most anything!" Of course, patience doesn't come in a bottle.

There are many foods for the spirit, but you will have to discover for yourself the ones you need. You are the one who has to find them and you are the one who has to use them. You can't get them from me. All I can do is awaken you to the need for them.

Look Within For The Truth

What I'm saying is, you have to work for the higher things. You have to search for them. One day you'll be finished looking for them "out there." Then you'll find that the higher things have to come from an expansion inside yourself, deep within yourself.

It is said that the kingdom of God is within. I suppose all of us go through a period in our lives when we just have to see if it isn't out there in the world somewhere. We go through that and we find out it isn't. Then we begin to look inside. It's so hard for a young person to accept this. Perhaps it's hard for everyone.

It seems to be human nature to think of God as being in some far off, difficult place to reach, like the top of Mt. Everest. But then Mt. Everest was climbed. What about the bottom of the sea? No, even its mysterious deeps have been explored by bathysphere. Outer space? Our NASA probes haven't found a trace of God out there. There is an old saying to the effect that if you really wanted to hide God from man, all you would have to do would be to put Him deep within man's heart. No one would ever think of looking there. To a surprising extent, I think, this is true. For some reason we are very reluctant to look for God in our own hearts.

We're always looking for some church that has the right God for us. We go to church to find God. Are you sure He is there? If He wasn't inside you in the first place, how could you hope to find Him in church?

When I started looking inward, seeking the inner help, I was working with a teacher who shed some light on a very practical matter. He told me that everyone needed a job to keep alive, to support himself, then he added, "But the job really doesn't support you — you support the job." That was a new concept for me. If we want to have a job, we are the ones who have to stay ahead of it. This is where we have to start.

I began to discover double meanings, double levels, always two in everything. There are parables that tell one story on the surface, with a deeper meaning beneath. In each person there is an inner self and an outer self. I began studying some of the ancient Greek plays in which the actors wore masks called the *persona*. If the same actor put on a different mask to play a different character, he had a different *persona*. The word *personality* comes from the Greek word *persona*.

I feel that a lot of people use their personality to mask the real person beneath it. Inside is where the real person dwells. "What he is deepest, he really is," Murdo MacDonald Bayne used to say. How deep do we have to go? We must go beyond the mask.

In the Greek plays I read about the laughter of the gods. I wondered if God ever laughed at my foolish antics. One day I said to myself, "My circulation isn't good." Then I took another look at what I'd just said. Who said, "My circulation isn't good"? If it is *my* circulation, *my* body, then who is the *I* who is doing the talking? For the first time in my life I was saying that *my body* was one thing and *I* was another.

When we say things like, "My circulation is bad," or "I'm losing my hair," or "My body is cold," we are measuring, we are evaluating something going on in the physical body. Doesn't this make sense? We have heard the saying, "To be absent from the body and to be present with the Lord." Are you understanding this?

Once I thought the "Lord" meant a man. Then I found that the "Lord" meant the Truth. It meant the Law, God's Law, by which everything is governed. I was present with Law and present with Truth. It all took on a new meaning to me. I started thinking differently. I started thinking as two people.

I was first of all in my body, and sometimes that was not comfortable. But did you know there is a place from which you can like everything? There is a place where we are right with everything, where we can see good in the bad, where we can see good in all mankind, where we can be a brother or sister to all our brothers and sisters in the world.

I found that there is no sickness in spirit. Can you see there are two things going on here all the time? I found that there is no hatred where love is. I thought that if my patients could only be absent from their bodies for a while and be present with God, there would be no more complaints, no more sickness. There is only sickness in the body.

Life Has Many Facets

After seeing these two avenues — the physical and the spiritual brought out in my life, I began to look back into some of the original work in the *Bible*. I found there was a medical side, a spiritual side, a mechanical side and a chemical side in the Old Testament writings.

Going back into the papyrus scrolls written around 3,500 years ago, we find a number of very interesting remedies. For instance, they would soak a donkey's tooth in honey, then apply it as a medication to a person's body. Dung was gathered, refined and taken internally for certain illnesses. The writings mention processes where horse's hair was concentrated or where the hoof of an ass was boiled down, dissolved and taken as medicine.

The people of that time also used lizard's blood, swine's teeth and old stinking fat that they cooked until it became liquid. Medicine was made from the excreta of various animals and from ground up dead flies. These are some of the ancient medical remedies people used to treat their ailments.

Then about 1,400 B.C. a very wise leader named Moses arose from among the Hebrews living in Egypt. Moses was a devoutly religious man, and he began hearing a Voice that would tell him what to do. He led the Hebrews out of Egypt. The Voice gave Moses the Ten Commandments and an additional set of laws and instructions that completely changed the way of life of these people. Moses heard the Voice say, "I am the Lord that healeth thee." They dropped the old treatments with dead flies, animal excreta and lizard blood.

When they began following the new laws and started cleaning up their minds, the Hebrews became a strong, vigorous and healthy people. They found that the body follows the mind when the beliefs are changed. The body becomes a willing servant of the mind. By following their new beliefs, the Hebrew people of this time were able to overcome many of the problems they faced.

Divine instructions were given to them. Here I can see "two" coming up again, the inner and the outer. On the one hand were the treatments devised by Egyptian doctors for the outer person, the body, and on the other hand were the Divine instructions given to Moses and directed to treating the inner person. As the Ten Commandments and other laws were adopted into the formal religion of the churches that sprang up, important changes came about in those people. There is a wonderful passage in the Good Book that says, "If thou wilt diligently hearken to the voice of the Lord thy God . . . I will put none of these diseases upon thee." You see, the spiritual side of healing goes back a very long time.

Would you believe that even leprosy could leave people? And that a lot of mental illnesses could leave people? About twenty percent of the people in mental institutions today could have prevented their problems if they had just followed good law with a little self discipline. Another twenty percent of those who are mentally ill would be healthy today if they would just follow good law and eat the godly foods. I could take another ten percent away from the mental institutions if they would diligently listen and hearken to religious law instead of the law of the barroom and the bottle. They could leave their alcoholism behind. That adds up to a total of fifty percent of those in mental institutions who could be taken out right now by following these laws.

Healing Is From Within

So we need to get into another level of existence by stepping up into a new dimension. As my mother used to say, "If your outlook isn't good, get a new inlook." We have to start from the inside and come out. I believe we live on what we pour forth. Do you know, the day is going to come when you are going to radiate health, and your body is going to feel it. Your body is going to have a good time — and it needs it!

Do you know what hatred can do to the kidneys? It can produce a phosphate crystal that causes great distress in the kidney tubules. What we think will finally have its effects in the cell structure of the body. If we would care for the spiritual side of life, many diseases would never visit us.

We are all seeking. We all have our problems and troubles. But right now, let's seek our way out of this confusion. I believe we can only do this when we step up into the next dimension, where all one's old beliefs and wishes are foolishness.

We have to find a place within ourselves where we can stand and nothing will disturb us. This is why we have to be absent from the body. Then nothing of an inferior nature can disturb us. We are all trying to tell right from wrong by means of our outer senses. You can't do it that way. You have to go behind the senses.

There is something on the other side of the fence that is green, that is gorgeous, that is godly, that is good for our health. I must tell you about this because some of you are unaware of it. Any physical problem we have to take care of is secondary. We have to go back into ourselves to heal the cause. You can't go outside to get it.

The higher state of mind is man's best nature, but we aren't always seeking that higher state. We see the earth and what's in it and on it, but this isn't the real beauty of life. A lot of people think they would feel better if they were married or if they had a car or if the mortgage was paid. But you have to feel better even without these things. If such things are affecting your health, they are keeping you earth-minded, earthbound, and you have to let go of worrying about them.

What Is Real?

When I look at these two facets, the physical and the spiritual, I begin to think that the spiritual is the only real value we have. Physical things, physical pleasures, come and go — in that sense they are unreal. These are the things that thieves can steal, that are tarnished by rust and time. All kinds of things can happen. What's going to happen to you if you lose your material possessions? Will you be able to stand it?

We have heard, "My kingdom is not of this world." When we go within, we start watching the unveiling of the Divine in our consciousness. We behold this beauty and hold it within ourselves. We have to be a witness to this wisdom. We have to look inside to find the real truth.

We have to go into this new dimension I'm talking about. We should have a willingness to look away from our old life, because there is something much better waiting for us. Of course, the human senses are going to hold us back to a degree, because unless we taste food we won't be satisfied. Many people gain satisfaction from sounds, colors, tastes, smells and feelings. That is not enough.

To get into the new dimension we have to build up our spiritual treasures. Greater bank savings don't mean greater security. Physical health isn't a sufficient foundation for eternal life. Physical necessities allow only an improvement in the outer person.

Spiritual peace is the source of health. The harmony of being only comes when we have harmony within. Recognize the good things you have and enjoy them, no matter how few they are. There is no limit to enjoyment in the spiritual realm.

And All These Will Be Added

We have been shown the way! "Seek ye the kingdom of God, and all these things shall be added unto you." Our physical needs will be taken care of as we learn to seek God's kingdom in the Inner Temple.

Now, when we build the Inner Temple, the physical temple becomes a double powered thing. It becomes the Temple of the Divine. If we want to change this temple, we can. If you want a new stomach, you can build one in seven months time. But what we really change in life is our spiritual concept. We change the physical self to the spiritual self, which never changes.

When you finally reach Truth you don't have to change. You have arrived. There's nowhere else to go and there's nothing more to get. Then we are one with all men. Then we have reached the state of all wisdom where we can harmonize with other people.

To do these things we first of all realize that the Temple is not made by human hands. As long as you hold on to the idea that this human temple needs only human care, you will be seeking a doctor to cure you.

If you could be a co-creator, if you could become one with the One who takes care of this Temple, you would start the rejuvenation. A human body is born after nine months in the mother, but when it first comes into the world it is not alive. But all at once God breathes a breath of life into the nostrils of this babe, and it becomes a living soul. The infant is not fully alive until it receives that breath.

There is no mystery about the inner life. The only mystery is in how you see God. That is the only mystery. There's no hope for man at the level of earthly things. I believe at this level men are primarily selfish, power hungry and greedy. You don't find these things in the place where all healing flows forth.

When we look inside at first, evil becomes less real. Sickness is less acute, partly because people increase the degree of sickness by paying attention to it, by nourishing its effects in their minds. If you leave the sickness alone and live your life, sickness will often correct itself.

Lose Yourself To Find Yourself

As the self disappears, every need will be taken care of. Our desires become less acute and our fears begin to evaporate. Our assurance and confidence become greater. We become more alert. A new keenness begins to show in our attitude. We call this an Inner Presence. We notice that its power immediately starts to work on the inside of the body.

The joy that begins to develop doesn't depend on the outside things. No outside stimulus is needed to keep it going. The light of the Inner Presence begins to radiate outward. When we have this power coming outward, then we have taken a giant step forward.

Here we find that life is without end and we begin to see with different eyes. We hear now with different ears and we hear things we have never heard before. There is something within that tells you, "This is right," or "This is wrong." This is the Voice I am talking about.

We understand truths not known before and we no longer have a separation between God and self. As we look to these truths we "consider the lilies how they grow; they toil not, neither do they spin." We fear nothing. Our Father takes care of us through all difficulties. You have no worries or problems because, "It is the Father's good pleasure to give you the kingdom."

But if we leave the Father's kingdom, disease and disharmony come about. I am convinced that if we keep our tongues from poor speech and our lips from deceit, if we do good and act as our brother's keeper, we will have begun to follow the most important commandment, "Thou shalt love the Lord thy God." We will know that we must love our neighbors as ourselves. We will no longer lay up for ourselves treasures on earth.

When we follow God's injunction to "Abide in Me," then we have the Life. If we go to the spiritual way first, all other things will be added unto us.

You are fortunate. You can learn from the lives of the seventeen men I spoke of earlier, the men described in Hill's book *Think and Grow Rich,* men who sought and found riches on this earth. They also found suicide, prison, exile and so forth — these were men without a life. You don't need to repeat their errors. You have another way and you will be taken care of.

So today I ask you to awaken, to arise to the finer things and start this spiritual life going. You can't just talk about it. You must move on it. It is ever ready for you, and now is the time. Now is the beginning of the rest of your life.

I asked God for strength
that I might achieve;
I was made weak
that I might learn humbly to obey.
I asked for health
that I might do greater things;
I was given infirmity
that I might do better things.
I asked for riches
that I might be happy;
I was given poverty
that I might be wise.
I asked for power
that I might have the praise of men;
I was given weakness
that I might feel the need of God.
I asked for all things
that I might enjoy life;
I was given life
that I might enjoy all things.
I got nothing I asked for
but everything I hoped for;
In spite of myself,
my unspoken prayers were answered —
I am among all men
most richly blessed.

— Author Unknown

Chapter 10

From Silence We Come Forth

Nothing will ever happen to you unless you give it your consent.

Have you ever watched alley cats? Living on the edge of survival makes them furtive, stealthy and fierce. They fight with and hiss at one another. They eat from garbage cans and they will grab any morsel of food left within their reach and run with it. They will utterly destroy the peace of a warm summer night with their howlings.

We have many invisible alley cats running around in our minds, and I can tell you (with all due respect for cats) that they are not there for any good or noble purpose. Two of the meanest of these creatures are fear and anxiety.

The human organism can be completely destroyed by the depredations of these invisible alley cats. You can cut out a tumor or cyst, things you can see and touch, but fear and anxiety are not visible to the human eye. Yet they are very real. We see their effects constantly.

When we have a certain thought, a blush will come to the cheeks. Fear, hate or anger can likewise bring consequences to the body — but, unlike the blush, these consequences can involve great suffering. Such emotions can cause congestion, resulting in an excessive amount of blood gathering in some part of the body. Fear can bring a blanched face. Where does the blood go? If the blood is held in a certain place for a length of time, a clot or embolism may be caused, perhaps even a stroke. That's why fear and anger can be contributing factors in high blood pressure. And, the effects are seen in the body, perhaps your body.

It may not be your first fear or the first time you have become angry, but like the constant dripping of water, the accumulated effects of anger, fear and anxiety gradually affect the adrenal glands and the thyroid gland, which is the emotional gland.

Eventually the whole body is changed. Today adrenaline is given to persons suffering from asthma attacks. Why has the adrenaline in their bodies been used up? It is possible that fear, hatred, anxiety, regret, remorse, resentment or resistance have produced an adrenaline lack in your body, years after you started hating a person.

There is an effective technique for overcoming fears and hates that I would like to share with you. The technique is to go into quietness. The technique is to be silent, to be absolutely silent, to go within.

What Causes Tension?

We can only come forth after going within. We can only come forth with the godly expression, and that is a quiet expression. Do you think God lives in disturbance? Do you think it is disturbing to do a godly deed? Do you think it is disturbing to do the truthful thing? I want to tell you, a lie will upset you. A lie will come forth in the body and will disturb you physically.

Revenge generates a good deal of tension, strain and stress. But that which is godly takes no strain. It is done peacefully and harmoniously, and the physical body is renewed and restored. Then we can say, "Amen, it is finished." Do you want the physical body to suffer more? No? All you have to do is recuperate and get well.

A wife has to release her husband from fear and give him freedom within himself. True love does not bind one person to another or coerce another against his will or trespass against another. One cannot go through life saying, "He is mine" or "She is mine." We must free one another to be about our Father's business.

Each and every one of us is on a mission of his own and each must perform that mission in his or her own way. We don't have to have possessions to be content. We should enjoy what we already have. We should give thanks for what we already have and not worry about what we don't have. We must enjoy the here and now! Then we will come to know that our lives will change through a spiritual concept, because all there is, is in the eternal NOW.

As we meditate, go into the silence, back into our deeper selves, we find we come forth with the spiritual knowing that was there inside us. Without spiritual guidance the physical body is ruined, ruined through vengefulness, hate and anger. Only the spiritual knowledge will show you the value of love, peace and the finer things in life.

When we put the spiritual concepts into practice we will be more joyful, more peaceful, more contented. We are sometimes prone to depression. We all have problems to face and to work out, but we can transcend them through faith and love — and joy will follow as day follows night. It is our birthright to be joyful and healthy. We can learn to rule and control our physical bodies, to master them. We don't want to just keep our bodies alive, we want to have healthy bodies, healthy minds and happy spirits. We have to have something with which to meet life with tranquility.

Pills Do Not Solve Problems

The experts say that if you want to "make a killing" on the stock market, invest in those companies that are manufacturing tranquilizers. Every year those stocks are increasing in value as more and more people turn to more and more pills as the answer to their problems. However, it is possible to toss the tranquilizers in the garbage can and do better without them. We know that tranquilizers do not solve anything, because they don't change the situations that give rise to the problems for which the pills are taken.

We can do better. The solution is already inside us. Better than any pills ever manufactured, peace and harmony await within us. We can learn to use them by first going into the silence within ourselves, finding that special place where they are, then bringing them forth. This may take practice in the beginning, but it is the only real way to get peace and harmony.

We should stop and think about the still, small voice that is deep within us. We need to be very quiet to hear it, for it never shouts. This voice will tell us how to measure things well.

For one thing, it will tell you there are no victors in fighting. There are only victims. There is no victory in life when it is necessary to live under constant stress and strain. Which way do you choose? The still, small voice will tell you to go the peace and harmony way every time.

In Silence Is Strength

Many of us have yet to realize that there is more to life than just the power of material things. We have to relax and enter into the ocean of peace. This is God's world. We find that the real miracle takes place in silence. It is in silence that we say, "Oh, now I see," or "Oh, now I hear." It is in silence that we *feel* the miracle taking place. This is where we understand how foolish we have been. This is where growth is taking place.

Regardless of the situation, the moment you find out how foolish you have been, that is the moment you go on to greater enjoyment. You go on to greater things. You will never quit smoking until you find out how foolish you are. You will never quit drinking until you find out how you are paying for it and maybe you'll have to pay for it twice. You find out when you have come to this place of realization that your life is your own, to be lived as it ought to be lived. It is the still, small voice that tells you these things.

How many times have you given advice to other people that hasn't done any good? It is like water rolling off a duck's back. It never does them any good. Why? Only an awakening helps us. When you have the awakening you begin to make decisions, you arrive, you begin to shine. At that moment you begin to overcome. This is not the same as hearing voices talking to you — this is quite another thing. No one is talking to you physically. If you can't hear your Inner Self you are not listening with the real ears of life.

Where are the real ears? Where are the real eyes? Where are the real feelings of life? Someone may say, "I am deeply touched." How is he touched? Is this a bodily thing? No, it is not. It is that which we are deep within, a very real place.

We must withdraw from all of our powerful temptations by going into the Silence, this absolute silence within. We quiet the mind as well as the body. We must rest from all the material and physical powers. We must realize that all the power of the universe cannot prevail against us, because we and God are one.

Jesus told how the rains descended, and the floods came, and the winds blew and beat upon the house, but it fell not, for the house was founded upon a rock. Isn't that the kind of person you want to be? One that is unmoved? One that is untainted? One that does not worry, fret and stew?

The body is always the effect, never the cause. You must realize that. Suppose I asked you, "How is your health this morning?" What would you say? You might have to say, "My health is all right, but I am sick." If I asked you about your ulcers, you might say they are giving you pain. But how is your health? Health is always all right. Are you understanding this? Your sicknesses are not all right.

The Mind Can Heal

In terms of health, there is no disease at the level of spirit. There is no dis-ease in good health. If you will follow good health principles, eventually dis-ease, dis-harmony and chaos will leave. All of your health thoughts will add up to health in the future.

If you want to be well five years from now, start right this moment. Too many of us are prone to look for the miracle that takes place in 2 minutes. But in the twinkling of an eye, we *can* change our *consciousness*, and the body will come right along. The body follows the mind.

How is your nervousness? "Well, I am nervous, but my health is okay. I am exhausted most of the time but I feel pretty good." Are you seeing this thing?

As the story goes, a man called the family doctor to find out what his wife's trouble was. The doctor said, "She has a malignancy." The man said, "Well, I don't care as long as she's healthy."

We separate things. Our mind separates things. We have an idea that a disease is separate from the body and the mind. I want you to understand that disease is *not* separate from the body and the mind. It is part of the person. It is the state you are in. Disease is a lack of good health, the state you *should* be in. It has come as a result of bad habits and bad thinking. It is an accumulation of lower level thinking and emotions. The body does not produce a disease unless you help to bring it into existence.

As Job said in the Good Book, "Fear came upon me, and trembling, which made all my bones shake." What you fear will come upon you. If you fear anything long enough, it will finally absorb you. If you keep your mind upon the fear of this and the fear of that, fear of tomorrow, fear of your husband, fear of your problem, fear of financial loss, fear of insecurity, pretty soon you will be lifeless. When you become negative enough, you just fade away. What is the answer? You must let those fears go. You move into security, peace and harmony. You change your mind and what goes into it.

Why don't we start another kind of epidemic? Let's start an epidemic of good will. Let's start an epidemic of smiles. Let's start an epidemic of good. Let's hope that an epidemic like this will sweep the world.

There is a little song that goes, "Little drops of water, little grains of sand, make the mighty ocean, and this pleasant land." Little thoughts, when we put them all together, add up to a mighty ocean. Health is made up of many thoughts, many attitudes. It depends upon exercise, breathing, personal habits, words, thoughts and deeds. They move us forward or draw us backward. Through strains and stresses, we can choke off the normal chemical processes that help sustain health in the body.

Many of us do not realize that we choose our own reactions. It is said that peace of mind is not based on what happens to us. The main thing is our *reaction* to what happens to us. If we don't deliberately take charge of our reactions, they take charge of us.

Our health is based on our thoughts and on our reactions, our reactions to other people, places and things. Good health requires that we remove all the old negative and adverse thinking. Working toward peace and harmony means controlling our reactions. Yes, this is work. It takes practice to reverse our old thinking habits.

We find that God is healing all the time; so we must go within and come out with a positive attitude, with a calm and serene feeling about ourselves, about the situation and problems facing us, as we slow down and let God heal the situation. No one can disturb us unless we consent to be disturbed—because we are one with God and we bring forth the steadfastness of the godly state. Then we discover that nothing of an inferior nature will upset us. We stand steady and let God take over. Then we will feel these finer workings taking effect in the physical body and in our human relationships.

"As A Man Thinketh"

To see the final result in your body, you have to work with causes. The things that cause change in the body are thought, feeling, food, drink and exercise. Positive thoughts and feelings permit the proper food, drink and exercise to do their work. But good thoughts must be emphasized as working the miracle.

You don't have to be religious to understand that good thinking is good for the liver. We know that sorrow has an effect on the liver. We know that humor, mirth and lightheartedness have an effect on the liver. Our moral concepts have very definite effects on our physical bodies.

For your own good you need to love. For your own good you need to take stock of your thinking. Every reality appears in degrees. For instance, between hot and cold there are various degrees. Do you want good health? You can only get it by adding more good to the body. Health is made up of many thoughts, and right thinking uncovers an abundance of health if you will put it to work in your life.

The definition of silence is "noiseless." Can you go where it is noiseless? "Enter into thy closet," we are told. This means we must go really deep within ourselves. We go into the Inner Self. Why do we go there? Why do we go into the silence of the Inner Self? The *Bible* says the kingdom of heaven is within. You have to go within. Now, we do not say this is easy. It is simple, but it is not easy. Often the mind is a chatterbox. The mind wanders, the mind daydreams, the mind thinks. Have you ever gone deep within and silenced the noisy mind? It takes practice. "Where silence is, is not given to any speech whatsoever," said a wise sage. There is no wandering. Everything stops. This is where there is absolute silence.

We practice silence. Then the things of this life can pass by, and we don't even notice. This is a place free of all activity, motion or disturbance. This is a place of calmness, of serenity. This is a place where you get acquainted with wisdom. "Know thyself," Socrates told us. This is where we go to know ourselves.

There is no explanation quite so effective as silence. If you are right, your life will do its own explaining. If you are wrong, you can't explain. So you go calmly on your way, forgetting everything except the business of right living, and you let time explain for you. It is in this quietness that you do the real living.

Many people who get sick believe they have to go to a doctor who has been in practice a long time. But God doesn't have to practice. He already knows. In the God Presence healing can take place within your body, your mind, your heart. It is only doctors who practice. So, don't you think it would be wise to go to the One who knows?

It is a mistake to assume that the first time you try it the body will respond immediately. It is just like when you step on the brake of your car. It doesn't stop immediately. The car slows for thirty feet or more before it comes to a stop, depending on how fast you've been driving. It is the same way when you press on the accelerator; it takes a while for the car to gain momentum. But when you keep on practicing, bringing forth the right thoughts, the right feelings, you will gain speed and momentum. After a time you will shift into high gear, and the desired effect will be reflected in your body.

To make a success of this physical body, you have to orient your goals with respect to eternity, not expediency. Expediency drives people to satisfy the short-term goals — physical pleasure, the accumulation of wealth, power, prestige. Some people tell me, "If I can just get enough to take care of my old age, that is all I want." This may sound modest, but modesty is not enough, either. You may not be able to enjoy your old age if you don't begin practicing the higher thoughts now. It is heartbreaking to see a person reach old age without developing the qualities he or she would really like to live in — wisdom, beauty, harmony, peace and good will toward fellow human beings.

Man must develop by carrying out his noblest duty. And what is that? To be kind, to be courteous, to be his brother's keeper, to help others become happy and fulfilled. But what is life? Is it just eating, sleeping and working? Is is just keeping the heart beating and the lungs pumping air? Is it just making money? For what purpose, I ask?

We seem to maintain our vitality and strength for the battle of life. What does this gain us for the future? Stop and think about this for a moment. If you were really interested in your future, you'd be living a better life right now. If you prepare a way now that is good for all eternity, you will have a better life today.

The Soul Must Be Fed

Harmony of the soul is much more important than harmony of the body. We try to provide food, clothing, shelter, comfort and plenty for ourselves and our families. But these are all temple duties. What do we gain from these in our eternal unfoldment? If we have only aimed to supply ourselves with the basic physical amenities, we may discover we have failed in life. The soul must be fed as well as the body.

There are many spiritual uses for this physical body. We have many bodies all in one. Man is passing through life, and if he doesn't perfect his soul in the process, he has not fulfilled his purpose, he has not lived the life more abundant. To know the joy of doing the right thing, to be honest with one another, to lift another person who needs help — these are the noblest aspects of our mission. These are the things upon which the soul is fed.

We Need Many Experiences

We must use the talents we have been given and enjoy them. We have to centralize all our energies. We must take up one path, follow through with it and make it a success. We must take care of our health. We must prepare ourselves for opportunities. We need much experience and we should thank God for all experiences that come to us. Each day we must start out right from where we are and grow from there.

What is to be done? We increase our vitality by discipline and practice. This is a part of our higher living, a part of the evolution of the soul. We develop habits of work, of industry, because we want to do what we have to do in this world with joy. Learn to work helpfully and constructively, accomplishing good in all that you do. These things are for your own good and for the good of your health. When we work we always work for noble ends. We then develop confidence in our abilities and direction. We get to the point where we realize that we are growing in harmony and peace; we are at peace with all people and with ourselves. We start with optimism — that is all we have — "half a glass of water." But if we know we have that, we have enough for this moment. We will be provided for.

We learn never to quarrel, never to argue. We find we must be honest in all our endeavors with ourselves and with others. We don't associate with negative people. We learn something from everyone we meet. We pick our companions with care and we work to bring out the best in them and in everyone we meet. In all of the opportunities that come before us, we select the highest and the noblest.

If you know that another human being needs you, use this opportunity to serve, but never lower yourself to that which is not good, that which is not best for you and for the other person. Select your partners, select the people you associate with. When you help people you have to be above the situation, you don't let yourself be dragged down into the situation. Never allow anyone to take you below the good that you have within you.

We must live the religious life. This is absolutely necessary for good health. Everyone has this longing within him. We all long for improvement within ourselves.

To achieve this you must go into silence. "The Lord our God hath put us to silence," the Good Book says of those who had departed from godly ways. To get back to the godly life we must go within, enter into the silence and come forth with finer, more noble ideas and thoughts. Then the body, a willing servant of mind, will become well.

We live on what we put forth. We live on what we give. You will never have in life more than you give.

So, as we release what we are at the deepest center of our being, we come forth knowing that all is well and with the feeling that " all that I have is thine." We lift our fellow man to a higher consciousness so that man may live with God.

The Winning Man

Think smiles, and smiles shall be;
Think doubt, and hope will flee.
Think love, and love will grow;
Think hate, and hate you'll know.
Think good, and good is here;
Think vice — its jaws appear!
Think gloom, and dusk descends.
Think faith, and faith's at hand;
Think ill — it stalks the land.
Think peace, sublime and sweet,
And you that peace will meet.
Think fear, with brooding mind,
And failure's close behind.
Think this: "I'm going to win!"
Think not on what has been.
Think "Victory," think "I can!"
Then you're a winning man!

—David V. Bush

From the Doctor's Pen . . .

We all have the potential of becoming more masterful in our expressions and technique. Surely, within our very soul we have the privilege of becoming greater than that from which we started. Certainly from the very low spots, there is a place on high to which we can look. We are like the flower, knowing that in our upward travel, and in our life growth, we can come out of the dust of the earth, out of the blackness, out of the mud, and be surrounded by the darkest cloud and yet we can always look upward. The flower is always seeking its light from above. The flower knows where to look for light—always above itself. Some have greater problems in their growth life—some are not so symmetrically designed as others; but the inherent spirit of all is to look upward and turn a lighted face to the source from which its light came in the beginning. If the flower did nothing but bring color to those who are in remorse or in sorrow, if it did nothing but bring joy to those who are unhappy and downtrodden, if the flower did nothing but bring happiness to the sick room, surely it would be worth its living.

To become the light of a rose, we must be all that it is possible to be, and not meet situations with resentment, resistence and stubbornness. We must live above these faculties. The rose, itself, is not interested in overcoming the black cloud, or in overcoming the dust of the earth. It wants just to become its sweet self—a beautiful rose. Its life was made easy and was used to uplift others because in its very self it represents the Light which brought it here. It is one with the Light that brought it here. It is the light. To become that light we have to become all that is expected of us.

Bring this beautiful light to the surface. Don't hide it. You should be known by the light you carry. Make this light your life. Living this life is being lit. Become that light.

Chapter 11

From Intellect To Spirit

Pain makes men think,
thinking makes men wise,
wisdom makes life endurable.
— TEA HOUSE OF THE AUGUST MOON

The word "light" is one of the greatest words that we find in our study of the spiritual things, the religious things. We speak of *enlightenment*. We speak of the *light* of understanding. Christ said, "I am the *light* of the world." We realize that we need light to find the right way to go. Yet, it is also written, 'He that dwelleth in the secret place of the most High shall abide under the shadow of the Almighty." When we think about it, we find that we need both light and shadow. Each is useful, helpful and comforting under certain circumstances.

When the Good Book speaks about living "under the shadow of the Almighty," we might give some thought to where this book was written. It was written in a land blessed by an abundance of sunshine. In the desert you are always looking for a shadow, a cool place. Similarly, after living in the heat of the world's problems and troubles, it is good to know we can find refuge in the shadow of the Almighty.

Most of the people I meet these days are seeking for something higher and better all the time. We may not always find it right away. Some of us have so many sentiments developed in one direction that we feel it would be going to extremes to develop further. What we strive for, really, is balance — physically, mentally and spiritually. Sometimes we even have to balance our activities within the spiritual realm itself when we have limited our explorations to only a single dimension or direction.

A Happy Life Is A Balanced Life

We should always seek balance and strive to know the truth. As you try to live your best and highest, your health will steadily improve. If your life is not right, it is time for a change. Man has been seeking the mysteries of God for a long time. Man has been and is being evolved from the lowest, most vulgar level to the highest ideals and sentiments that lead to the highest levels of consciousness.

In some ways it would be good if we were

all on the same level of consciousness, all of the same mind, so we could see things alike. But we are not. We are all free to make our own choices. That is why we forgive those who don't know any better. Though we are all on the same journey, we are all on different paths and different levels. We are all free to search for the truth and to rise to greater heights.

We must all take time to grow. We will all eventually come to the right path for ourselves as we grow. If you let this world push you around, your growth will be slower. Wouldn't it be wonderful if we could, through searching, right thinking and wisdom, direct our lives so that we could live at the highest level all the time? I believe this is possible.

I remember my son Art falling out of a tree and breaking his arm. His brother David was standing beside me and remarked, "Daddy, he didn't use his carefulness." Art is more careful now. Wouldn't it have been better if he'd had his "carefulness" developed to the point where he didn't have to fall out of the tree at all?

Often we live such muddled lives, such lives of sadness and sorrow, that it seems we should be able to do much better by developing a more intelligent and noble viewpoint, a sense of "carefulness." What prevents us from doing this?

A person who gets all tied up within himself is responsible for tying himself up. This is the "little self" at work. It is the 'little self" that seeks temporary relief from problems by taking tranquilizers, then takes a nose dive right back into the same problems. You can lead a tranquil life if you cut yourself loose from this "little self."

The world has a lot that attracts the little self. Through ambition we can have it — but ambition can kill us. You can jump on that treadmill of endless wanting, but the effort of running after things will sap your vitality, the energy you could be using to enjoy life. Instead of actually enjoying life, you would be spending all your time getting the things you think you have to have to enjoy life with. It just doesn't work.

Remember, God Is Everywhere

It would be lovely if you came to a point in your life where you could just BE. That's when you arrive. That's when there is no more trying, no more seeking, no place to go and nothing to get.

I once had a woman patient who cried for three months when her son was sent to Alaska by the army. She didn't realize God was up there, too.

There's a story about a little boy talking to the minister after church. The minister offered the boy a dime if he could tell him where God is. The little boy said, "I'll give you a quarter if you can tell me where God is not."

You see, we start limiting things in life and we get to the place where we live on just one side of the fence — the selfish side. The activities of the "little self" produce physical ailments because its entire focus is limited to the physical body and its desires. This isn't enough of an outlet. If we center our minds, our thinking, all our activities on ourselves, we produce a kind of energy congestion in the physical body that leads to an intense feeling of frustration. We all know people who are frustrated. They have no outlets for their energy. They have it all bottled up inside.

I used to work with a psychologist in New York City. Many of his patients were filled with hate. He had a solution for this. In a back room he had some rubber heads set up. He would have his patients go in there and pound those rubber heads with all their might, so they could get the hate out of their systems. Usually when a person hates, he has been hated or abused by someone else and he lives in that hate. He is saturated by hate and has to get rid of it. Sad to say, people tend to express that hate toward others instead of simply letting go of it.

Why live in hate? When my patients are lacking calcium, I give them calcium. When they lack love, I'd like to be able to give them love. But, unfortunately, I can't pour it into their hearts with a funnel! Hate can be replaced and healed by love. But the person has to be open to receive love and has to be willing to release the hate. Love is often what we are lacking. The best way to receive love is to give love. Then it comes back to you.

Thoughts are things, and people can become heavily burdened by their thoughts. We say, "That person looks like he's carrying the weight of the whole world on his shoulders." Have you ever seen a person like that? They show it on their faces, too. It can be seen in their eyes. The person who lives in vulgarity, the person who lives in low sentiments or the person seeks to out-do another person doesn't have a life-giving magnetic quality in his eyes, does he? They just don't go together.

Are we talking about health and disease? Yes, we are. We are talking about health and disease of the mind — disease of the mind and lack of ease. When I talk about disease of the body, you may think of cancer or high blood pressure. But it really is lack of ease in the body. Lack of ease in the mind and lack of ease in the body go together. When there is dis-ease in the physical body, there is dis-ease and dis-harmony in the mind. So let us reason this out and find which side of the fence you are on.

A Fence Or An Ambulance

'Twas a dangerous cliff as they freely
confessed
Though to walk near its crest was so pleasant;
But over its terrible edge there had slipped
A duke and full many a peasant.

So the people said something would have to
be done.
Their projects did not at all tally.
Some said, "Put up a fence around the edge
of the cliff."
Some, "An ambulance down in the valley."

But the cry for the ambulance carried the day,
For it spread through the neighboring city;
A fence may be useful or not, it is true,
But each heart became brimful of pity.

For those who slipped over that dangerous
cliff,
And the dwellers in highways and alley,
Gave pounds or gave pence, not to put up a
fence,
But an ambulance down in the valley.

"For the cliff is all right if you're careful,"
they said,
"And if folks even slip and are dropping,
It isn't the slip that hurts them so much
As the shock down below when they're
stopping!"

So day after day as the mishaps occurred
Quick forth would the rescuers sally
To pick up the victims who fell off the cliff,
With their ambulance down in the valley.

Then an old sage remarked, "It's a marvel to
see
That people give far more attention
To repairing results than to stopping the
cause
When they'd much rather aim at prevention.

"Let us stop at its source all this mischief," cried he,
"Come neighbors and friends, let us rally.
If the cliff we will fence, we might almost
dispense
With the ambulance down in the valley."

"Aren't we picking up fools just as fast as
they fall?
And shall this man dictate to us? Shall he?
Why should people of sense stop to put up a
fence
While the ambulance works in the valley?"

But, a sensible few who are practical too
Will not bear with such nonsense much
longer.
They believe that prevention is better than
cure,
And their party will soon be the stronger.

Encourage them, then, with your purse, voice
and pen
And while other philanthropists dally,
They will storm all pretense, put up a stout
fence,
On the cliff that hangs over the valley.

Better guide well the young than reclaim them
when old,
For the voice of True Wisdom is calling.
To rescue the fallen is good, but 'tis best
To prevent other people from falling.

Better close up the source of temptation and
crime
Than deliver from dungeon and galley
Better put a strong fence around the top of
the cliff
Than an ambulance down in the valley.

—Joseph Malen

Many people come to me to take care of their ailments. The man who can do it the quickest, the man who can do it now — he is considered the miracle worker. But I wonder if those who seek a quick cure realize that they will wake up one of these days and have still another disease or discomfort.

They will come down with another health problem because the doctor who gave them the quick cure the first time never dealt with the cause of the problem. We are constantly working with causes and effects. I see people coming to me and I wonder, "What started all this?" They have so many problems, so much sadness in their lives, so many memories they are carrying around with them. It is wonderful to see people change their lives just by changing the direction of their thinking.

To Improve Yourself, Start With Your Head

A long time ago a woman came to me and spent a half hour telling me about her problems — how her husband had run away leaving her with two children, how she had to live with a sister who didn't want her. She had tried to get a job, but none of them ever lasted more than two days. Now she felt there was no use any longer in living. She just couldn't go on.

I didn't hear her mention a single good thing about her life and I was getting to the place where I was fed up. I wanted to shake her. Finally, I said, "You know, if I were going out with a girl tonight, you'd be the last girl I'd go out with." She said, "I didn't come here to hear that sort of thing!" I said, "I know, but I thought I'd shake you up a little bit. I don't think you are going to change your husband or your sister or your boss. But you can change yourself. Until you change yourself you will never have a pleasant life. You have to start with yourself. You have to go within and come forth. You have to arise and shine!"

Then I told her, "I know there is a beautiful rose inside of you, but you don't see it. You are carrying it around, and you are the closest one to it but you can't see it. If you could just see the beauty within you, you would express this beauty, and the boss would like to have you around even if you didn't work hard. Your husband would never have left you if you were a beautiful soul. There are beautiful thoughts that you could bring to yourself if you could change yourself. Go out and get a job and be a beautiful person. Walk out of this office like a queen. Walk out like a rose. Everytime someone sees you on the street, don't let them point a finger at you and say, 'There goes a poor soul.' "

"How much do I owe you?" she asked. I said, "Well, darling, this visit won't cost you a cent, because you couldn't pay for it. It is worth a million dollars, and you couldn't pay me. But I expect to see you back one of these days when you have changed."

Some time passed, but I was working in my office one day when in came this same lady. She didn't say a word about any troubles. Instead, she said, "I feel wonderful, doctor. Is there something I can do for you?" She had been bound up in troubles of her own making but she had worked her way out of that mess. She looked beautiful. She now has a husband who adores her, one that she admires. She has never experienced this kind of love before in her life. But she didn't deserve it the way that she was. She had to learn to love herself, she had to express love, before she could be loved. We all get caught up in this self-ness at one time or another and we have to get away from it.

Some people have the idea, "You have to love me the way I am whether I'm mean or not." It just doesn't work that way. If you are mean, you attract meanness. You can't be loved until you give love. You have to change your life, you have to change yourself, then your life becomes different, and the whole world looks different.

Another lady came to my study one day. She told me where she had been staying, then said, "You know, I was tied down in bed for three days." When I asked her to explain further, she said, "There were three old 'battle axes' there, three old ladies. I had a nightmare and I guess I started saying things that weren't very nice, because they thought I was losing my mind or something and they tied me down in bed. The more I tried to get out, the more straps they put around me to keep me down. For three days I've been trying to get out of that situation. Then the first thing I did was to come here."

I didn't understand what she expected me to do or why she had come to me so I asked, "What seems to be the trouble?" She said, "Those three 'battle axes' . . . " And I interrupted to say, "Yes, those 'battle axes' will have to be taken care of — but what did you come here for?"

"My kidneys — " she finally got out. What interested me was that the three 'battle axes' had been foremost in her mind, not the kidneys. So I told her, "Your kidneys will never be well until you love those people."

"Love them?" She seemed almost stunned with surprise. "You wouldn't love people like that, would you?"

"Yes, you will have to — for your kidneys' sake. You have to for the sake of your physical condition." It is very difficult to show a person that there is a direct relation between their intellect or thinking and their physical condition. She asked what she should do, and I suggested that she send a nice gift to the ladies.

She was horrified. "Me? Send a gift to those 'battle axes'? That's just too much! That's the last thing I'll ever do!" I hear that from a lot of people — "That's the last thing I'll ever do" — but they usually do it. I said, "Oh,yes. You're going to send them a nice gift." She stubbornly refused again, so I went out, bought a nice tablecloth and napkins, had them wrapped and brought them back. I insisted that she sign the card I'd bought to go with the present.

She sent the gift to the ladies — the 'battle axes' — and, do you know, she received a lovely letter from them five days later. And there was a nice check in it! The three 'battle axes' said, "We can't believe that we had such a wonderful person staying with us! To think we missed recognizing what a fine woman you are! We're sending you a check because we feel we owe you an apology."

This lady cried. She couldn't believe that such a thing could happen just from giving a gift. Then I said, "Now we can take care of those kidneys."

People make wrecks out of themselves mentally, and the kidneys, the stomach or something else breaks down shortly thereafter. When the thinking is distorted, distressed, disturbed, an excessive strain is placed upon some part of the body. Fear does this. Where does the fear come from? "God hath not given us the spirit of fear." says the Good Book. It is your "little self" that creates these fears. We make them ourselves.

When you finally see the relationship between the mind and body, you will want to root out the fears, hates and other negative thoughts that are bombarding you so you can turn to higher and lighter thoughts. Thoughts are things, and they come to us as vibrations. A hateful thought is so powerful that it rips through the nervous system like a bulldozer, causing havoc as it goes through the body. Hate really shakes you up. When we learn to be humble, peaceful and harmonious, our brain cells are calm and we don't get "all shook up."

We hear people say, "Boy, did that hit me," or "You give me a pain in the neck," or "You make me sick to my stomach." These are destructive thought reactions and they become imbedded in memory in the physical system somewhere as stress. Then there are later problems as these memories pop out over and over to haunt us.

When bad memories come back, we tend to work the whole episode over once again. You find yourself thinking about it and finally saying, "What does she think she's trying to get away with?" Or "I'll get even with him." You begin thinking about revenge and what happens? The hate reaction comes again in full force and that powerful vibration shoots through the body again. When that vibration goes out, you are the one who sends it out. You are the one who sends it out with your God-given vitality and energy. Sending out destructive thoughts is like throwing a rubber ball against a wall. They bounce right back and you are the one injured by them.

We have to go in another direction. We try to reason these thoughts out through intellect. But if you try to reason out emotionally loaded thoughts from now until the end of time, you will never get anywhere. The intellect can't help us with the emotions.

It's even worse to talk things over with a friend. The friend will suggest a way to solve the problem, then you'll be going from pillar to post trying different methods. Your friend's intellect isn't any more helpful than yours. There is a way that works, and you have to go that way. It's the spiritual way.

We can fill ourselves with love until there is not a crack or cranny left in us for hate or revenge to hide in. We can insulate ourselves, so that no adverse vibrations can penetrate. We can educate ourselves so that we are only receptive to thoughts and vibrations of love and harmony.

Man does not live by bread alone, we are told. You may not have bread on the table but you won't starve. There is another kind of bread that feeds us — the "bread of life." It makes no sense for people to starve themselves to death emotionally and spiritually when the bread of life is right at their elbow, so to speak. You can kill yourself with destructive thoughts, when right next to you are the good thoughts, the valuable thoughts. All you have to do is change your thinking and you can start from where you are right now.

There is a story about a man who had been paralyzed for thirty-eight years. He was lying by the pool of Bethesda at Jerusalem when the Christ saw him there. Now, when he told this man, "Rise, take up thy bed and walk," suppose the man had said, "No, I can't. I've been paralyzed for too many years. I can't do that." He would have been using his intellect if he'd said that. But, you see, the moment he was told to arise, he took no thought. He stood up. He was even able to walk away carrying his bed, according to the scriptures!

How many times do we say, "I can't," or "I won't do that"? We *could* do it if we didn't take thought.

Look Inward For Happiness

The point I want to drive home is that we live on what we give out. Some try to live on what they take from others, but you can't do that. You can't live on what people give you. You can't expect happiness to come from other people. What do you do when you've come to depend on someone for your happiness, and they don't give it to you anymore? You will be in a sad place if that happens. Do you try to make anyone else happy? That makes you happy, doesn't it? You can make yourself happy or you can make yourself unhappy. The choice is yours.

Where the Bible says, "Whatsoever a man soweth, that shall he also reap," it really puts the responsibility right on your own doorstep. It tells you that you can have the abundant life and how to get started.

All of these great lessons tell you to do certain things starting right from where you are. Are you going to start by asking favors for your "little self" or are you going to ask in behalf of your "higher self"? There is a life that is truly happy, but it isn't the life of the "little self." The little self is never satisfied. Nothing is ever quite good enough for it. The little self always wants the things of this world, and that is not enough. Can the intellect get us on the right path? No. Unless the intellect is directed from a higher level, it will serve the little self.

Now, Solomon said, "With all thy getting, get understanding." I am not saying the intellect is worthless. I am not saying that we must disregard the intellect. We find that our understanding will help us in many ways throughout life. What I am saying is that the intellect is not enough. The intellect is a servant, not a master, and when we try to make the intellect the central authority in our lives we may find that life becomes increasingly empty, increasingly frustrating.

We find mentioned, "the peace which passeth all understanding." You don't have to understand wholly and completely. You'll never be able to understand all things. But when you develop spiritual trust, you will find that there is nothing to get, nothing to strive for intellectually. It is the spirit that quickeneth. You will be delighted to find that the intellect is the willing servant and will follow right along where you direct it. All the churches — Jewish, Christian, Buddhist — teach the same thing: It is the spirit that quickeneth.

Christ said it very well: "If ye had known me, ye should have known my Father." Then Thomas came up, saying, "Shew us the Father and it sufficeth us." The Christ simply replied, "He that hath seen me hath seen the Father."

But you have to see double, you have to see the two-in-one. If you can see that, you will understand that, "It is the Father in me that doeth the work." That is as true for us as it was for the Christ. The Father doeth the work. Let it be that way. Let this spiritual power express itself through you when you talk, walk, sleep, and in every moment of your life and work. You will find it is good for your body. But the thoughts you express in your "little self" are harsh and hard on the body.

It was Paul who said, "Think on these things." Perhaps you have been thinking intellectually for a long time. But you have never thought away your problems. And there are always new problems. Then Christ came along and said, "Take no thought."

Do you understand the double levels here? We get, "Think on these things," and then, "Take no thought." It is when you think not that you repair and rebuild your body. We have to think, but when you are thinking, you are using the body's vital energy. We have to have a balance. Some of us are just "thunk out." It is often our stinking thinking that gets us in trouble.

To be one with God we leave the intelligence alone. We leave the intellect alone, we let go of it. We allow the "little self" to die of its own accord and we take up our life on the spiritual path. The intellect, then, becomes the servant of spirit. Now we have chosen to live the spiritual life, and the intellect follows along. We no longer try to "figure out" a person. Instead, we look to the spirit in that person and we see a beautiful soul, a beautiful life. We see the world afresh through new eyes. We don't ask "why" questions any more because living the spiritual life fills that intellectual emptiness with joy.

I believe that our purpose here is to kindle life with Life. Wouldn't it be wonderful to be all aglow with the Spirit and to go around like a lamplighter setting others aglow? You would really be a magnetic person.

The intellect never gets us into the spiritual kingdom. Consider the difference among the intellectual, the physical and the spiritual kingdoms. When we are in the intellectual and physical kingdoms we have unrest, strife and confusion. There is no confusion in the spiritual kingdom. You really can't find confusion when you look at the way God put the earth, planets and stars into the great space of the universe. We are sitting on a speck of mud that is whirling through space. Isn't that wonderful?

There is no strife, confusion and unrest in the spiritual kingdom. Stop for a moment and think about your life. Are you on the fence side or the ambulance side?

The "little self" is always the center of the physical kingdom and the mental kingdom. When you come out of that and enter the spiritual kingdom, you are reaching for the "higher self."

You Cannot — God Can

You can think of many intellectual experiences and find that you can use them for spiritual good, but your problems can never be worked out for you by the intellect alone.

For instance, when you eat your meals do you ever stop and think what proportion goes to your heart, your liver, your arms, your legs or your eyes? If you tried to work this out in the thinking mind, it would never get done. We have to leave that to God. After all, He created you. We eat food and we trust it to go to the proper places. We should also trust spirit to put us in the proper place.

A lady came to me in great distress, confusion and disturbance and said, "I want you to put me back together." Put her back together? Now, I cannot do that. When Humpty Dumpty fell off the wall, not all the king's horses and all the king's men could put him back together. If we are so broken up that we need someone to put us back together, we will have to bring that problem to the Creator. That's something only He knows how to do.

Our intellect must be the servant of life, the servant of spirit. If you try to let intellect run your life, the "little self" will quickly take over the job and run both the intellect and your life.

When you leave the "little self" behind, the spirit will know more than all the trained intellects put together. We become reborn — reborn of the spirit. We need faith in the law of life and we have to LET the good life flow through us. We can never *make* life happen. We have to stop struggling and resisting. The Good Book tells us, "Resist not evil."

I treat people who are all tired out from resisting evil and fighting evil all the time. The resisting I am talking about is the struggling in the intellect. We become afraid to let go of the "security blanket" of the intellect and grow up to live the spiritual life. Of course, the intellect can't understand what it is to "arise and walk," or how we perfect our lives from a spiritual standpoint. We realize that we have to use our mind and intellect but we must use them as servants.

There is no security in the intellectual world. You have to build yourself a faith, a spirit of faith and faith in the spirit. You have to build up your faith in the Law. The laws of life set down by Moses are still the laws of life. He told his people that if they would come out of the "little self" and live in obedience to God, they would have no diseases. The self will leave us alone only if we trust in Spirit. Then the higher life will come to us as our true inheritance.

People say, "I picked up this characteristic from my mother's side of the family," or "I was born with this problem and I just have to suffer with it." We must get away from that. When we say things like that, we don't even know what our true inheritance is.

The Good Book says, "All that I have is thine." Wouldn't you rather have that than all your thoughts, all your understanding? My mother died of tuberculosis at the age of thirty. When the doctors gave me up to die at the age of twenty, I thought, "I have to just give up, because my mother died young, and I will too." Is that how we have to think about our inheritance? Are we going to place more belief in the inheritance from our parents than in the inheritance from our heavenly Father?

The Good Book says that it is the Father's good pleasure to give you His kingdom. Could you take it? That is what you have inherited! I can tell you, that is why we have to be obedient. We have to be almost childlike — innocent and eager to receive.

You may go to a hundred different doctors to get a hundred different diagnoses and a hundred different treatments, but you may still have your stomach trouble. Nor are you going to reduce your weight unless you do the right thing. You had better decide what the right thing is.

If you start doing the right thing, what is right for you will come of itself. Perhaps you don't realize this, but it is true. This is one of the laws of life.

Claim Your Rightful Riches

Health is not the natural birthright of man. This may seem strange to you, but health is reserved for those who learn to live correctly. Health is a reward. The ignorant person may never be well.

We talk about the eye being the window of the soul, and it truly is. When I use iridology (iris analysis) in my work, sometimes I see the black in the iris of the eye, and when that person starts living correctly, I see the dark spot fill up with white lines. I almost glory in this because I know that person is living The Life. In the spiritual life we put light in dark places. The Good Book says, "If thine eye be single, thy whole body shall be full of light." Single? It means of one purpose. "But if thine eye be evil, the whole body shall be full of darkness." You can't give God lip service and serve the world's purpose. If you see darkness, darkness will come to you. If you see light , light will come to you. You get what you see; you live in what you see.

I see that the sick need more than intellectual understanding. We find that muddled lives and sad experiences always bring sad results to the physical body. What do intellectual seekers want? They must find the answer. They want to be satisfied in the intellectual world. Like the physical being, the intellect is greedy too. If it finds the answer to the $100 question today, it will drive you to search for the answer to the $1,000 question tomorrow. The intellect is never satisfied. It can never find the spiritual answers for us.

Materialism always fails. Even the instinct within us is wiser, because it knows the creation. It knows there is something in creation that is good to us, that feeds us, that takes care of us through thick and thin; whether it be in the garden, the rain, the sunshine, the sunset, the colors, the friends. The creation has provided us everything to work with.

To solve the riddle of the "self," we must find the mystic way that leads to God. But some people are not spiritually minded. They have been side-tracked by the intellect, saying "I can figure that out for myself." But we find that we don't have to try to figure everything out if we follow the wisdom of the Good Book. "Seek ye first the kingdom of God and His righteousness, and all these things shall be added unto you." You are richer than you realize. You'd give your heart a much better time if you knew how rich you really were. How thankful we should be!

The universal disease of mankind is ignorance, and wisdom is the only remedy. When we live by the laws of life we become wise. Keeping these laws is the only way we can be happy. When we break them we die. It is essential that we live by the laws of life.

Unless you know how to live, you can fall heir to one disease while you're trying to cure another. We must seek out the causes and do something about them. Then the effects will take care of themselves. Which is your choice — the fence on top of the cliff or the ambulance down in the valley?

Miracles happen today just like they did when Christ was healing people. And today, as then, it is because people change their lives. People turn around and go the other way. They change from within.

Look To The Better Life

We hear a call in our soul that tells us we want the finest there is for ourselves. I know you deserve and want the very best. Delight in cleanliness and in song and laughter. Study beauty and learn that it belongs to the people who are having the most glorious experiences. This makes you feel good, and in this good feeling you live. Your feelings can make you or break you. You use words to express beauty. You make your home into a beautiful place. You desire to become a better person. You will always have goals to strive for and to reach, and as you travel along the path each goal will be higher than the previous one.

If you already have all these things, if you already have this great joy, then you will seek the perfect balance. In England when someone becomes an extremist, they say, "He has gone to the edges." Don't go to the edges. Balance your life and put all these ideas together.

We take an interest in all creative life. A great character has a warm feeling for humanity and his fellow man. This is the basis of all religion, that we find our own good and turn to help others find theirs.

Moses taught the people of Israel the Ten Commandments and other laws of life. Christ expanded upon many of these, and all true sages teach these laws of life. If we would only use them every day in everything we do, our bodies would follow along with this livingness, and we would be free.

You find people who actually resent their own bodies — the temple of the living God. No wonder they get sick. When you get discouraged, distressed and disturbed, you have to take your "self" in hand, so to speak, and turn to the higher values. Your body will always respond to this kind of loving care.

"Fear not, for I am with thee," it says in the Good Book. Fear not, God is with you. There is no fear in God; there is no fear in perfect love.

I have given you the key to the lovely ways in life. If you could only realize this, you would leave your "self" to live in the light instead of the darkness. The plan is already worked out for you. You just sow the seed, and the harvest will come. Drink your teas, and the body will respond. Don't be impatient. Don't worry about time. Don't try to arrange these things according to a schedule or timetable. Leave the whole thing to God and to the nature He created.

But we must decide the course we are going to take. We must walk forward, not looking back. I walk with a good partner. I am in business with God. That which has to be taken care of will be taken care of by the Father and me, because the Father and I are one.

There is no disease and no ill health in God. He frees us from those ways that give us tension. We are powerless to work out these problems ourselves, so we accept God and we are made whole.

We are changed people. We have changed our thinking as we change our clothes, and the garment of our mind is as soft and beautiful as the rainbow. We live in love, beauty and harmony and we get our inspiration from the Father's creation.

I know that my supply is from God. I need not depend on human beings, or on my intellectual self, but "I will lift up mine eyes unto the hills from whence cometh my help." I will go forth with God, silently, because in the silence God does His greatest work.

I am now living in the Higher Self and I know that God will never let me down.

"His eyes were too pure to see iniquity. His countenance outshone the sun."

Chapter 12

Be Filled

All the flowers
of all the tomorrows,
Are in the seeds
of today.

"All things come to him who waits," says an old proverb. Sometimes things come to those who don't wait. We would hardly picture ourselves as waiting for problems and troubles, would we? We try to avoid them. Yet, they come anyway. Many of us spend far too much of our time trying to patch up the holes in our boat. We get so busy plugging up holes so problems and troubles won't swamp us that we don't look up and see the beautiful ocean we're sailing along in. We don't see the beautiful things in life. Mother told me years ago that we should pay attention to the roses and ignore the weeds of life. It is possible to become so busy pulling weeds that we miss the roses. We deserve the best in life.

I remember when I was young my family would always put up a barrel of apples in the fall to last us through the winter. Every two weeks we would go through that whole barrel, looking for apples with bad spots on them, because we had to remove them before they started the good apples rotting. I can still see my family — my brother, sister, dad and myself — carrying all those apples upstairs. Then we would sit at the kitchen table, cut out all the bad spots and eat the apples they were in.

Do you know, out of all those apples in each barrel, year after year, I don't remember ever eating a single good apple? I was always eating apples with bad spots cut out of them!

Now, we can have wonderful lives if we don't spend all of our time cutting the "bad spots" out of the experiences that come to us. We can see much that is good and beautiful in life if we look for it instead of turning our attention to what is bad, what is ugly. You are the one who decides where to turn your eyes and how to spend your time. It is up to you.

Would A Mental Operation Help You?

A lady called me the other day and said, "My daughter is desperately in need of courage." I wonder what chiropractic adjustment could be given for courage. I wonder what kind of drug would be appropriate in this case. Perhaps a mental operation is needed here. If something is

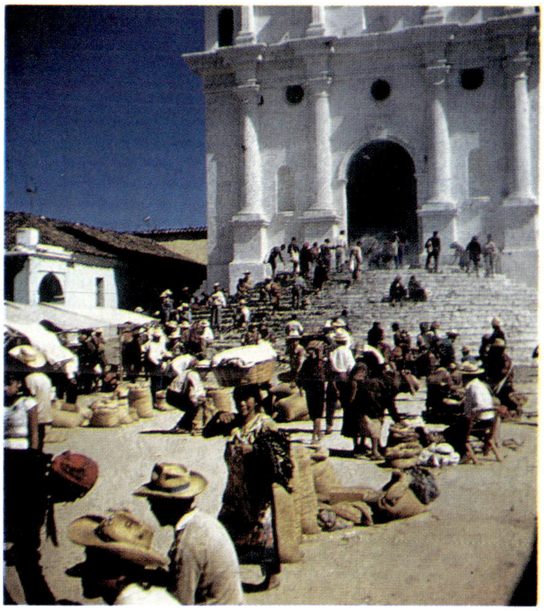

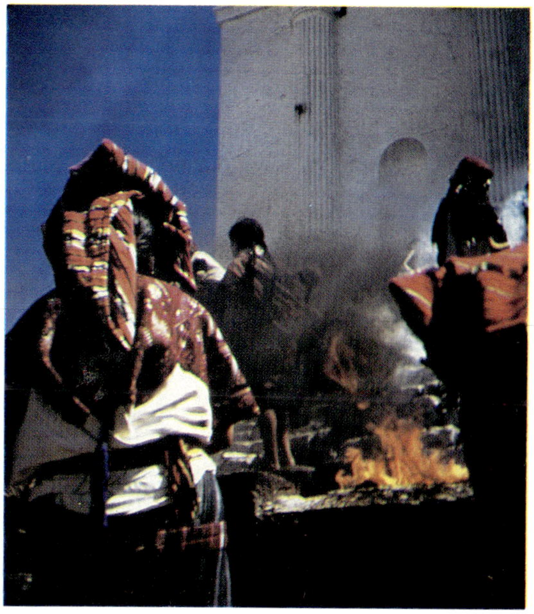

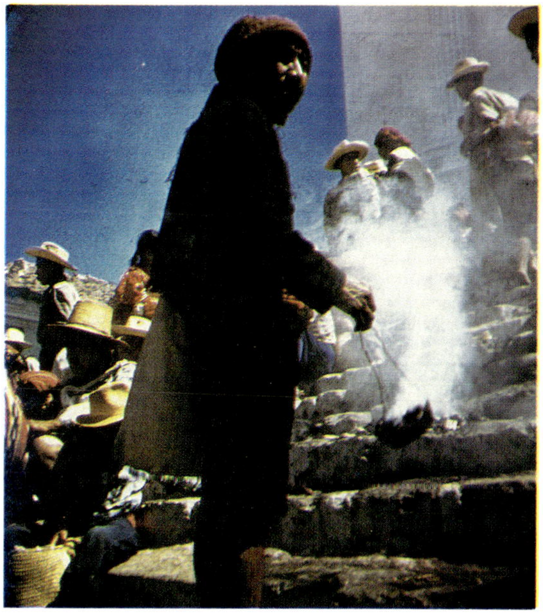

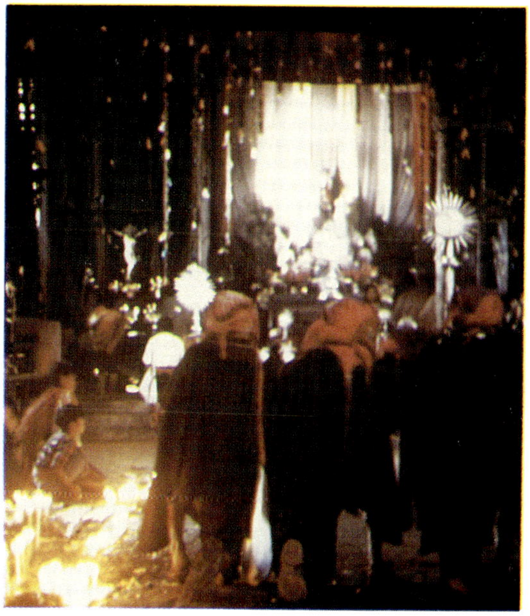

Upper Left: View of the church in Chi Chi Castenango. Upper Right: On the church steps people burn prayers in urns so the smoke will carry them to heaven. Bottom Left: In spiritual matters, we have to go as we see the way to go, whether by smoke, water or statues. Bottom Right: Candles burn among rose petals inside the church, a ritual of the local Indians.

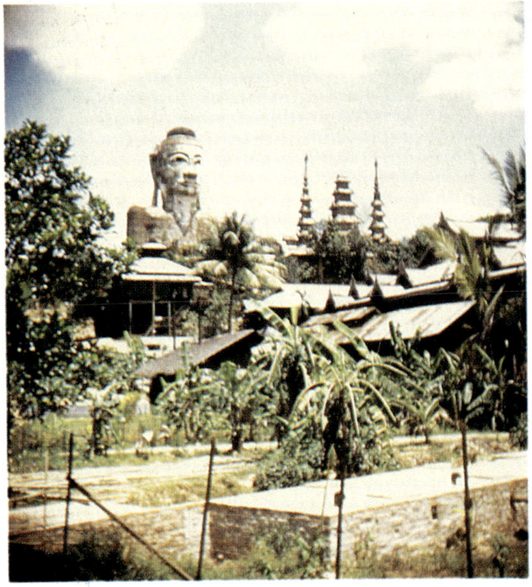

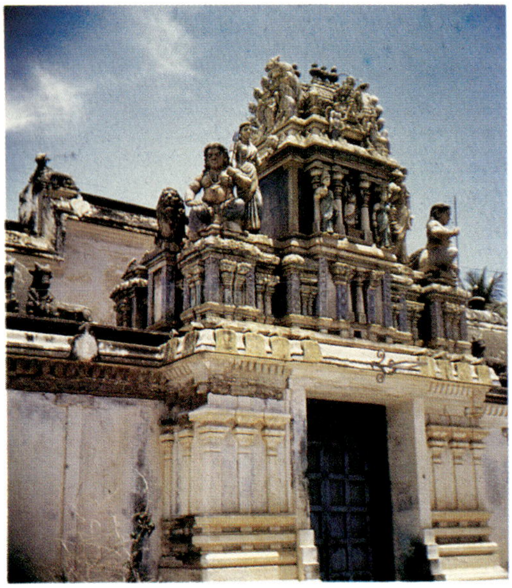

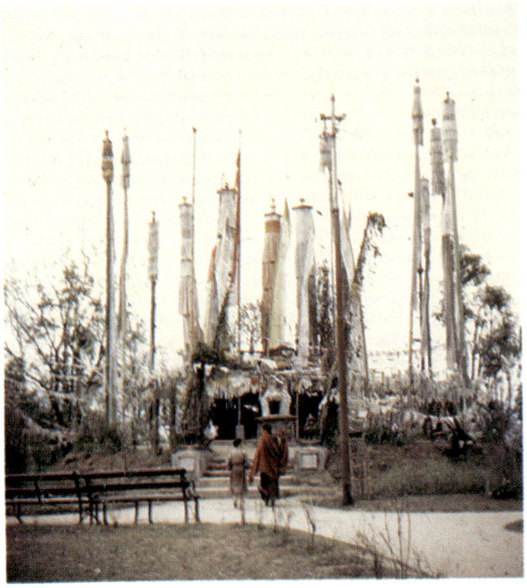

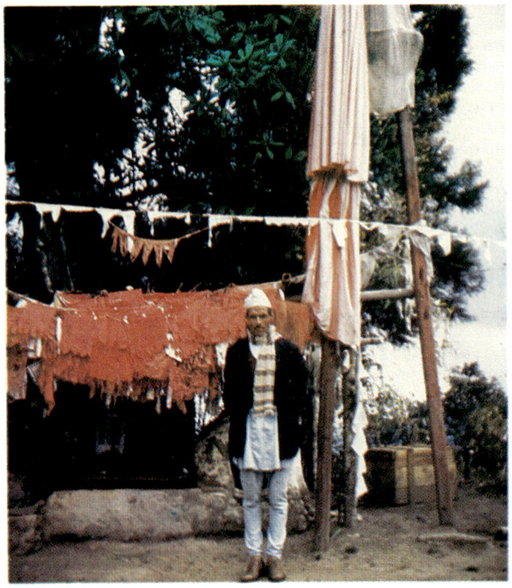

Top Left: The lying Buddha is over 100 feet long, and we saw this is in the southern part of India. Bottom Left: Here are the prayer flags where people would write their prayers, believing that as the wind blows them it carries the prayers into heaven to be answered. Top Right: The temples are all different according to the religions they follow. Bottom Right: A close look at a line of prayers hung with clothes pins so the wind can carry the thoughts of man to the gods. This was in northern India in Nepal.

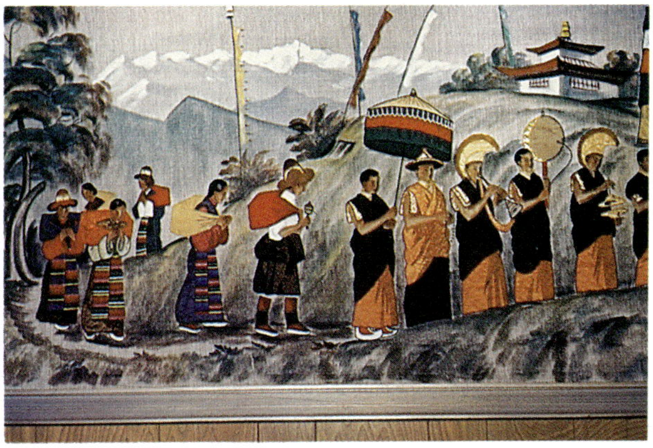

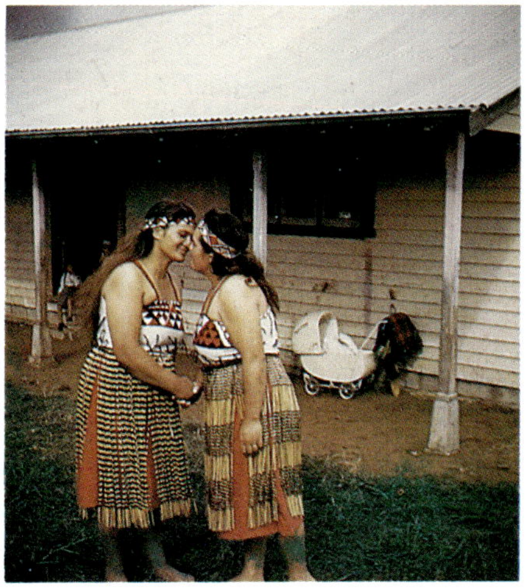

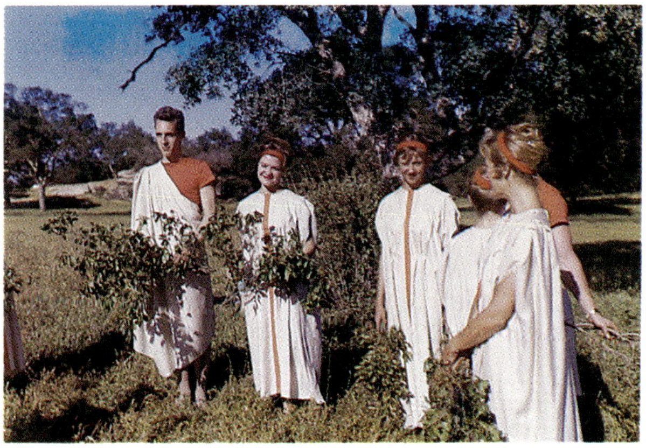

Top: This painting depicts the families and groups traveling to the temples in Darjeeling, the northern part of India and in Tibet. Our visits show that the colorful attire and the peoples' simple means of going to the temple is no different than the simplicity found in Mexico or any other country. Middle: To greet a person, I often say, "I feel wonderful," but rubbing noses is the greeting the Maoris share with one another. Bottom: An Easter morning sunrise ceremony at my Ranch.

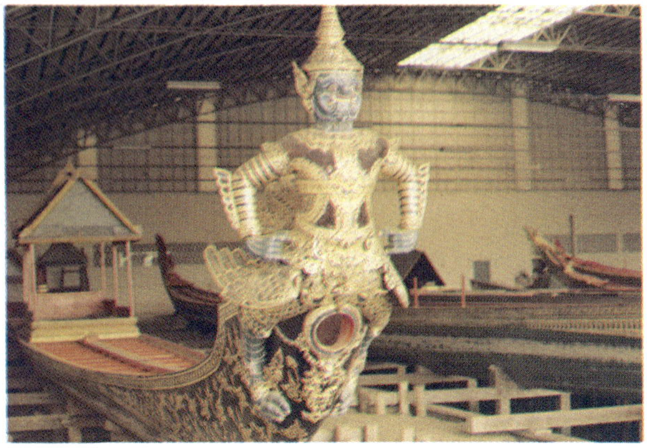

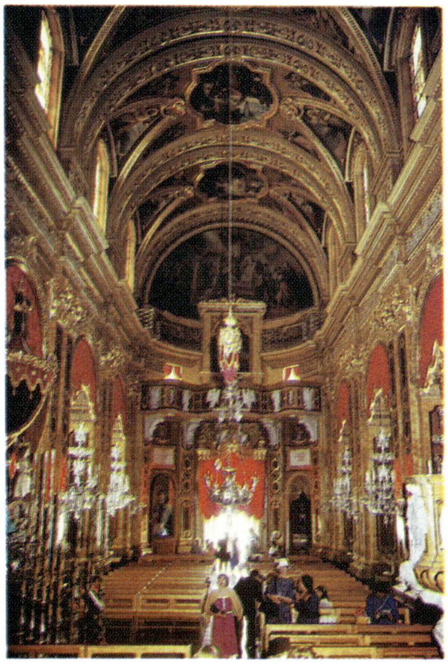

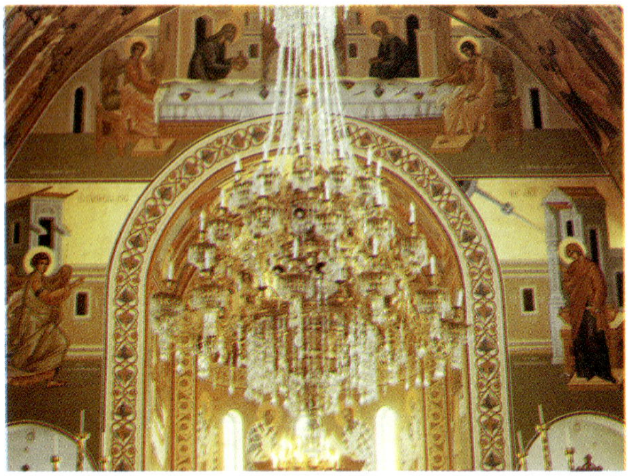

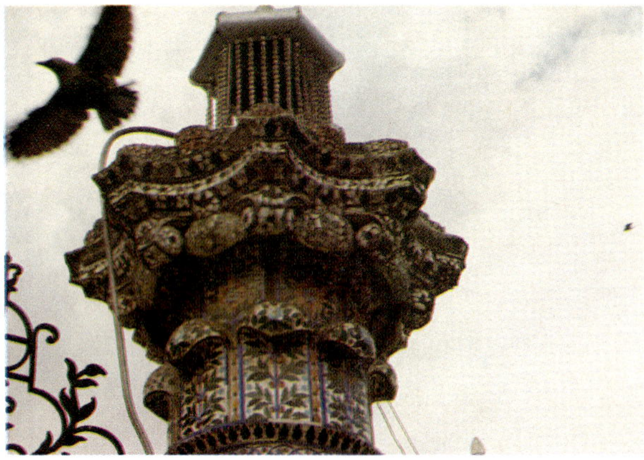

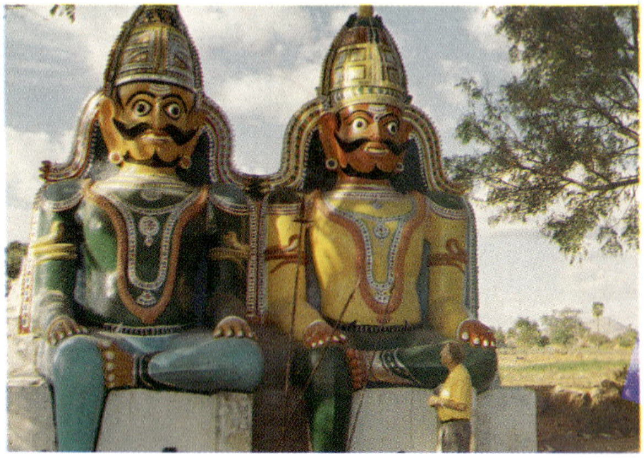

Top Left: Figurehead on the royal Thai boat represents a good luck spirit. Top Right: Cathedral on Malta where Dr. Jensen was dubbed Knight Commander. Center: Greek Orthodox Church. Bottom Left: Beautiful monuments and architecture all over the world show that beauty was in man's mind from the beginning, that beauty is in the mind and eye of the beholder. Bottom Right: Two protective spirits like many of those we found in India.

wrong in the mind then we have to go to the mind to correct it, don't we?

It is possible for the mind to become stagnant. It is possible for the thinking to become stagnant. Sometimes when a stream begins to run too slowly in the summertime, algae begins to grow on the rocks and the water tends to become stagnant. Then when the rains come, the algae is swept away, the stream is fresh and clean and sparkling again. Things have to move along. When we are really disturbed and nothing seems to be changing, we need a good spring cleaning inside the head. We need a mental massage to get good fresh thoughts circulating again. Otherwise, we reach the end of our rope. Then what do we do? Tie a knot in it and hold on. You have to do something. You can't let go. You can't let things just slip.

When nothing seems to be going right, we have to turn to the spiritual values and look again. After all, life isn't just a barrel full of "bad spots." There are good apples in the barrel, too. We have to lift our vision above the physical level. Life isn't just in the heartbeat or the bowel. Life isn't just the breath in the nostrils. If there isn't some happiness with every heartbeat, you are living like a vegetable.If there isn't some joy with every breath you take, you are going through life like a machine. There is more to life than this.

Can I share one of my health secrets with you? Many times I can't help you physically until I have helped you remove the problem that is plaguing you mentally. You will improve wonderfully at the physical level if you will "let go" and release the mental problem. If I could only get you to let these problems go, you could get well. But you make it very difficult. A lady once came into my office and wanted me to pray with her so she could have more patience. I said, "All right, let's pray that you have tribulations." She said, "But that's not going to help me." Then I told her, "Well, darling, when you have had enough tribulations, you will learn what patience is."

I think we all realize that wisdom grows as we get along in years. Wisdom comes at the end of our experiences. But too often we try to avoid experiences. We want life to be pleasant, easy, effortless. Don't wait until you are about ready to die to say, "Look at all the things I've missed! I could have gone on trips! I could have taken time out to really enjoy life!" But what do we do? We are too busy. We are busy-bodies, jumping from one pot of troubles into another. Don't go around looking for trouble all the time.

Why can't people let their tensions go? Patients ask me, "How am I supposed to do that? Tell me what to do." Do you want to know something? I can't make you release your tension. Your tension belongs to you. I can show you that it is there. I can tell you it is causing problems. I can awaken you to what is going on, but that is all I can do. The rest is up to you.

Do you think I can give you joy? Well, I can't. I can help you find your way in the world, but if you don't respond by moving your feet you will stay right where you are. Many times your own mind is causing the problem. One of these days you are going to come to the conclusion that you have been your own worst enemy. I'd like to help you turn that around so you could become your own best friend. Wouldn't that be a marvelous change?

Why couldn't you become a friend to yourself, right now? Why go on living with misery that you produce yourself? You don't have to stay in misery. You can get away from it. But you have to move. Make a friend of yourself, and the enemy will disappear.

It is time to realize that we can change our lives. If *you* will change your life mentally, *I* can easily change your life physically. Physical tissue is easy to repair.

You must recognize that whatever you are looking for in life is also looking for you. If you want to find the higher thoughts and the nicer things in life, they are there. If you knew that something you really wanted was in a shop on Main Street, then that's where you would go, isn't it? If you look for problems, you will find them. If you fear problems, they will find you. What you fear will come upon you. What you develop in your mind has already begun to take shape in reality. If you find yourself picturing things you don't want, then get rid of those pictures!

It is very easy to let the problems that come into your life take you over, but you don't have to let them. A problem isn't the same kind of experience as a spider bite, or a kick from a horse. But your reaction to the spider bite or the kick from the horse is what you have to take care of inside your head. It's what you have in your head that needs to be fixed.

When Will You Start Living?

A lady said to me the other day, "My arthritis I have learned to live with. My dentures I have learned to live with. My eye glasses are just fine. But if you lose your mind, you've lost everything."

We must realize that we are vessels. We have to fill our vessels with as much good as possible each day. I see some people filling up their vessels with fighting, resistance, misery and other things that aren't good for them. They are filling their vessels with destruction — with jealousies, hatreds, fears and disharmonies. In one of Christ's parables He directed us to gather "the good into vessels, but cast the bad away." That is what we should be doing with our vessels.

When I look at you I look for the good but I usually see it only in brief flashes of light that escape through the cracks and crannies of layers of negative thoughts and beliefs that you have surrounded it with. It is there, ready to be harvested, but you have to let those negative weeds go first. If you cared about your life you would put it in order. You would reorganize it. You would "cast the bad away" and gather the good into your vessel.

In order to have the good life, we have to begin seeking it. This is one of the keys to getting well. The Good Book says, "Seek ye the kingdom of God." This is what we have to do first. If you have been seeking all the bad and harsh things in life, you will have to learn to avoid them; and if you want to avoid them, you must seek the higher thoughts and better experiences. This is the only path that will lead you to harmony and happiness. The only path that will do you any good.

When we have made the higher path the main priority in our life, the next thing is this: We must learn to be thankful for every experience that comes to us. If you stub your toe — yes, be thankful for it. You are not going to do it again. When Thomas Edison mentioned that he had done 4,000 experiments before he invented the electric light, someone remarked, "What a waste!" Mr. Edison replied, "Yes, but now I know 3,999 things not to do any more." We should give thanks for the hundreds or even thousands of mistakes we have made. We can wake up now and not do them any more.

The next step is to get away from the attitude that we are unjustly treated, that we are underprivileged, when certain things are taken from us. People who are overweight come to me for help, and because I take away certain foods from their regular eating habits, they act as though I am picking on them. I tell diabetics that they can't have bread. So they hide it under chairs and in their rooms to keep me from seeing it. You have to get away from this idea. You need to realize that under circumstances like these, something better is being put in place of what you were doing before.

If we have a persisting physical problem like asthma, diabetes or obesity, we have to change our concepts or we will have these problems the rest of our lives. I am leading up to one thing: You have to let go. These are mental concepts, and if you don't let go of them, you will continue to suffer. Many of you have emotional ties to things in your life that aren't good for you. You think, "If I can't have this, what am I going to do?" Find out what to do. There is always another way to go. Find a better way. I know people today who live the healthy life just because they *like* feeling healthier!

Many people who have come to the Ranch have given up coffee. I'm telling you, for me to give up coffee was a job! People talk about coffee substitutes. There is no substitute for coffee. Coffee is the real thing as far as I'm concerned. On the other hand, I had to find another concept. What did I do? I put something better in its place.

Put Something Better In Its Place

Speaking of coffee, we had a man twenty-nine years old here at the Ranch, and he had a blood pressure of 240. He averaged thirty cups of coffee a day. I told him he would have to give up coffee. He said to me, "Doctor, I'd rather die than give up coffee." And, do you know what? He is dying.

The primary job we have is to replace what we are doing now with something better. There is a good replacement, and this is the basis of our work. But you will never accept a replacement until you get tired of the old habit, until you decide to let it go in order to seek the better, the higher. Can you understand that? The secret is in that seeking.

"Seek ye first —" Yes, you know the rest.

You know what to do, and the job is put right on your doorstep. It starts with you.

Some people are even afraid to laugh. These people must think, "It isn't dignified to laugh." Have you ever seen someone like that break out in a laugh despite himself? At first he tries to stop it by pressing his lips tightly together. Then the corners of his mouth turn up anyway, that frozen mouth opens, and laughter pours out like a dam has broken. I think a good belly laugh sometimes helps more than anything else. To hear a good old-fashioned laugh in a family — isn't that a wonderful thing? But you know we sit and fill up our vessels with moping, doping and hoping. We don't have anything in this vessel that we can squeeze a good laugh out of or a good life out of. I want this life to be a good one.

We are too often fighting. When there is no one around to fight with, we imagine ourselves in an argument. We fight with ourselves. The *Bible* says, quite simply and to the point, "Resist not evil." You are resisting life, you are resenting, you are fighting — and it is tearing you apart, draining your energy. You say, "I don't like him. This isn't right. I wish things were different. I hate my job." All day long you resent, you resist, you rip and tear at yourself. You wake up tired in the mornings because you resent going to work. You don't want to be full of life. Why? Because you choose to see the miserable things instead of the good things in life. You wouldn't be half so tired if you had a better concept of seeing.

A doctor in Chicago once told me about an occasion when her nephew wouldn't go to work one morning. She decided to go over and see him in order to find out what the trouble was. "I just don't want to go to work," he grumbled. "What's wrong?" she asked. "I'm tired," he said. "I don't like that job." So she said, "If you don't like that job, that is no reason why you have to stay in bed." "There's nothing to get up for," he said. She promised to buy him a new suit if he would go into town. You should have seen him jump out of that bed! Of course, this didn't solve this young man's overall problem. But it did show him that attitude, a change in attitude, can make all the difference in the world.

A similar experience came to me while I was attending a university. It was announced that *half* the class had to stay for a three-day series of examinations, while the *other half* would be dismissed, free to go home. Those who were dismissed walked out with joy; those who had to take the examinations stayed there in misery. "Why did it have to happen to me? Why should I be on this side of the fence today? Why is it that I have to take the exams, and the others don't?" We often go through these resisting concepts.

We Don't Have To Be Wall Flowers

Have you ever seen a girl sitting on the side of the ballroom wishing and hoping for a dance? When someone asks for her for a dance, her face brightens up and she is all bubbles. I've known people to sit at home moping, but when someone comes by and asks them to go out for a little fun, they are all joy. If we already had the joy inside us, we would never have to feel alone or neglected.

Some people are looking for a doctor to help them, but you need to know that most doctors have been trained in the medical schools to look for physical symptoms and to prescribe a certain drug or treatment to get rid of those symptoms as quickly as possible. You'll find that many people look for the kind of doctor who will give them "quick, speedy relief" from symptoms. But symptoms aren't the real problem.

Usually when people come down with an illness, you have to look in many directions to determine what is causing the problem. And this cause is not something that can be treated with pills, tonics and carrot juice. This cause is the thing in your life that started from the mind and worked its way out to the physical body. Most doctors won't take the time to look for this cause. Most medical doctors don't want to listen to your problems.

Now, there are psychiatrists and psychologists who will listen to your problems — often for fifty dollars an hour and up. There are movie stars who travel around the country and take their psychiatrists with them. This is very expensive listening, I'll tell you! A psychiatrist told one actress, "You have to get away from acting for awhile. I want you to change your outlook and your job." What do you think she did? This lady became a drygoods clerk in a department store, and now she is as happy as a lark. It was a big change for her to give up the celebrity life, but it was something she had to do to be happy.

In England a lady inherited a considerable sum of money, enough to retire and do anything she wanted. But she said, "I'm so happy doing housework, I'm going to continue." Could you do that? Most people have the idea that if they had a great deal of money, they would do something different from what they are doing now. They think happiness is always somewhere else. We have to be happy with or without money. This is very important.

"Well, just tell me how to get well," many people say to me. Of course, I have heard about the keys to the kingdom. I'd like to give you the keys for getting well — the keys for unlocking your situation so you could come into something new. I could talk to you about new foods and I could tell you about getting away from diluted foods and refined foods that are not good for you. There are things I could tell you that would help you tremendously, but the first thing you should do is seek the higher thoughts in life. Above all, realize that you need to be enlightened. When you become enlightened, you get out of your problems.

We may think of our country as scientifically advanced, but really, we are living in the Dark Ages. We live in the Dark Ages when we think we are catching a cold or when we think we are coming down with some disease. We think the world is full of germs and viruses ready and waiting out there to grab us, to invade our bodies. We think we have to be afraid of them. This is part of the Dark Ages.

When you're in good health, you can go any place and not "catch" any disease. When you live the more abundant life and believe in something that is of an enlightened nature, you can go through hell and it won't even singe your clothes. You can stroll through the "valley of the shadow of death" feeling peaceful and confident.

Enrich Your Life With Good Thoughts

You are on a mission of your own and you are on your own path to work it out. People are hungry. What are they hungry for? They are hungry for love, for kindness, for happiness. I think you should study these things, bring them into your life, express them. We live on what we give out. We live on the joy we give out. We live on the love we give out. This is the kingdom that has to be changed in our lives.

Many people realize that they have to change but they don't know what to do. They are handling much that is negative in their lives. If they would bring in more of the positive, the negative would be left behind. Then their lives would change.

A little girl was criticized by her grandmother for being dirty. "But grandma," she said, "I just washed my face and hands!" And the grandmother said, "I still see a lot of dirt." The little girl replied, "Grandma, I am clean, but there is dirt on your glasses."

Often the dirt is how we look at life. We have to clean our glasses. We have to change our concept at the very beginning.

People come to me and say, "Doctor, how many units of this shall I take? Should I take three teaspoons a day? Should I take a cupful?" Do you know what I'd like to tell them? I'd like to say, "You can only use worry one-half hour a day between eleven a.m. and eleven thirty. I want you to take a big dose of joy between two and three p.m. I want you to have a good laugh between five and six p.m., and when you come to the dining room table I want you to come with a 500-unit smile. Do you want me to write the prescription for you?" That's what I would like to say. Are you following me here? When I tell you to grow up and wise up, I mean you should do it now.

It is said, "A merry heart doeth good like a medicine." Do you have a merry heart today? Are you glad you're here? Are you glad for the beautiful morning? Are you glad you have good friends? Are you glad you only have twenty cents in your pocket? (I have to work very hard to feel glad when I only have twenty cents.) In the morning, do you raise the window and say, "My God! Morning is here again!" Or do you say, "Dear God, a wonderful morning is here again!" How do you look at it?

Can you see that a merry heart means a glad heart? It is a light heart that does us good. It is the heavy-hearted person who needs to change. I would like to lift the burdens from your heart but I can't do that by operating on your body with a scalpel. I am trying to operate on your mind with the truth. I am trying to operate with suggestion. I am trying to operate with concepts. I am trying to operate by replacement — replacement of new thoughts for old.

A lady came here to have her health built up so she could have a surgical operation. When she was built up she didn't need the operation! We falsely accept the concept that life is in the breath, but we have to have our concept in the life that precedes and generates the breath. We put our trust in the surgeon's scalpel and not the concept of life that moves the scalpel. If we could recognize that trust in the concept of life is the most important thing we have, life would change for us.

Live Beautifully Every Day

When I speak of joy, I think of it as something we wear. I think you should buy some new clothes, some new garments. You should wear nice clothes of lovely colors. A new hairdo always does something good for a woman because other people tell her how beautiful she is, and then she is helping to bring out the best awareness in these people. Why shouldn't you live to bring out the best in others? Why shouldn't you live so that other people come along and say, "Gosh, you look great today! It's nice to see you looking so good!"

People can be funny. The other day I received a letter that said, "I am enclosing twenty-five cents. Please send me information on how to cure the itch." For twenty-five cents! A thousand different things could have been causing her itch. But all the money in the world can't cure some kinds of itch. There was one lady who developed an itch every time her husband went on a business trip. Eventually, the doctors diagnosed it as shingles, and it became so bad she had to be hospitalized during her husband's absences. It happened so many times she decided to get a divorce.

One of the most unusual cases I have ever had was when a man came to me with swollen ankles. I gave him a thorough examination. I couldn't find anything wrong with his kidneys. I checked everything but couldn't discover the slightest clue to what was causing those swollen ankles. So I had to sit down with him and get him to go over all of his living habits from morning until night.

We started with what he had for breakfast and continued until I had a long list of foods he ate, activities and other miscellaneous items. At that point, we were still getting nowhere. Finally, I asked, "Well, what do you do in the evenings?"

"Oh, I play poker," he said. Sometimes from nine in the evening until five or so the next morning." But he hadn't offered this information when I was making up my notes. I had to dig it out of him. When I had him cut out the poker playing, the swelling in his ankles disappeared. You have to stop what is causing the trouble, even if it is poker playing.

The Best Medicine — A Merry Heart

We have to learn to let go. "A merry heart doeth good like a medicine," the Good Book says, and there is a world of good in this. We have to develop mirth all over again if we have gotten to the point where life is nothing but seriousness. We have to develop joy. You may have to do this by practicing, just as you exercise to loosen up and strengthen the muscles of your body. It may take you three months to laugh well, just as it takes three months to develop a muscle. I see many people who are negatively charged these days. They have spent their lives taking care of negative things and they have forgotten how to have a good laugh. It is difficult even to get a chuckle out of them.

You have to stop this. You can't live the good life when you are always dwelling on the negative things that cause tension and stress. You have to learn to cope with your problems with a positive attitude. Your attitude is your altitude, and a good laugh can do wonders in lifting that altitude.

The wise person has a merry heart, a good sense of humor. You have to recognize that you are becoming a wise person as a consequence of your experiences. Experiences are not meant to drag us down but to teach us lessons. Every experience teaches you something, and in this sense, it is a good experience. How many times have you burned your fingers? How many times have you eaten green apples? How many times have you bumped your head? You learned something, didn't you? Now why can't you realize that all of your problems and troubles have led you to the point where you can now begin to live the good life? You can enjoy yourself, relax and get on the higher path.

What prevents us from using our experiences to become wise? You go to a doctor who tells you to cut out starches from your diet. You go home and do it but you still live the same old life. Do you see what I'm getting at? Why don't you find out what to do?

The body follows the mind. The body is an effect of the mind. So you are going to take the good path, the higher path. You won't talk about your troubles any more because you have learned to gain wisdom from them. Believe in joy, believe in good health, believe in the good life, and these things will follow naturally. "As thou hast believed, so be it done unto thee," said the Christ.

Many of you don't know that your beliefs belong to you. They are yours. You have to be careful about telling people your beliefs because there are so many people who will try to get you to "unbelieve" your beliefs. You can't go and seek wisdom from the ignorant. You can't go and seek good health from those who are sick themselves.

How do you find a starting point on the higher path? Go inside yourself and pick out something very lovely. Let go of the negative things and go forward with this one lovely thing. That is a start.

The spiritual concept of healing involves arriving at a point in life when we recognize that we ourselves can overcome all our problems and troubles. If we have a Creator who can put millions of stars in their proper paths in the sky, then we have a Creator who can put us in our proper path. If we have a Creator who allows us to sit relaxed in our chairs while our planet is flying through space faster than a bullet, then we have a Creator we can trust.

Everyone Must Learn For Himself

If you haven't let go so that God can guide and help you, you are still following man's ideas and man's inventions—and these are what have been getting you into trouble all along. You haven't yet learned where to go for your health. You haven't yet learned what the higher path is.

The higher path leads to the real joy of life. You will find this path when you are wise enough to look back at your problems and laugh, when you have that merry heart that doeth good like a medicine. You have to have mirth. You have to go through life light-hearted. You have to greet life with pure joy through your trials. This is the attitude to have toward problems.

In the physical world we have natural laws that govern the behavior of all physical things. The physical body would get well in a hurry if we would cleanse ourselves of the old thoughts and let new ones take their place. The law of cure I follow is that all cure comes from within and moves out, from the head down and in reverse order as the symptoms have appeared in the body. This is Dr. Constantine Hering's law of cure.

Good health is an inside job. If you want to get well, you start from the inside. Where is your understanding? In a book? No, it is inside you. What I ask is that you go to your understanding and recognize that you can expand it. When you become a better person within, the people on the outside will enjoy you more. You will enjoy life more. You will enjoy people more. You will enjoy your children more and you will be better able to help them grow and develop.

You can do this when you let go and let God work through you. When you let go and let the good life flow through you, then you are ready for a new body because the body follows the mind. The body is the willing servant of the mind.

If you will recognize this, then you will fill your life with light. You are not going to try to eliminate all the miseries. You are not going to spend all your time cutting the "bad spots" out of the apples. You are going to let the light shine through.

As Lavater said, "Whatever we do, all eternity will feel it." Our body is affected by each single change, and our position in life changes as we change our thinking. Remember, thoughts are things. It is in the thought world that we create. It is here that we become a co-creator with all that is good. As we keep our minds close to God, we begin to live the life abundant. We are drawing from Him who is on high.

We look within for our outlook. We look within for the passage to follow. This is because as a man is within, so he is without. As the law works above, so it works within the man. As God moves and has His being today, He fills my every thought, every cell in my body so that whatever I do is acceptable. When I have the acceptance of God, I will have the acceptance of man. When I am right with God, I am right with man. When

I get to this point, I realize that I have let go of this world and I live in another.

Do Not Conform — Be Transformed

"Be not conformed to this world: but be ye transformed by the renewing of your mind," says the Good Book. This is so true. The whole lesson is in that. If we could walk in health and truth, we would find that sickness leaves of its own accord. You are spending your life running after a cure. Why don't you just do what is expected of you? Why don't you just get on the right path, and then the right will come forth and assert itself.

We have a God of good consequences. You must recognize that good health comes from doing what is good, whether through food, through the people you associate with, or through the attitude you have toward your job and your personal finances.

Your purpose here is to grow and to serve. But you serve well and with good compensation when you become wise. Our growth should reach the point that whatever we have to give should be the wisest truth possible. I am looking for wise counsel but sometimes I don't recognize it because I haven't grown enough. Wisdom is the last thing that comes to you. You should be happiest at the end of your life. Happiness is an outgrowth of wisdom.

Be tired of being tired. Be bored with being bored. Be sick of being sick. As Scripture says, "He that getteth wisdom loveth his own soul; he that keepeth understanding shall find good."

My Wish

For you to have
Enough happiness to keep you sweet
Enough trials to keep you strong
Enough sorrow to keep you divine
Enough hope to keep you happy
Enough failure to keep you humble
Enough success to keep you eager
Enough friends to give you comfort
Enough faith to look up to God
For He never lets you down.

From the Doctor's Study . . .

One reason why many doctors are unable to reach the patient is because they so often ignore the deep mental concerns and problems that go along with physical symptoms.

It is easy to work with a knee problem, a stomach pain or a shoulder out of joint. But, when a patient has a mental problem, or is mentally "crippled," few doctors are perceptive enough to see these things. Many times such problems may be hidden by a patient's notion that "such things shouldn't be talked about." Unless the doctor sees something wrong and delves into it, the mental problems underlying the physical symptoms will not be taken care of.

We have to take care of symptoms, but if we don't take care of the patient on the other end of a symptom, true healing will not take place.

Chapter 13

Healing The Nervous System

Nature is slow but thorough;
Nature cures,
but she needs an opportunity.

Most of us think we work pretty hard at our jobs, at the many tasks small and large that are part and parcel of life. We know that we have to eat the right foods to keep up the body's vital energy. But still we grow tired, and if we work too long and too hard for too many days, especially if worries are crowding in on us, the body breaks down. Now, we don't call this an "energy breakdown," do we? No. We call it a nervous breakdown. The nervous system has become depleted. It no longer does what we want it to. We have to stop what we are doing so that a healing can take place in the nerve cells, the nerve structures. We may have been working hard, but the nervous system was working harder.

What is this nervous system that works so hard for us? We know that a fine network of nerve fibers runs throughout the body, connecting the muscles and organs with the brain. We know that electrochemical messages are constantly traveling from the various parts of the body to the brain and from the brain back to the body. This is going on every moment of our lives. We know that many parts of the body operate automatically — we don't have to think to make our liver function or to get our lungs to breathe or to tell our stomach to digest its food. But our thinking *does* have an important effect on all bodily processes such as these, as we have already mentioned. And it also has an effect on the nerves that carry the messages. We can build the body up or we can tear it down by what we think.

The human brain is made up of ten billion nerve cells that are constantly evaluating and adjusting what is going inside your body as well as what is going on outside our body in the immediate environment. If you are looking at a beautiful rose, smelling its delightful fragrance, admiring and enjoying it, every cell of your body is in some way aware of what you are doing. In the same way, if you are at the garbage dump looking at ugly litters of junk, wrinkling your nose at the stench, your cells are aware of this, too. The nerves get the word around, so to speak.If you think "rosy" thoughts, the nerves are uplifted and soothed. If you think "garbage" thoughts, the nerves are dragged down along with the rest of the body.

My mother once told me something I will

never forget: God will forgive you of your sins, but your nervous system never will." It is the nervous system that I treat. I have to take care of the nervous systems of those who come to me with a health problem. How are you taking care of your nervous system? What thoughts have you put into it today? As you go through life, if you are living in confusion or vengefulness, if you are living on that ragged edge, the nervous system is going to break sooner or later.

God will forgive all you have done, but the nervous system just goes on. It doesn't know about God. The only one who knows God is you. The nervous system is your servant, and its job is to follow you through life.

You are the creator of all that goes through your nervous system. You are a co-creator of the spiritual power that relieves the nervous system. Your nervous system responds to how you think and to what you give it to do. If you give it loving things to do, it will respond to that, too. Your nervous system needs to have a good time just as you do. If you choose the higher path in life, if you seek perfection, it will have a good time.

Many of you are well off materially. You have money, clothes and companions. You can buy this and you can buy that; but this is not giving the nervous system all it needs for good health. "Getting" things is not what gives the nervous system a good time.

In the advertising industry they say that the one way to sell people on a product is to put the word "get" in the advertisement, because everybody is interested in *getting*. They say the greatest advertising gimmick is to give people the idea that they are going to "get" something special if they buy this or that.

I read an article once that only had about a hundred words, but the word "get" was in there twenty-four times! They claim it was one of the most effective pieces ever written to sell people on an idea. Now, getting is important in its way, but to get money you must have something else first. Money is an effect, the end result of doing something else. So when you open up your business on Monday morning, the idea of getting isn't the most important thing. The most important thing may be giving or sharing. It may be loving. It's what *you* have to offer your customers. You have to give something good to get something good in return. You don't deserve more in return than what you give out. You cast your bread upon the waters, and what is rightfully yours comes back. You can't expect your neighbor's bread to come to you. And this is just as true for the nervous system as it is for life. You have to give it a little something. You have to give it something good.

You Earn Your Health

Many of us expect what we want to just come to us. We don't realize we must earn what we want. People have the idea that they can come to me, and I will give them health. That's not the way it works. You must earn health. You work for it. Let me give you an example.

A thirty-five-year-old woman came to see me with her head bowed down to her hips from arthritis. She'd been told she would spend the rest of her life in a wheelchair. The arthritis spurs on her spine were as big as thumbs. As we looked at the X-rays of this lady, I said, "The first thing we are going to do is to go after this from a physical standpoint. We'll put her on a special diet. We'll emphasize the sodium foods. We're going the hit this arthritis hard physically."

I went after that lady's arthritis with everything I had. I prayed for her. I wanted her to get well. It wasn't a matter of business at all; it was more of a dedication. At the end of a year, her spine was perfectly straight (a picture of her is in my cookbook), and I received a report from Magnolia Hospital that there were absolutely no arthritic spurs on her spine!

As I look back on that work, I can say truthfully that it was a work well done. But I was so ignorant in those days that I didn't realize what actually had happened. You expect certain things to happen in life even though you don't know all the "whys" and "wherefores." You go where you have to go. You do what you have to do. You just love and share and suddenly something wonderful happens, right before your eyes! You make a success out of your life, make a success out of your health, only according to what you give. But back then, I didn't know that. I thought the healing had come from the physical work.

Everyone who had seen this lady would come to me and ask, "How did you do it?" Everyone thought I was wonderful. To tell the truth, I didn't see those arthritic spurs dissolve. I wasn't sure what had dissolved them. But then when I got together with this little lady in my office, I said, "You know, a year has passed, and a wonderful thing has been done."

"Oh yes, doctor," she said. "I would have crawled all the way from Long Beach to see you in Los Angeles. I would have crawled the whole way to your office!"

Can you understand what happened? She earned that healing! Without that attitude, no dissolving would have taken place! She wouldn't have taken the care to eat the right foods without that attitude. She had brought a dedication along with her. It was something within her that did the job. It was what came forth from her that made that healing a success!

In another case, a minister of a Religious Science Church asked that I go see a lady with a breast tumor. When I entered her room she was lying in bed and weighed less than sixty-five pounds. Paralysis of the larynx prevented her from speaking.

I pulled the covers off her feet and noticed the toes were beginning to turn blue. Circulation is very important. When a patient is extremely ill, I always look at their toes, because when the toes start turning up and getting blue, I know I have a very serious case on my hands. This lady's toes were as cold as ice. No circulation! I put the covers back on and I suppose my face revealed my concern for her.

I was thinking, "What have I been given here to take care of? What can I possibly do for this lady?" On the surface the situation really looked hopeless. But I was not going to give up.

So I stayed up all night with that lady, feeding her just a teaspoon of broth every half hour. I helped her get the broth down because she was unable to take anything on her own, and she had to have something. We had to make a start somewhere.

In the morning we found she was a little bit brighter. Do you know what I mean by "brighter?" There is one thing in life above others that expresses the spiritual coming forth. When we are a little bit brighter, we begin to shine. Light only does one thing, and that is to flow out. You don't make light. Light is. The Christ is the light of the world. And, we saw a little brightness glowing in this woman's face.

We had to have light coming from this little lady because this is the energy that heals. After that she steadily improved, and in three months she was well. When she went back to her doctor, he examined her and shook his head. "I must have made a mistake in my diagnosis," he said.

Later, at a lecture, this lady stood up and said, "I remember Dr. Jensen coming in and pulling the covers off my feet. I saw the look on his face — and it wasn't good! My doctor had given me only three weeks to live. Others had given up on me. I was looking for hope. I was looking for a door. I was looking for an avenue." Something important had begun in this lady's mind. Can you tell what it is?

You Must Shine — To Arise!

Remember, I've said you have to have a path. This lady was looking for a path. And she said, "When I saw the look on Dr. Jensen's face, I thought, 'Oh no, I can't have another man give me up. I'm going to show him.' " And she did!

Right here is the crux of the whole thing. You live on what you give forth. If you haven't anything to give forth, you're dead! You have to lift yourself above this idea of always having somebody give something to you. You have to shine! You have to arise! You're going to have to do it! Don't talk to me about intentions. Intentions are wonderful, but deeds are much better. These things must come out of the body.

Now, the point of these wonderful healing cases, as far as the nervous system is concerned, is that the instructions for the body to heal, the instructions for the cells to repair, must come through the nerves. That is why we must give our nervous system a good time.

People come to me and say, "You know, that woman is really shot," or "This man's nerves are gone." Gone? Shot? What does this mean? It means the nerves are depleted. Do you know how a nervous system becomes depleted? You wear it out from anxiety, fear, jealousy, hatred. You wear it out from worry, fretting, vengefulness. Then you can't direct your body and its activities because the nervous system that takes care of that for you is exhausted, shot. You've worn it out. You're ragged. You're on edge and your nerves are on edge. You have pushed them too far. You have become an extremist in the negative thoughts, the negative emotions.

You can't do this and expect the nervous system to take care of business as usual.

The nervous system has to be taken care of. If it is going to work properly and to keep you in good health, you must take care of it. How important is the nervous system? To some of you the stomach is the most important part of your body; getting food in that stomach is the most important thing in the world. But if your nervous system isn't right, you cannot digest that food properly. The nervous system is the directing force for every activity in the body. It has to be powerful. The directions for every cell to repair, to rejuvenate, to rebuild have to travel along the nervous system pathways. The nervous system is the most important center for your relationships, your work, your sexuality and everything in life that requires responsiveness.

If your nerves are shot, the body is more or less helpless. I have to start out with many patients who come to me with health problems by first taking care of their nerves.

Now, we find that nature does the healing here. I call this the healing of the motor force in the body. It is said, "It is the spirit that quickeneth; the flesh profiteth nothing." That flesh will stay there as long as you leave it there, but if you are going to move it, you must have incentive. The dust of the earth knows nothing of incentive, of spirit.

"For dust thou art, and unto dust shalt thou return," it is written. We are talking about the physical body. But we are also talking about soul quality, something that the dust and the body know nothing about. When we speak of these qualities, we have to think in other terms. I mentioned incentive. I mentioned inspiration. Now I am going to talk about spirit. There is the world of dust, this world of effects — but there is another world beyond this one.

We hear people say, "He is a genuine person!" Is that because of a good looking physical body? "He put his whole heart into the job." Does that mean he just worked harder than usual? No. The qualities we are talking about are soul qualities, inner qualities, that have nothing to do with the dust of the earth.

We Must Feed The Nervous System

I want you to know that it is possible to destroy the nervous system, the good in our nervous system, physically. We can lose the value of this system through the winds that chill us. Hot baths can be enervating. Some people stay so long in these hot baths that they drain away the good energies in their bodies.

We have a need for phosphorus. Vitellin is a phosphorus rich brain and nerve food that is found in egg yolk. We need the lecithin it contains more than anything else to build this nervous system. Lecithin is a brain and nerve fat, an oil, and it is essential in the building of the brain and the nervous system. We need the nerve fats found in animal products, and for this, we have to turn to the animal kingdom. I don't mean that we must eat meat, but we must have lecithin, which is not found in vegetables and fruits.

But you could pour vitellin into the body and still wear out the nervous system faster than you could build it up. An overanxious person does exactly that.

"Be anxious for nothing," the Good Book says. We go through life in overanxiety, overworrying, overfretting and overstewing. Unless we put the spiritual values to work, unless we make the necessary adjustments inside the head, all that God can do for you through foods is wasted. God's program is more than just the foods for the body.

We must use the whole program. You can't live on the dust of the earth and simply forget your own soul. Your motor system, your nervous system, needs the higher things. Some of you are neglecting the lovely things in life. Some of you seem to think that just breathing is enough. But to marry a person just because he or she takes sixteen nice breaths a minute isn't enough. We don't choose a companion just because his heart beats regularly seventy-two beats a minute, do we? That isn't enough.

What makes for good companionship? Those things that are found deep within a person. My teacher used to say, "That which you are deepest, you really are." This is the genuine part. This is the part I see in you.

Rest is necessary for the motor system. Nerve stretching is wonderful. That is why yoga (such as Hatha-yoga) exercises are especially good for the nerves. They are wonderful for tensing and relaxing the nerves. Massage is also good.

Exercising out in the open is marvelous for the nerves — living in air that is fresh and active, getting out of humid weather, going to a high altitude, all these things that involve movement and activity are always good for the nerves. We have to avoid exposure to cold, loss of sleep, overexcitement, long hours of work, night work and irritability of any kind. Impatience can deplete the nervous system, as can unnecessary thinking and worrying.

From a health standpoint there is a close relation between the mind and the body. We manufacture acids in the body every time we think. Of course, joy doesn't produce the same type of acids in our body as hate. But whatever the acid may be, sodium can neutralize it. Sodium is stored up in the walls of the stomach and bowels and in the joints. If your thinking gets to the place where it is unnecessary thinking, harsh thinking or thinking that begins to crush you, this produces acids that draw the sodium from the stomach and from the joints. Is it possible, then, that such thinking can result in arthritis? Oh, yes!

Things To Avoid

Spices, such as pepper, are among the harshest things in their effect on the nervous system. Pepper is seventeen times more irritating to the liver than alcohol. Spices of all kinds destroy the nerve ends in the body. Salt, nutmeg, ginger and condiments of all kinds can have bad effects. There is no food value in them whatsoever, and they do not belong in the human system.

Diseases are hard on the nervous system, as you would expect. We aim for health and avoid disease. We need a clean body. We need to live a clean life. We must live according to nature's laws and God's laws.

Sunshine is a wonderful tonic for the health—when taken in the right doses. Sunstroke damages the nervous system. I have an uncle who was blinded from sunstroke. The eyes are actually extensions of the brain and as my uncle's nervous system broke down in the extreme heat, he was blinded. We have to be careful of extreme heat.

It is necessary to know all these physical things about the nervous system, but they can't help you if your mind isn't right. My dad used to say, "God helps those who help themselves, and God help you if you don't help yourself." You have not been helping yourself to all the godly things when you are sick.

Recreation is very important. Vacations are important for the nervous system. "Vacation" comes from the word "vacate" — get out of there! Get somewhere new! Get into something refreshing, something lovely, something you like to do! Do something stimulating, something inspiring, get away from the old routine! This is a vacation. This is what renewing of the body and mind is — to get away, to vacate.

Gentle friction rubs are good to protect the ankles. Keeping the ankles warm helps the nervous system very much, especially in the young person.

Work with your beliefs, not against them. I am not here to sell you on some different belief. You have to be good for your health's sake.

The problem today is that we are all separated. She is this, and he is that. We think somebody has something different or better than we have. Or we think that what is, just *is*. We have to stop going around, looking at people's things and ways of life, and mentally putting little tags on them that say "better than mine" or "not as good as mine." Don't compare. Everything has its place in the world.

God's Church Is Without Walls

We should get to the place where we all believe in what is good and what is right, and live so that we could all go to God's church, the one church, and believe in the same thing — truth. Then we would come out with the same wisdom and we could walk together. If we don't walk together, we are going to have problems in life. A person who cannot walk with his fellow man is at odds with him, and from this there is friction that grates on the nerves. So we have to be agreeable.

When we are looking at lack of nerve nutrition, we have to consider tension, excessive tension. Now we are getting close to the mental cause. Now we are closing in on that point where we have to let go and let God come in and take over. Then we have to appropriate more of the good in life. We have to go a quiet pleasing way. We even have to live a care-less life. It is all right to live a care-less life if God is flowing through you, caring for you and in you. There is care, but you don't have to concern yourself with it; God is doing the caring for you. You just let go of the physical things and let God work through you. This is good for the nervous system.

Outdoor work and the mountain life are always good for the nervous system. The person who always quarrels, always sees the negative things in life, is tearing down the nervous system in the body. We need to get rid of this contentiousness, throw it away. We need to get our tongue working so that we say only what uplifts us and those around us. When we are very tired, we can't speak or think properly. The love essence of the body is drained away when we have dissipated this nervous system.

At-One-Ment With Nature

As we talk about these excesses and negative things, we have to recognize there is much good in life. Let us turn to it. Too often many of us are depending upon mother. We don't do anything on our own. We have come to depend on her so much that when we get out on our own, we look for somebody else to play her role with us. We become keyed up. We become emotionally upset. Then we look for someone to mother us, to comfort us. That is not the answer. You feel tense because you are not in agreement with life. You are not in at-one-ment with life. It is your responsibility to take care of these things.

If you are not in at-one-ment with life, if you are not in at-one-ment with nature, you become depressed, you begin to live with "the blues." You worry and you are touchy, miserable, unhappy and irritable. This is the reason why you are tense. When the tension leaves, when the attitude changes, your nervous system recuperates and gets well.

Some people even worry about worrying so much. Things look blacker than they really are. You lose your sense of proportion, your sense of judgement. You know how to make a mountain out of a molehill but you don't know how to make the mountain back into the molehill it really is. You don't use the mind for corrective purposes but become caught up in destructive thinking. You are always patching the holes in the boat of life, afraid it is going to sink, instead of guiding it in the right direction and admiring the view. As my mother said, "Nourish the roses and ignore the weeds." You're not going to get anything good out of those weeds, so why nourish them? Why waste your attention on the negative things of life? You can't afford to be afraid of the unborn, the unseen things. We need to spend our time looking after and appropriating the good in life.

We Need To Get Along With Others

Some don't have the knack for getting along with other people. Why is this? What keeps us from getting along with them? We can't seem to get into agreement with them. We want them to believe as we do. We want them to look at life as we do. We can't let them go their own way. You will have to set them free before you can be free. That is the secret. Let them alone. Let them grow. If you have a good idea and they refuse to accept it, shake the dust off your feet and let them go.

We have to look for what is lacking in life. Many of us go through life carrying a chip on our shoulders, or we go through our lives critically examining ourselves. We set standards we can't measure up to. Then we get into the "poor me" way of thinking. "I haven't got this. I don't know how to do that. Poor me." We get into that rut and we go through life poor in purse and poor is spirit.

I recently saw an article in a London newspaper. Fifteen persons, most of them doctors, attended a dinner at the British Medical Association headquarters and later collapsed with food poisoning. Fifteen doctors! Perhaps they were "practicing" on themselves. A doctor should know better than to eat something that could make him sick!

Do you know that ninety per cent of all ptomaine poisoning cases in California used to come from church dinners? This is according to the health statistics from Sacramento, California.

Who are we? Where are we going? What do we have in life? I often wonder about people. I would love to give you a system. I would like to say, "Take step number one, then step number two, then steps three, four and five." But this doesn't work. I can awaken you, but you have to find your own path in life. You have to do it yourself.

People Won't Make You Happy

As you begin to grow in life, as you begin to discover what you can believe in, you will find that you cannot expect complete happiness from another person. This is the secret of a happy marriage. This is the secret of good friendships. Don't expect too much from the other person. You can't center all your plans around another person because he may not be able to fulfill your expectations. He has his problems too. Then, again, if you seek advice from someone, you may find that his conclusion is based on experience that amounts to less than half of what you know. You may have more experience. You may have better opinions. I believe the best opinions are the ones we develop within ourselves.

When I tell people to go back to God or to get close to God, they often ask me, "What is God?" Who is God? If you can show Him to me, I'll believe in Him." I have struggled with this one. I have struggled to find out who and what God is, and I have found that if you have eyes to see and ears to hear, He is there.

One time I drove up through the desert and into the mountain slopes of Blythe and Bishop, California. I had driven quite a way that day and I stopped to go to bed early — right at sundown, in fact. As I spread my sleeping bag out and climbed into it, I noticed I was surrounded by lots of bright orange poppies. Just as the sun began to set over the mountains, the poppies closed up. I thought, "Well, this is funny. I wonder who is doing this!" I was curious about where the power to close all those poppies came from.

It wasn't just one or two poppies closing now and then. All the poppies around me were closing up. Nothing small at all. Perfect coordination, perfect timing. It seemed to be a Law that was running through nature. It seemed to be a Principle that was taking care of all nature. I closed my eyes and fell asleep.

The next morning I awoke bright-eyed and bushy-tailed. I was refreshed and ready to go! As I rubbed my eyes and admired the sunrise, what do you supposed happened? That's right. Those closed-up poppies began to open and to spread those lovely, delicate orange petals to the early light. I lay there wondering — who was opening those poppies?

I had to give the credit to God. I thought if He could open those poppies every morning, if He could recharge and rejuvenate me through the night, I had a lot to be thankful for. I believe that by thankfulness and gratefulness you are going to do more for your nervous system than anything else. If you can't thank God for all the good you receive and for all the wonders of nature around you, you are not going to get all the good you should have for your nervous system.

The more I look to God, the more I find — the deeper He is, the bigger He is, the wiser He is, the more powerful He is. I believe that God can only do as much for you as you are able to open yourself to receive. I notice that God seems to do very little in some people, and the reason why is not hard to discover. Mother told me many years ago, and this is something I believe, that God can only do *for* you what He can do *through* you. The secret of the whole idea is exactly that.

How To Get Rid Of Nervous Tension

Do you want to get rid of nervous tension? Start thanking God for all the good things you have in your life. A minister in Washington, D.C., prayed before the United States Senate not long ago, saying, "Oh, God, a lot of things are wrong, but give us the light to see all the good things as well." This is the attitude we have to take. We have to see the good things as well.

To be grateful is "having a due sense of benefits received," according to the dictionary. We have to see the benefits given to us and take pleasure in them. It is a treat to have something of a pleasant nature go over the nerves.

We have discussed anxiety, resentment and resistance. Now we need to replace them with something pleasurable. Then we won't wear out the nervous system. We'll restore the vitality of the nerves. If you keep your nervous system in good working order, then I won't have to treat it. If you keep your nervous system up, your ulcers will improve. Every condition in the body will improve, because the nervous system affects every cell and every organ in the body.

I don't know where you can find understanding except on the inside. We have to be delighted with all of life. We have to accept life with joy. It has to be good for us as it comes to us. It is all there for a purpose, a good purpose. So we have to go the joyful way, the way of agreement. And where can you get more agreement than in nature? Where can you get more agreement than in the garden with the birds and the flowers? Where can you get more agreement than with God?

To have that refreshing moment, to have it welcome, to have it acceptable, to have something worthy of acceptance — this awakens the feeling of gratitude within us. We must have good feelings because feelings are what arise and flow in this motor system, this nerve system. We are always going to have some kind of feelings in it, so we might as well choose the best. A pleasant face arouses pleasurable sensations and gives the possessor an agreeable companion. We must avoid things that aren't helpful to us.

We have to be thankful. We have to make formal acknowledgment and we have to express gratitude. We have to give thanks and we have to give credit, too. Then we are thankful. Gratitude is good for the nervous system. There is an art of thanking. "I am thankful for this moment. I am thankful for what is yet to come."

Can you be thankful for what is yet to come? If you have all of your money in the stock market, you may not be. So, you see, you cannot put your thankfulness in this world. That is why I say you have to thank God for what has happened, for what will happen.

Giving Thanks Is The Best Prayer

We should thank God for all the good foods and all the knowledge that we have in order to keep our bodies well. We have to be thankful in all things that we are doing. This is a gratitude that is expressed, and we have to manifest thankfulness. To manifest means to bring into being, to bring into existence. It means "man-I-feast." We do not leave our thanks unexpressed. We bring our thanks into being; we manifest thankfulness.

Why should we manifest thankfulness? We are rich. We are joint heirs to the kingdom. It says in Scripture, "It is the Father's good pleasure to give you the kingdom." If it is the Father's good pleasure to give us all this, it should be our good pleasure to receive it, to be thankful for it.

Where is this kingdom? It is within us. Are you looking on the outside? Are you going to be happy only when you get things, when you have things? Perhaps you already have it and you don't know it. You have to count your blessings. You have to express this good and godly principle because, "He that hath, to him more shall be given." You must acknowledge what you have before you can receive more. Do this and you will have a good nervous system. You won't be frantically running to and fro. You won't be as anxious as you were before. It is your relationship to this Deep Within that embodies all the supply, all the abundance that God has given you. This is the only way you can regenerate a nervous system that has broken down, one that has become dissipated.

Should we expect it to come from the outside? It won't. It comes from within because this is where your real understanding is. I already have all that the Father has because of my oneness with the Father. I am one with the Father. "The Father that dwelleth in me, he doeth the work." We have been told that "The works that I do shall he do also; and greater works than these shall he do." The Christ did not depend upon himself, do you know that? He depended upon the Father.

Was Christ rich? Would I like to have what the Christ had? Really, I would love to have it! What did He do? Was He able to heal? Was He able to change water into wine? What a power there is when you let the Father do the work! These are wonders of life!

We should look upon our innermost being as a fountain where all good is flowing — it is where God pours forth out into the world. Are you getting close to the truth? You have to live on what you pour forth. If you pour forth the godly power, the nervous system will rejuvenate very quickly.

Within us is an endless supply of what we need. You don't have to try to make the supply. It is already there. It is manufactured for you. It is complete. You will never have to attempt to build up a supply because you already have one. You just have to go within yourself, and all is well. You have been supplied with everything you will ever need.

The point is to let it flow. You let this supply flow out of you, and wherever you are, God is. This is complete release of our anxiety; this is complete release of our tension. When we have released, we become a giver, a giver of good. When you are a giver of good, do you know what comes back to you? At that point you don't have to worry about getting any more. Once you begin to give, you can live on what you are giving.

This, I think, is one of the greatest secrets I can tell you: You live on what you give. It is that simple. You haven't any more than what you can give. This may be difficult to figure out by man's reasoning, but if you can accept it, you will find that you are a very rich person. Everyone comes bearing gifts of some kind. You should look for these gifts, and above all things, you should be a bearer of good gifts to your fellow man, to your employer and your work, to your children and to your family. The kingdom of heaven is within us, and it must flow out from us. Don't try to block it. Don't stop it. Don't think, "Now, this person wouldn't appreciate it." We are not to judge. Giving is enough. If other people don't understand this wisdom, let them go their own way.

You Are Responsible For Yourself

We can't be responsible for others just because their parents didn't bring them up right. We can't be responsible for those who don't yet understand. We can't be responsible for them because that would deprive them of the blessing of learning their own lessons in life, of growing and accepting responsibility for themselves. That is one of the greatest blessings in this life — taking responsibility for ourselves and rejoicing in that.

I might say that we carry this truth out into the world. A lot of people have the idea that we go into this world to preach the truth or to hear someone else preach it, but I think the truth is within us. We are very worldly human beings. Sometimes I think preaching to others is unnecessary. I think the truth should be preached in our words to ourselves — then be expressed in our deeds. The most a preacher or teacher can do for us is to awaken us to the truth within.

I spent some time with a teacher named Emmet Fox in New York, and he said, "You know, to work this truth out is very simple, but it's not easy." Sometimes a particular truth may be so simple that it lies just under our noses for years before we discover it. We don't say it is easy. What I have to tell you may be simple, but it may not be easy.

The Good Book tells us it isn't easy when it talks about the way being straight and narrow. The way can be hard to find, hard to follow. It was easy for Christ to give to the multitudes, but you find that the simple truth is that it was hard for the multitudes to pass it along.

The average person creates sickness — not good health. The government tells us that ninety per cent of the people in this country are sick. Now, that is quite a multitude!

Out of this multitude, a few will get well. I don't know if that is going to include you or not, but it could. "He that hath, to him shall be given." As you have this wisdom and you use it and give it out, you will find that this is an expression of your abundance, an expression of your supply.

Use The Power You Have — Or Lose It!

This is a principle of life: "He that hath, to him shall be given, and he that hath not, from him shall be taken even that which he hath." Even if you only have a tiny bit of something, if you don't use it, it will be taken away from you. There are many people who work for me, and I can't expect more from them than they have to give. All you can get from me is what I have. And what I have I must give, because if I don't give it, it will be taken away from me. In my experience, I have found this to be so.

From him who has much, more is expected. We may not have silver and gold, but such as we have we must give. This may be required of us in such simple ways as encouraging others or in expressing a talent or gift that brings pleasure and benefit to people.

If we believe we are lacking, if we hold back in our giving, we will demonstrate lack in our lives. Believe in abundance, and abundance will be supplied to you. We must let God impart through us. God can only do for us what He can do through us. We have to grasp this principle. If we can get this "flow consciousness" and experience this flow continually moving through us, then the oil will come for our lamps, and bread will come for our tables, and we will constantly have the good coming to us.

You have been blessed. The flow continues like a great river. There is no stopping of God's supply. We must demonstrate that which we have. Then more will be given.

Many people are barren, not bearing the good fruit they should be manifesting. But if we could be filled with the Spirit, the fruit will come, good health will come. The Good Book says, "The spirit of man is the candle of the Lord." When we let the Spirit flow through us, we are aglow with the Light and we can find our way.

We Don't Get Blessings — We Earn Them

Now, I want to emphasize the fact that we have to earn our money, we have to earn our health, we have to earn our happiness. Money is not given to us. We earn it. The same principle applies to health and to happiness. We are not given a supply. We earn it. If wisdom is embodied within us, then we have done the inner work. The next step comes when we begin to pour out. To hold it within is not fruitful and is not going to bring you good health or anything else. It has to be pouring out.

You are an instrument. This instrument is kept alive by what you pour out. This is the secret of the whole lesson. This instrument becomes alive when we pour forth, and supply comes to us.

We Have More Than We Know

Something has to flow through you, or you are dead! Death is inactivity. Death is stagnation. If you are alive, you have something and you can get started putting it to work. You must have the good flowing out, but you first have to establish the good within you so that the supply can come. We give because we have abundance, but if you don't have this abundance within, you have nothing to give. That is why you have to know God. You have to go with Him. You have to develop this God-sense within you, and this is God consciousness. Being grateful for what you already have will start something within. Then the power will come. Then you will have the power to reveal who you really are.

There is no place in the *Bible* where you can find Christ asking for help. There is no place where it says He asked for payment. There is no place where He even hinted that He wanted gratitude or thankfulness from anybody. He didn't want anything. What was supplying His needs? What was supplying the abundance that He shared with others? The God within. He was supplied and abundantly supplied. Did the Christ want wealth? Satan offered it to Him, and He refused it. Did He want power and recognition? Again, Satan offered Him these things, and He refused them. No, He didn't need these things. He was well supplied from within.

Christ didn't do anything but shine! "I am the light of the world," He told us. He gave through His life what the Father gave Him. He lived on this flowing forth. The life is ever flowing and is an expression from within. One of the greatest things that can come from you is Light.

Of course, the human side of us is always wanting to have something. And we have been told how to get it. It will come when we cast that bread upon the waters. The bread will come back, sometimes with a little jam on it!

Perhaps your cup will run over. Perhaps you will receive more than you expect. There are times when I have been given a gift. I just feel like I can't do enough for that person because they pleased me so much. Have you ever been pleased? Have you even been enjoyably taken care of? Don't you feel at the moment that you want to give something?

Bring Out The Best In Others

Have you ever heard someone say, "I bring out the worst in him"? We must learn to bring out the best in others. We have to live with other people, so why not make them happy by bringing out the best in them? Don't we all want to live in a happy world? But you first have to make your world happy by establishing happiness within yourself. Then you can pour it forth. You can live in that feeling. But I love you, and I'm going to live in that feeling. From that point on, the body feels good. I don't want to moralize to people, but I can't understand why they would choose to live in hate. I can't understand why they would choose to live in jealousy. I don't understand why they continue to worry and fret. There are wonderful alternatives right at hand, but the best I can do is to point out those alternatives to people. They have to make their choice. I can't do it for them. I have to drink the broth I cook myself.

We are told to pray for our enemies. You

have to have a lot of love in you to pray for your enemies! It took great love for Christ to bathe the feet of Judas when He knew that Judas was going to betray Him. I know what the average person would do. The average life is built on "getting even." Ordinary life is built on revenge. But, " 'Vengeance is mine, I will repay,' saith the Lord." The Lord is the Law. The Law is a Principle. You cannot have revenge on anybody without paying for it sometime in life.

I don't like to say that the principle of life is that we are complete within ourselves, but the potential is there. We are much more complete than we think. We can have all the good we need if we will go within — and as we permit it to flow out, more flows back to us. Whatever you are seeking in life is also seeking you. If you are working on that wavelength, that is what comes to you. If you are on that level of consciousness, that is what comes to you.

I almost have to laugh at the belief so many people hold to that we must run around all our lives, wearing ourselves out, trying to find the kingdom of God. It lies within. The kingdom is the King's domain. When we walk in the Light, we share that kingdom. There is no reason in the world why we shouldn't walk like a king or queen instead of a pauper.

When I said you are only an instrument or vessel, I know that this instrument is physical. But this instrument feels, and when you have rested, when you have been released, when you are assured that everything is all right, the body recuperates and gets well. The nervous system recuperates and gets well. The cup of joy runs over, and all that the Father is and has flows forth into expression.

I would like to share some thoughts I wrote many years ago.

All Roads Lead From You

God has made you the hub and the center
of the world in which you live;
All roads lead from you.
We are the center from which all things develop.
You are the hub of the wheel.
The world is built around you.
There is no world without you.
It takes many people just like you to make the world.
But you are the one who represents your world.
You have within you the privilege
of seeing any kind of world you wish.
You can put on glasses that qualify and refine
the world's expression, actions and reactions.
You can see things in beauty,
see them in joyful activity,
see them in the hands of the Divine.

You and God share the act of creation.
He creates beauty; you are a joint creator.
You may share it and represent it for him,
or you can drop to the lower spheres of living
where things can become horrible, terrible,
mixed up and confused.
And if you become attracted to these things,
you will automatically represent them.
You can look at the world through "rose-colored- glasses,"
glasses may be speckled with dirt
so that you see spots on everyone on whom you look.
Your glasses may be blue, dark and dreary,
or they can carry a beautiful light
that will bathe everything with a peaceful softness
that illumines and shows all things
are working for your good.

You may possess health if you recognize
that you alone are responsible for yourself,
for keeping your mind alert,
for giving your body the proper exercise,
choosing proper foods,
seeking proper company,
breathing proper air,
believing in the proper God,
A God of Love, a God of Harmony and Contentment.
You are the one to decide whether you live
with the downcast or the uplifted.
You are the one who chooses melancholy or ease of mind.
You must make your agreement with the finer things
with which you want to live.

Knowledge and culture are here for our higher good,
but you must reach for it.
You must realize

that even you may be covered with darkness.
There's always a light shining that says,
"Be still and know."
It tells you to stand where you are and be somebody —
to be in the image and the likeness of God.
You look for the healing.
You must recognize healing.
You must recognize that deep within you exists
the beginning of all feelings,
of recognition
and awareness.

You must recognize your oneness and completeness
in the One Trinity,
the Father, the Christ and You.
You must recognize that good health is your responsibility
and it is necessary for your complete trinity with the Father.
It is to love thy neighbor as thyself,
but it begins with you.
You may forget,
but the Divine in His creation never forgets.
He has made white the lily of the field;
He remembers even the fallen sparrow.
He needs you even to the marrow of your bones.

Surely,
if we are unhappy,
if we feel neglected,
it is our lack of faith
and our lack of holding on to the one thing
that never leaves us — our Father.
You have the privilege and the power
within you
to mold one with God
or to stand alone.
What will it be?

Let us think about it for a moment. Each morning let us go forth and give freely of all the good that we know. And as we give forth, we know that we have the approval of our heavenly Father. We make friends through our giving. We achieve through our giving. Our ambitions become great through our giving.

Our love is godly as it comes from Him. The heavenly Father has given us all. We are each a child of God. We have received from a loving Father. To impart that which is loving and part of Him is to be one with Him. This whole world is in need of spiritual enlightenment.

Life Returns Good To Us — As We Give

As we go forth to make this world a better place to live in, let us realize that soul expression, the understanding from the Deep Within, is the wisdom that we need most in life. Freely I give, not thinking of what comes back, for I know as I give of Him, my supply is ever coming back to me.

I have been grateful for all that God has given me. I have been good to others, and that included me. We are one with Him, and as we are good to one another, we are good in spirit to Him — because as we have done unto the least of these, we do unto Him.

I know that as I care for the other person and make that person happy, I become happier myself. To see you uplifted, I become uplifted myself. You need me, I need you. To recognize that we are all children in this kingdom is to recognize that we all have the same Father, that the same Father takes care of us all.

So as we go together, let us give wholeheartedly of all that is good. Let all our needs be good. If you will receive this, you are right. You are the richest person in the world because you have the Father's kingdom, and in expressing it, you will be cared for.

The Father who takes care of the fallen sparrow also takes care of that which is created in His image, and that is us. We are His sparrows. We are His beauty. We are His life. We are His children. We have the opportunity in this lovely family to be the influence that can help those who are downtrodden, those who are sick. It is our business to go about doing good.

I know as we go about doing good and uplifting our fellow man, we are serving our purpose in life, for our purpose is to serve in life. As we serve, we do it from within — because God is within.

Only a life lived for others
is a life worthwhile.

—Albert Einstein

Chapter 14

The Divine Plan or Man's — Which?

As you change your consciousness,
you change your body.

To a great extent this world is a world of man-made troubles. I have never met a person who didn't have troubles. I have never met a person who was completely well. All of us have some sickness, some problems and troubles. We have to face the truth even when it is not particularly pleasant. We have to start from where we are and grow from there.

You see, we have both the challenge and the privilege of overcoming these things. We have to overcome all the way through life. The *Bible* says we can even overcome death.

What do we overcome as we go through life? We overcome all that which is truly of a miserable nature. The more we overcome of this, the more negative things we can leave behind us, then the more good we can take into ourselves.

As we gain experience, as we gain vision, we gain in wisdom. I feel that the more vision we have, the more wisdom and discernment we have, the better we become at choosing the right way. Greater wisdom gives us increasing ease and confidence in dropping the old and taking on the new. This is an inner strength we begin to develop.

What Do You Need Most?

Many people live in a world where every thing is physical. Unless they can touch it, hold it in their hands or put it on the table, they refuse to believe it is real. Unless they have something they can put in their mouths and chew, they feel they are not getting fed. They feel that only the physical things can satisfy them.

But some people are hungry for love. Some people are thirsting for kindness, which is a little different from the physical side of life. We have needs that go beyond the physical level, the worldly level, and we must take care of those needs.

On my bookshelf I have a book called *The Poisons in Your Mind.* Of course, we have all heard of people being poisoned by such things as arsenic and strychnine. But, have you ever heard the expression, "His mind is poisoned"? Or, "She has a venomous tongue"? A person who has a destructive mind is poisoning himself and perhaps others.

But we must also realize this: The person who is close to someone with a poisoned mind can never be touched by it unless he gives his consent. Nothing can ever harm you unless you give your consent. The poisoned mind primarily hurts the person who has it.

In the same way, the only thing that can help you is the good you have within you. We have to start from a helpful point within ourselves in order to have a good body.

I can go through hundreds of formulas and recipes for building up a good body with food. Food will do unbelievable things toward a cure or correction. The blood can do much when it gets the proper chemical elements. The mind is important to the body just as the blood is, but we also know that the mind supervises the blood. We can say, then, that there is a mental body that supervises the physical body. And it is just as important to have the mental body taken care of as it is the physical body, perhaps even more so.

It can be difficult to take care of the mental body. The physical body is relatively easy to take care of, but have you ever tried to give advice to someone? Have you observed how difficult it is to get past a person's mental barriers, to get a person to see life a little bit differently? Often it seems impossible. Taking care of the mind is harder than taking care of the body. The physical body doesn't know what to do and will mold to your will. But to mold one will to another will is another story altogether. I think many of us are built of stubbornness. We find all sorts of excuses for not taking good advice. We analyze it, find something wrong with it and reject it. By doing this, we miss much that could work to our benefit.

Our minds have a built-in analytical ability. We also have a will that can put our analytical ability to work in destructive ways. We criticize. We tear things down. We become so highly skilled at analyzing what is wrong with our friends, our families, our employers and others that we can't recognize good advice even when we are suffering from a problem we can't solve on our own. We don't realize that at least occasionally it is better to follow someone else's will than our own.

Are You Will-ing The Wrong Results?

I wonder why each of us can't realize that there are times when our own will is not the best will to follow. I wonder if we are capable of recognizing that our will has brought us many troubles in life. Think for a moment. Is there a time, yesterday or today, that your will has caused you trouble? As we have already seen, what goes on in the mind affects what goes on in the body. Is it possible that by changing your will you could change your body? The body is a servant of the mind, and the mind is often a servant of the will. Can you see the connection here?

We could have a wonderful servant ready to do God's will if we could get that stubborn will of ours to move over. Our will is pushy, but it isn't very wise. It doesn't know much about causing things to happen. We have to work with causes. We have to start with causes, because causes start the chain of events that bring us good or harm. It's like playing dominoes. We stack the dominoes in a nice row. We push the first one, and the rest tumble down. Sometimes, mentally, we don't know what or where that first domino is. The will gives it a whimsical push, so to speak, and down goes the whole row of dominoes — at the wrong time, the wrong place or in the wrong circumstances. Then we are in trouble.

Wouldn't it be nice to know what that first domino was doing? Wouldn't it be nice to be able to control how, when and where we push over that first domino? That will of ours can spoil a whole day by just knocking down one domino at the start. Then every other activity the whole day long goes wrong. God's will is different. In God's will there are no mistakes.

We are going to look into and compare the physical body, the mental body and the spiritual body. We are going to examine certain ways in which they work alike. We are hungry in all three bodies. We are serving in all three bodies. When we do not have harmony in all three bodies, we have trouble.

Many people are destroying their physical bodies out of ignorance. They don't know how to keep them up. And many people need a tonic, not only for their physical body, but for the mental body as well. There are certain tonics for special functions in the body to take care of the kidneys, the lungs, the heart, eliminations and so forth. There are also certain tonics to correct conditions in the mental body, conditions such as depression, fear and hate.

There are sicknesses in the mind just as there

are sicknesses in the body. You can take carrot juice if you have an infection of the eyes, but we must realize that the mind may be infected as well. We may have taken thoughts into the mind that touched a sore spot. What did we touch? We touched something we didn't like. We touched something that reached through the mind to affect the physical body. I am giving you this comparison so that you will look for tonics for what is wrong with you mentally as well as physically.

We have foods that will beautify. We have foods that will stimulate. We have foods that are nervines, foods for the digestive system and foods for the glandular system. There are many foods that help make up the physical body.

We also have to take care of what goes into making up the mental body and the spiritual body. We have weaknesses of the mind as well as weaknesses of the body. I think it is well for us to work on our weaknesses whatever form they may take. They say a chain is as strong as its weakest link — and the body is as strong as its weakest link. What about the mind and the spirit? Aren't our thoughts as strong as their weakest link? Isn't love only as strong as its weakest link?

The spiritual body is the most subtle, the least assertive, and the most powerful aspect of man. It never forces itself on the mind or body. It never overrules desire, passion or will. It only takes charge when we invite it to be in control. The mind is intermediary between spirit and body. When we bypass the self and go to the Great Within, we find spirit. And it is through our spirit that we commune with Divinity. What nourishes spirit? What releases the power of spirit? Love of God and our fellow man. Prayer. And faith. In return spirit nourishes the mind with joy and peace. And when the mind is experiencing joy and peace, the body is at its best.

Whence Comes Help?

We reach out for the healing tonics, praying and hoping that they will assist in the way that is needed. If you came to me with a health problem, do you think I would try to build up your body with potato chips and pie crust? Could you get strength from those foods? Do you think you could get strength from scorched foods? Spaghetti? Dumplings? No, of course not. But the problem is we only begin questioning the value of the foods we have been eating *after* we are sick. In a similar way, after we have become depressed and downhearted, then we begin looking at what we have been putting into our minds. And that is the time we begin looking for a way out. We know we must change our foods, and it is wonderful to know that it can make a difference. We can be healed.

But no one hands you faith. It starts from within you. No one hands you good health for your stomach or kidneys. Again, it starts from within you. Health is within. You must start within whether the problem is physical, mental or spiritual. I can assure you of this. As we work with health, we have to realize that we can't simply have an offending organ cut out and say we are well. And it is just as foolish to think that we can cut out this thought or that thought and expect the mind to be well.

Do you want to get well? Do you want to correct the problem? Then let us put something better in its place.

Most people have this idea reversed. Most people are chasing after the outside cure — looking for the right doctor, the right treatment. But the cure is within. That is why Christ said, "The Father that dwelleth in me, He doeth the works." He does the job. Otherwise, how could we expect to do it?

Stop and think about it. Where are you going to find foods that will give you spiritual peace? In the kitchen or cupboard? No. They are only found in the kingdom — the King's domain — God's country. Where is that? It's like hidden treasure. You must seek it. The kingdom of heaven is within.

Down the street are a grocery store and a drugstore. You really don't have to seek very hard to take care of the physical needs. The physical needs are easy to care for. But that doesn't mean we do it properly.

A lady I know went to the drugstore and bought a bottle of a hundred aspirins because they were on sale for twenty-nine cents. Will the aspirins correct her problem? Will they elevate her thoughts? Will they build new tissue? No. She was simply following a standard that many people follow in this life.

Many people are on a path where they lose a little energy every day. They have been doing this for many years. But we can build back this lost vitality by eliminating the negative thoughts, the depressions and anxieties that are sapping our strength. Eventually the body will come back to good health. But, mark my words, you can't do it through physical peace alone.

The Good Life Begins With Understanding

The best dividends in life come when you realize what is right, what God's plan is, what the good plan is.

We know that many invest their money in stocks. But the dividends that you get from right living are treasure of a different kind. Good health may not be everything, but without it, everything else you have is worth nothing.

If we are going to learn to take care of our bodies, we have to begin with understanding. One of the first things we have to understand is that we must practice accepting change. You have to constantly practice that. Most people live a life of disappointment because things don't happen today like they did yesterday. They are unwilling to accept change. Many of them are afraid of change. We must realize that in life we go through cycles. We are going to meet different people. People change your environment.

People can produce problems. You are going to have to meet these problems, so you may as well learn to greet them with a good attitude. We must learn to get along with people. If we don't, we start a dis-ease program, a dis-harmony program. The dis-harmony program will really get us into trouble.

Everybody Needs A Guiding Purpose

To change our lives we must have a purpose in life. What is your purpose in life? Of course, many people would like to have a new Cadillac. Many people would like to have a new car or new stereo. But if your nerves are in bad shape, you might not be able to drive. You might not be able to sit down, relax and enjoy nice music. Wanting things is not what I meant by having a purpose in life.

When you live in anxiety, nothing seems to harmonize with you. Everything is wrong. Everybody is wrong but you. An Irish mother standing on the sidewalk in New York was watching a parade go by. Her son, marching in the band, was out of step with the other boys. Proudly she pointed her son out to the other bystanders and said, "Do y'see, now? Everybody's out of step but my Pat!"

How do we see things these days? Does everything seem to be going wrong? There is a possibility it is all starting right within ourselves. Perhaps this is where we need to make the change.

We need a purpose, and this purpose has to include taking care of our physical body. The physical body changes when the mind changes. The mind changes when the spiritual attitude changes. Now, I am not saying the spiritual body can bring good health all by itself. I don't care how much you pray, if you live on coffee and donuts, it is going to be perfectly natural for your body to work out a disease.

God may take care of each of us in a personal way, but that doesn't mean we can violate His Law and get away with it. He works through foods. He works through right thinking. He works through the teachings brought to us through the *Bible*.

You must have a goal in your mind. Your goal is your image. You must have a perfect image from a health standpoint, or the goal cannot come to you. Let's put this whole picture together. Can you change illness to health or poverty to riches? Remember how we used to read all those books by Horatio Alger? All his books were about how some poor boy rose up through the ranks from "rags to riches," finally owning the business. What a wonderful experience it was to read those stories! What a wonderful dream to put into our minds!

You must have a dream. To have this dream come true, you must work for it. You must reach for the sky. You may not touch it, but no matter how short you are, you must reach out and try.

Let's look at what having a life purpose is all about. Many people don't understand that there are two plans to choose from. There is man's plan. And there is God's plan. There are two ways to go.

A Good Body Begins In The Mind

Many of you would like to have a good physical body. If you knew that it starts in the mind, that would be a good beginning. I have never been able to help a person who didn't have good desires. I've never been able to help a person who didn't want to do good things. People come to me and say, "You're the doctor. What do you think you can do?" What do you suppose they would think if I said, "Do you know that I have quite a job just taking care of myself?" I have a big job just keeping my own house in order.

The body is the dwelling place of the Most High. You can make this body a temple of the living God. This is your house, to be taken care of as you will. Be careful of that "will." If your will directs you to drink too much coffee and to eat too many donuts, your dwelling place will hardly be fit to live in.

It is the Father's good pleasure to give us His kingdom, where perfection is the standard. Yet, we can choose not to accept His gift. We can choose to remain sick physically, mentally and spiritually.

We Ought To Have A Law!

Of course, nobody wants to remain sick. Then how do we get on the right track? Where should we seek health? Who is going to be our authority on right living? Our legal system is designed to steer us away from wrong living, isn't it? I have heard there are 385,000 federal, state and local laws on the books in the United States to enforce the basic provisions of the Ten Commandments — laws against killing, stealing, property destruction, cheating, perjury and so forth. Are these laws successful at guiding people into right living? I think you know the answer. I think you know that we will never have manmade laws that are going to give us good health. The various plans of man throughout the history of the human race have failed us.

We want a tonic that doesn't fail. I know of tonics for the physical body that will not fail you. For example, grape juice and an egg yolk are a marvelous tonic for the nervous system. But I want you to know that there are infallible tonics for the mental and spiritual bodies as well as the physical body. And these tonics are drawn from higher ways than man's ways.

This Amazing Body Of Ours

This body is wonderfully and fearfully made. Your body heat is kept precisely regulated at 98.6 degrees F. no matter how hot or cold it is around you. In a desert or tropical jungle with the heat sweltering at 115 degrees, your body temperature would still be 98.6 degrees. At the North Pole amidst ice and snow and temperatures dropping farther than 40 degrees below zero, your body temperature would still be 98.6 degrees. When the body is cold, a built-in mechanism starts us shivering to help maintain body heat. When the body is too hot, we automatically begin to perspire to cool the body.

God has designed the human body in such a marvelous way that many of its processes function automatically. The brain and nervous system are organized to take care of these processes as well as those that we exercise voluntary control over. The eyes, which are actually extensions of the human brain, are equipped with rods and cones to allow us to detect colors. From each eye an optic nerve containing 1,250,000 fibers leads to the brain. In each ear 24,000 fibers in the basilar membrane pick up the voices and different sound frequencies that come to us. When you stub your toe, nerve impulses tell the brain about that event in one-fiftieth of a second. Then you say, "Ouch!" Messages pass through our nervous system at rates of up to 224 miles per hour. God has given us wonderful bodies, but we don't take care of them.

Half of the ailments that people have today result from medical treatments they have received. Many people leave hospitals with more problems than they had when they went in. Think about the drugs and pills that people take today, chemical substances that medical scientists realize have undesirable side effects.

There is a lovely way out of this mess — a beautiful way to go. I am wondering if we are wise enough yet to choose this way. I am wondering if we have learned our lesson.

Let The Spirit Take You Over

Spirit and body have a definite relation to one another. Charles Lindberg demonstrated this beautifully when he made the first solo flight over the Atlantic Ocean in his plane, the *Spirit of St.*

Louis. After he had flown about thirteen hours, this big six-foot-six man became terribly cramped in the cockpit which was jam-packed with all the things needed for the trip. Later, describing this experience, he said, "After thirteen hours I became so numb that I actually bent down to pinch my legs to see if there was any feeling left. I could not even feel my own body when I pinched it. But at that moment I let *Spirit* take over." That is the secret of the whole thing — "I let *Spirit* take over." You can read this in Lindberg's autobiography. It is wonderful. To me it is the most remarkable passage in the whole book. When the physical feeling fails, "let the Spirit take over!" It is a secret well worth noting, because some of us have failed miserably at the physical level. Some of us can't feel this body and don't want to feel it.

Some people are ready to give up on this world and get into another one. That's when it is time to let the Spirit take over. There is no sickness in Spirit. There is only harmony in Spirit. There is only peace in Spirit. When you once come to this place, your body will have a good time. Most of us give our bodies a difficult time. We don't realize that we have to go a new way for the body to have a good time.

We have to recognize that the spirit has supremacy over the mind, but we have to *let it* have that supremacy. The spirit isn't a naturally dominating thing, like desire or will. Spirit doesn't make anything happen. It has no place to go, nothing to get — and this is the wonderful thing about it. If the body follows the spirit, there is a very slow but steady refinement. Time only exists at the physical and mental levels. There is no time as far as spirit is concerned. Spirit can wait because it has all the time in the world and more — eternity, in fact.

We Are Living In Eternity Now

Eternity is here now. We don't have to worry about eternity because we are in it right now. We should live as eternal beings but we become caught up in the pressures of time. So we separate ourselves mentally from the eternal values. Many of us think we are going to heaven when we die. Those who believe this usually think the nicer things are coming later. If some people went to heaven as the sour-pusses they are right now, they would make a hell out of heaven. These same people could change their hell on this earth into heaven right now if they could only understand.

If you want to get into the kingdom of heaven, you will have to start to work right now. You must become a seeker. You must use the spiritual power for mental and physical balance. Once you get a toe in the spiritual door you will say, "It *is* possible!" But you will have to make a start. It takes studying and seeking. Many people who get into spiritual studies have a problem with belief at first because they think they should be able to change water into wine right away. Spiritual work is more subtle than that.

To develop spiritually requires much studying. As the Apostle Paul said, "Earnestly desire the greater gifts, and I show you a still more excellent way." We never really finish but in each path we take we reach a higher level.

We have dominion over all God has given us. What a wonderful thing it is to take all these lovely things and to use them according to God's plan. This is right living.

You know, many people are interested in using spiritual power for getting money or for personal gain. But God's purposes have nothing to do with selfishness. His purpose is entirely impersonal, and it applies to everyone, not just an elite few.

A Divine Law has been provided for us so that "all these things shall be added unto you." But, you see, it only comes after you have set something into motion. The action that comes from the spiritual level is found through rising above. Don't hide your light, let it shine!

If you will rise to a level of spiritual consciousness, your body will love going along with you. Your body only becomes an antagonist when you are not letting it live in harmony with God's Law. The divine way reaches through the spiritual and into the mental, through the mental and into the physical.

What does it mean to look forward to a new day? It means we need to let go of our yesterdays. We need to be born anew. We don't really have a new day if we persist in trying to make it just like yesterday. Welcome change into your life. Go with this one thought in your mind: *now is the beginning of the rest of my life.*

Healing Thoughts — The Twenty-Third Psalm

We are constantly coming out of darkness. Perhaps the greatest healing way I know of is in the twenty-third Psalm. When it starts out by saying, "The Lord is my shepherd," many people interpret this to mean that the Lord is a man. The Lord is Law, and the man that might have been the Lord is only bringing the Law to you. The Christ said, "The Father that dwelleth in me, he doeth the works," and "He that hath seen me hath seen the Father." You see the works of the Father!

Now, since the Law is our shepherd, that is the plan we should follow. We must follow God's plan. The Law and the shepherd are to be instilled and practiced in our lives. These laws include the laws of life and the laws of nature. If you will find and follow these laws, which are all parts of God's Law, they will lead you.

The Psalm says, "The Lord is my shepherd, I shall not want." When you establish within yourself the law of good foods, the law of right thinking and the law of spiritual values, you will need nothing more because you will have good health at the physical, mental and spiritual levels. You will have good friends, a good family and a good marriage. You won't be bothered with violence or lesser forms of negativity. You won't be upset by man's plans. This is replacement therapy . We replace the bad with the good. This is why I say to follow the Law — then you "shall not want." We are all in need. We need food, drink and shelter. If we follow the shepherd we shall not want.

"He maketh me to lie down in green pastures." Green is the greatest color we have for healing, for relaxation, for letting go. Green is a tranquilizer in our life. When you go out to a green orchard or to a green pasture, you feel good. Our shepherd tells us to lie down in green pastures, to take it in, to breathe it in, to let that green run through us. In this way the healing comes to us.

"He leadeth me beside the still waters." Can you turn off your old motor which has been going putt-putt-putt-putt? Can you lie down beside still waters? Do you know how quiet still waters are? Have you ever seen a lake without a ripple, so smooth that it mirrors the trees around it and the blue sky and white clouds above? Rest is one of the healing qualities, one of the greatest healing qualities. You will never repair, rejuvenate or recuperate until you become very, very still.

"He restoreth my soul." Believe, for once in your life, that you can get close to God. You have been living close to people all your life. Now, try God. Go within, find God and ask Him to restore you.

"He leadeth me in the paths of righteousness." Do you think that a God of good can produce evil? Do you think you can behave unrighteously and expect a God of good to give you righteous results? You can't live on coffee and donuts and expect God to give you a good body. It doesn't come that way.

"He leadeth me." God didn't spoil the Garden of Eden. We did. There were no packaged foods in the Garden of Eden. There was no French chef in the Garden of Eden. No violence. No violent thoughts. We invented these things and we make ourselves sick and ugly with them. We will never straighten ourselves out until we follow the paths He shows us.

"Yea, though I walk through the valley of the shadow of death . . . " We constantly walk through the valley of the shadow of death. Death isn't bad, but the shadow is. Most of you look at these shadows and see them as fearfully dark. But with the Shepherd you need not fear. He knows the way out, the way into the light.

"I will fear no evil." No evil can happen to you unless you give it your consent. There is no evil unless you think of something as evil. Evil is made in the minds of men. When we become too pure to see iniquity, our bodies will become pure. Every cell in our bodies will respond to what we think and believe.

"I will fear no evil, for thou art with me." People are running to doctors, moving to the mountains, taking ocean cruises to find tranquility when the God of tranquility is right within us.

"Thy rod and thy staff, they comfort me." Thy staff — the staff of life. You think of the staff of life as bread, don't you? Perhaps whole-wheat, made in a bakery? When Christ talked about the staff of life He wasn't talking about bread at all. He was talking about the truth that we take into ourselves that gives us spiritual consciousness.

"Thou preparest a table before me in the presence of mine enemies." What a wonderful idea — to have a lovely moment in the midst of enemies, to let them see how God provides for us under all circumstances. Any enemy needs a good experience to lead him out of darkness. He may have a long way to go if he hasn't learned to forgive and forget. But he will come to that, just as we have. We must learn to look at those who would harm us and say, "One of these days you will find the truth, and the truth will free you of hate and vengefulness."

Much depends on us when we are in front of our enemies. That is the time the enemy changes — when he has the right influence before him.

Once when I held a class in Pittsburg, I was telling a lady this, and she said, "In this class we have to learn to bless people. Just bless them. I don't mean go out and bless them physically. But inside ourselves, just bless them constantly. Say the nicest things about them. We have to lift them."

That night she went to take care of her son's coffee shop, which was one of those old dining cars from a passenger train. While she was there, a burgular broke in. He waved a gun at her and said, "This is a stickup. I want your money." This lady said, "Well, son, help yourself, and bless you. May you use this money and bless other people with it."

"Mother," said the burglar, "I can't take it." And he left.

We may have a lot of enemies or we may not. But our greatest enemy is often ourself. So we have to change that. Love everyone, including yourself. When we are good to others we should be good to ourselves as well. So always prepare your table in such a way as to show care for yourself.

"Thou anointest my head with oil." If you go back into history, you find that oil was used in holy ceremonies. Oil was used by priests. It was used to anoint the heads of new kings. So this oil is a holy potion. When your head is anointed with oil, you can walk as a king or a queen. You have been blessed.

"My cup runneth over." Are you thankful for all the good that you have? Thankful for this body? Thankful for friends? Thankful for your food? Thankful for each morning and day? Are you thankful for what is yet to come? "My cup runneth over." Give a little and watch twice as much come back. Cast your bread upon the waters and have it come back. Are we glad for each other? Are you happy that you are happy? Let your cup runneth over with good thinking, with joy, with happiness.

"Surely goodness and mercy shall follow me all the days of my life." How much more could we want? "And I will dwell in the house of the Lord forever." We have a physical body, a temple of the living soul, which enjoys the Spirit that is within us.

What More Could Anyone Want?

This is the day that the Lord hath made. All that I have, son, is thine. Let us think about this a little bit. God is a God of generosity, of abundance, of power, of love. And He has offered to share all He has with us. Take a new look at life. Recognize that man in his plans has failed repeatedly. God never fails.

I will go forward recognizing that what I have to do will find favor in His sight. Whatever I have to accomplish today will be done with His will, not mine. Let me recognize that I can sit at the table prepared by Him with the food I need for all the cell structures of my body, the good of my mind, the humility of my spirit. And as I come to Him, as I come closer to Him, I realize I can let go of this world and its problems — in Spirit I have peace and harmony. Now I will let my worldly efforts go.

I can be born anew. Now I can take on the better things in life. I can eat with Him. I thirst no longer, for I recognize that what I give, I have. He that hath, to him more shall be given. We may not have bread, but we will always be provided for.

Those who are starving need God. Those who are thirsting need God. We need God's plan for our physical health. As we seek our physical body's welfare, let us raise our minds to Him. Let us rejoice that we are beloved of God. We are one with Him. It isn't necessary to chase after good health or anything else, since the Source is within us. There is nothing to get. We have it. The kingdom of heaven is within us. We are never without it. We are thankful as we go through life blessing whoever and whatever comes across our path. Then we have the law of good health working through us. This power flowing through us is the only influence we need with other people.

We know that He has worked His wonders through us. People will see that this is the life.

It is *this* life that we want to have flow through us. It is not our way to try to make life happen, but to find out what the good life is and to let it flow through us.

Every cell in the body responds to the peace and harmony we have in our mind. The tensions in the abdomen dissolve as we become aware of the deep relaxation in the mind. We relax in Him, knowing that we are perfectly cared for, that we have been provided for and have everything to be thankful for.

How happy I am! What joy it is to live! In this wisdom we are certainly blessed!

I would like to share with you a poem written by one of my employees at the Ranch.

Lost Horizon Found

There's a place in men's minds
Called the Valley of Dreams,
Where life as we know it
Is not what it seems.

Surrounded by mountains
Of deep peace and calm,
This Shangri-La Valley
Soothes care like a balm.

In the Valley of Dreams
An eternal spring dwells,
And Love is the music
That temple bells knell.

The River of Hope
Finds a happy home here,
As it wends through a land
Parched by doubt, despair, fear.

Its life-giving waters
Refresh and renew,
Giving strength to the weary
And heartbroken, too.

Plants of Courage spring up
Where this river has gone.
Soon sweet blossoms of Faith
Will burst forth like a song.

But to find such a valley
Requires much care,
One must search far and wide
To find happiness there.

Yet, when once it is found,
There is great peace of mind
And is that not the one thing
We all seek to find?

— Judith V. Koopman

Chapter 15

Walking in Obedience

A long life lived
is not good enough;
A good live lived
is long enough.

We want to find out what our place in the universe is and we want to find out how to mold ourselves to that which is perfect. To move toward perfection in our lives, we must mold ourselves to that which is perfect.

Most people would like to learn how to get well and stay well. We seem to understand the physical aspect of getting well but the moment we come to the spiritual, it becomes abstract. It seems beyond us. Very few people realize that what we do not see, the spiritual aspect of life, is the most valuable power we possess.

This may sound strange to you, but think about it. We live in an already created world; but that which does the creating seems far above it all, far beyond. It was there before that which was created. But we, living in this created world, think it is everything.

If we will align ourselves with the Creator, we will come forth, not with disharmony, not with disease, but with good, with happiness, with peace, with all the things we have been searching for.

Spiritual Values Are Hard To See

When I stop and think about the spiritual truths, there seems to be something about them that we cannot fathom. Many of us give up even trying to get hold of it because we haven't had a teacher. That is why we notice so many people running to India looking for a guru, looking for somebody who can teach them. That is why we have Maharishi over here with so many people following him. He was once in Squaw Valley, California and had over 600 people in his class. Now his students and student-instructors number in the thousands, and even some of our businessmen and U.S. Senators are beginning to wonder if they might find some guidance from his teachings. They are all seeking.

Man must have a God, or he will invent one. He must have something bigger than himself. Man has always searched for something bigger than himself.

Let us think along these lines and see if there isn't something useful we can attach ourselves to that will help us make a more lovely soul. In the soul's expression, it either gives the body a good time or a bad one. The soul is struggling very hard to make itself felt and known — to find its rightful place in the eternal struggle.

The soul gives the young body a hard time, trying to teach it the proper lessons in life. If we do not learn those lessons, if our minds stay childish as our bodies grow to adulthood, things go from bad to worse, affecting every cell of the body. Now, I am not talking about our ideal of the child, the one who is true, who is clean, who is pure. I am talking about "childishness" in a different sense, the qualities of the self-ruled child — the grabbing, the whining, the howling, the "give-me-that-right-now," the emotional tantrums, the selfishness. I make my living from adults who lead a child's life. It is not our work that kills us but the aggravations we give ourselves in response to our work. It is the aggravation I would like to study for a moment. To cure this aggravation you have to handle the mental situation, just as you handle a heart problem through physical care.

You nourish the body. You give it air. You breathe. You drink. You eat. You even dress this body beautifully. How many of you people go around a mental wreck, a cripple, as far as the mind is concerned? Why shouldn't we dress up the mind?

One lady said to me that she was born with sunshine in her blood. This is what we should have! If we could have this sunshine in our body and in our mind, letting the rays of that sunshine work through every cell of the body, every thought in the mind, we would be soothed, uplifted, refreshed — from the inside out.

People are funny. Often we will go to great lengths to hold on to unhealthy life patterns when we could just as easily change for the better. I know of a man who was taken to his sister's home very inebriated. The fellow was an alcoholic. His sister told him, "We want you to see our doctor." So he did. When he came back to his sister's house, she wanted to know what happened.

"The doctor told me I would have to quit drinking," he said.

"What are you going to do?" his sister asked.

"I'm going to change doctors."

We usually follow what we want to follow. We say, "My will be done, not thine." We get into trouble with our will and we don't know what a good will is. We don't know what our true inheritance is. We don't know what the godly power is, nor how to align ourselves with it.

Let's Open Our Eyes

We need to open our eyes and look again. What a wonderful thing it would be if we could align ourselves with this godly power and then go forward. And you *could* go forward, because there is no sickness in spirit. There are no tensions in the spiritual Kingdom — only peace and harmony.

There are many ways we could teach this truth. I have listened to many teachers who teach spiritual truth. some teach it by appealing to the intellect. Some do it with emotion. Some even teach with fear, trying literally to "scare the hell out of people." And they say that if a man doesn't do the things he knows are right, evil will come to him. We have to lead with the good thoughts. I would like to reach your understanding, the kind of understanding that dwells in the heart. I would like to touch you where the deeper things are, for that is where understanding exists. The spiritual values are sometimes hard to see and hard to understand, but we must awaken them by going deep within.

I do not say that everything within is good, that everything within is spiritual. War is found in the hearts of men. No one ever pulled the trigger of a gun until something inside told him to move that finger. But there is a *place* deep within where spirit dwells. Peace is there. Harmony is there. We must go beyond mind. It is deeper than that. The mind just flutters through life. Our minds get pushed around, caught up in the concerns of this minute. The mind never really rests. It thinks constantly. It never grows old. Our thoughts can grow old, but mind never does. People may say they are getting old, but they mean that their bodies are growing old. The mind can remain young, growing in wisdom, even as the body deteriorates. We can let the mind deteriorate, we can let it degenerate, but we don't want to let that happen. We want the mind to be strong, vigorous, alive and alert. We want it to serve us well.

You will never realize the lovely possibilities within you until you start using them. There is a genius within everybody. We are all different. Our faces are different. Our chromosomes are different. Our bodies, souls, desires and purposes are different. There is something within you that is unique. If you would seek this out, it would make you very happy. That which is within is yours, yours in a special way.

In my home I have some big wall panels on which are displayed spoons from all over the world. Each one is different. There are spoons from Switzerland. There is an umbrella spoon from Japan, a spoon with a bone handle from Alaska, a spoon with a turquoise handle from Arizona. Every place you go the spoons are a little different. Each craftsman put something original, something special into each handle. We are like those spoons. We are unique. Each of us is made differently.

We must express this uniqueness in our living. That is what it is for. You could make yourself very happy if you would just unfold some of the wonderful qualities you have within. You have to be yourself. You have to draw yourself out. You have to push yourself at times. You have to take time out to open your eyes, go within and equip yourself with those things that are uniquely yours in your journey upon the higher path in life.

Each Road Reveals A Higher Road

The Apostle Paul put it wisely when he said, "Earnestly desire the greater gifts, and I show you a still more excellent way."

I am trying to show you a map of how to get there, but this map is a map of the heart. It may seem very difficult for you, but each day you must move along. Each day you get a little higher. Each day you accomplish some of the things you are seeking in life.

One day you will have learned to take care of the mind just as you take care of your body. Both are taken care of in the same way; we have to illuminate the Great Within. It is said that God is within. It must be great if God is in there. Let us illuminate this wisdom and seek our direction from it. Then let us walk in obedience to that wisdom, letting it come out and letting it come forth.

We have to ennoble our character. How do we do this? It starts within. We have to develop self-confidence. How do we do this? From within. We overcome our bashfulness and timidity. We have to train our nerves. We have to quicken our senses. We don't buy any methods on the outside to do these things, because there are no cheap short cuts or gimmicks that can help us do this.

It has to come from within. This idea of reaching for the higher path in life should begin with brain building. We should build up our brain structure. Just as we build up our stomach so it can digest well, so we should build up our brain to think well. That is what it is for.

We have to be thankful for what is yet to come, for the good of our nervous system. If you are going to meet that problem with aggravation, despondency or discouragement, you will break down your brain cells faster than you should. Then you will have to take time to repair them.

It is remarkable how nature supplies us with all the natural ingredients to do everything we should. But we have to put it together, we have to make a life out of this idea. When we take care of the physical needs, we make a body. When we take care of the mind, we make a life for ourselves.

There was a famous singer who had poor health because he couldn't control his physical desires, especially his appetite for food. He could gain as much as a hundred pounds in four months time. He died from a heart attack. His wife couldn't go through life without him, and in six months she committed suicide. Two mistakes were made. One did not know how to live physically, and the other didn't know how to live mentally. We must learn how to take better care of ourselves.

Life Is More Than Physical

A surgeon separated Siamese twins successfully. He did a beautiful job in a most difficult operation, but he recently died of an overdose of barbiturates. What is this? We know the physical, but we don't know the mental. Where are we short? Maybe it is teaching that we lack.

I've heard of a young actress who can't work unless she has "pep" pills. Doctors have warned her that she has to cut them out or she will become "hung up" on those pills, addicted.

How do we live this life? How do we get

relief? Is this a life more abundant? Is this a life of shortage, of lack? Is this a life of balance? Stop and think about it.

A well known movie actor was told that he would have to quit working so hard and take a rest. He said, "I've saved nine million dollars and I have made up my mind that I'm going to save ten million. I am not going to stop until I get it." I don't know whether he will live to enjoy his ten million dollars if he gets there.

We persist in our demands upon life and upon ourselves, even when we know we are endangering ourselves. There is a story about a little boy who was in his bed upstairs. He yelled down, "Mommy, bring me a glass of water." So mommy brought the glass of water. In half an hour he again yelled, "Mommy, I want another glass of water." Mommy brought him more water. The third time when he called, "Mommy, I want more water," his daddy got into the act. His daddy called out, "You've had enough, you can't have any more water." The boy repeated, "But I want more water!" Then the father said, "I'll wring your neck if you ask for another glass of water!" There was a pause before the boy said, "Well, when you come up to wring my neck, bring me a glass of water."

I'm bringing these things out because many people go through life killing themselves mentally even though they may do some wonderful things physically. You can't sustain good health unless you respect and nurture the mind that makes it possible.

To live in the higher consciousness gives you freedom, and freedom is a very, very wonderful thing. Some people, after getting married, begin to experience this state as a loss of freedom. The wife says, "He won't let me do anything on my own." The husband says, "She always wants things her way." This is not a good marriage. Even though married, each must be free to live so that the nerves are working properly. We hear "She is mine," or "He belongs to me." This is constantly being drilled into us in so much of our popular music and in films and television. We find that belonging can become like slavery. But the individuality of each human being must be respected. We must be free and we must respect the freedom of others.

What Really Heals Us?

They say there is no cure for birth or death, but only for what happens in the interval. You are here between birth and death, and it is for you to take care of that.

Now, a doctor should be an artist. But is he? He handles all of the raw materials that nature gives him. If he only works on the physical body, he doesn't understand that matter is wed to the spirit and spirit works through this matter. It is the life in the doctor that must do the real work. The spirit in the doctor must do the real work. Christ said, "The Father that dwelleth in me, he doeth the work." Christ didn't claim to be healing anyone.

Doctors can be artists, but they should also be healers. A physical healing comes when old tissue is replaced with new. But when we replace old thought with new, the healing takes place on a deeper level, and we send people on their way happy and seeking a higher way of living. That is healing.

We should develop a strong and harmonious personality — a richer inner life. We develop this from our experiences. We use them for higher good. We use them for advantage.

You have within you the power to choose and the power to act. But you should realize that all the things you do produce consequences, and if you want good consequences to come, you have to start with the right thought. What do you turn to? Many people will turn to diet to change everything. Some people turn to drinking because they can't handle life.

Others turn to religion. Many scoff at religion, but deep down inside they are still seeking it. The religious person tries to find the right thought in church, but he will never find it there if it isn't in his heart first.

You don't have to tell me what your faith is. I can tell what your faith is from the way you live, from the deeds you do. Your faith may come first, but we live by what we believe. It makes no difference what church we go to if we are doing that which uplifts our fellow man.

Most people are seeking enlightenment. They might not call it that, but that is what they are seeking. A patient once came to me and said, "Please tell me how to do this."

I thought about it for a moment, and here is what I told him: "You keep practicing the higher and better way in life, the kinder way, say-

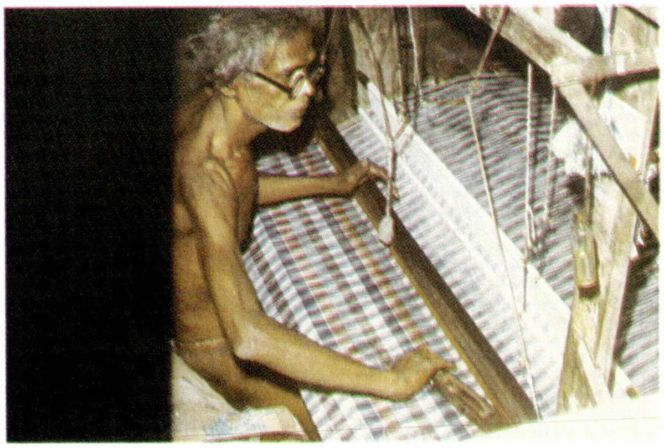

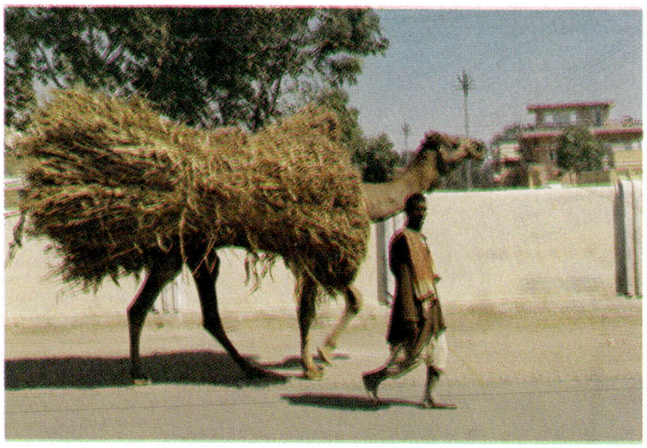

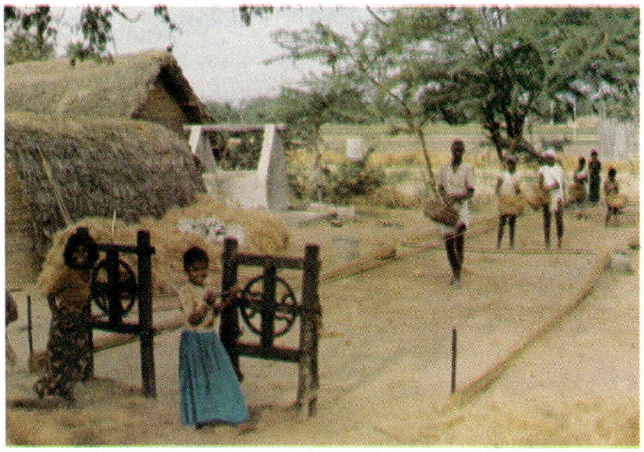

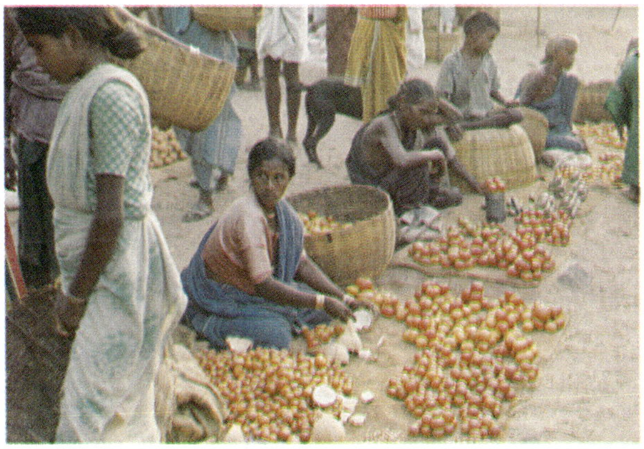

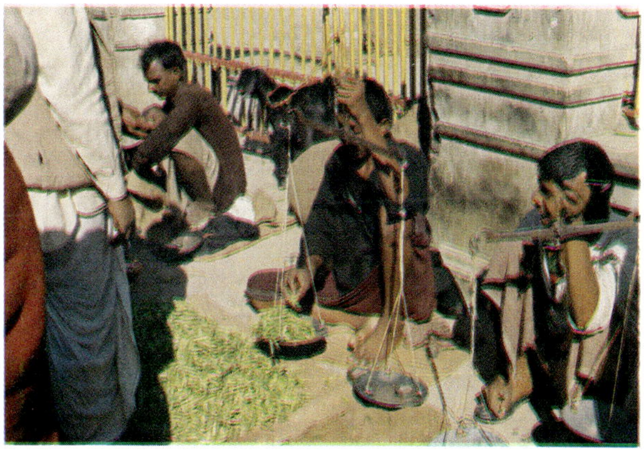

Upper Left: Weaving cloth in India. We must bring into our lives the weaving necessary to make a better world. Lower Left: A specialized market in India where merchants were selling tomatoes. Upper Right: This beast of burden was an unusual camel. I was charged 50 cents to take a picture of the camel's face because the owner considered it such a beautiful one. Lower Right: A man weighing out string beans on a balance scale. Center: Hemp rope is made in the outskirts of one of the big cities in India.

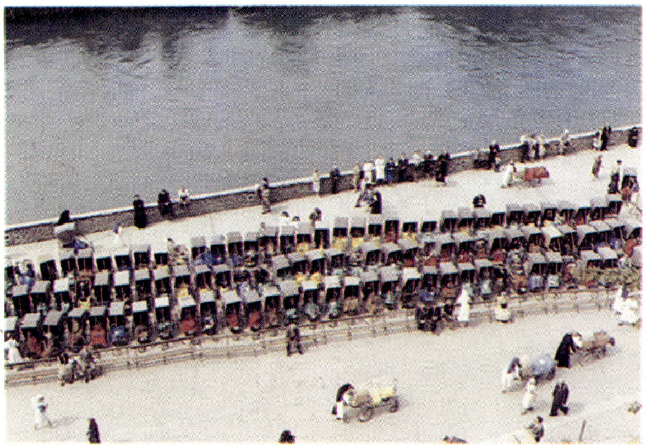

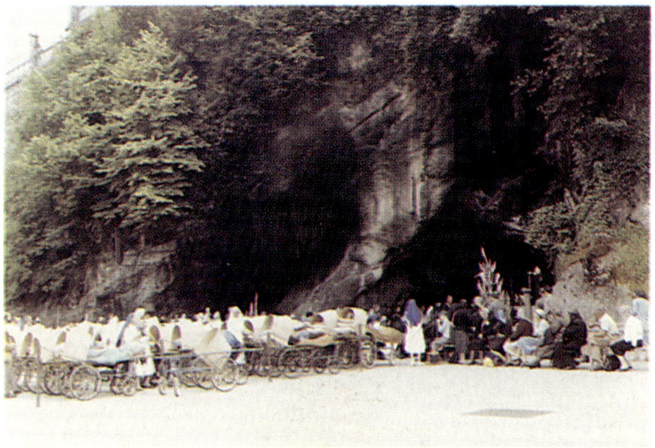

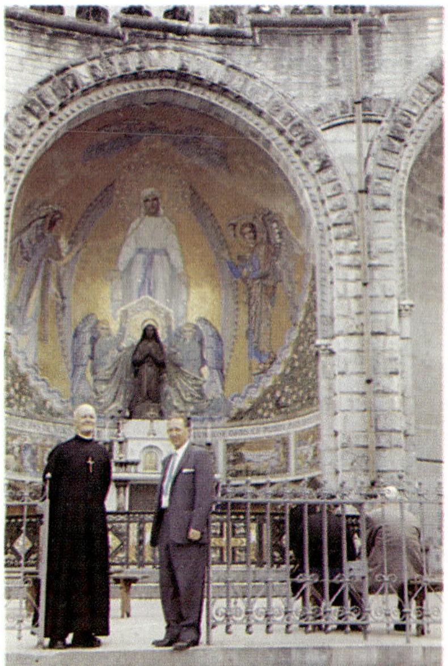

Lourdes, France. The day we were there 16,000 people were wheeled in their canopied wheelchairs and brought to the shrine for healing. At Lourdes, many are given solace for spiritual needs. Just to come and partake of the waters of Lourdes brings them satisfaction and a great inner peace. This can be the means for healing. I believe a peaceful heart brings healing.

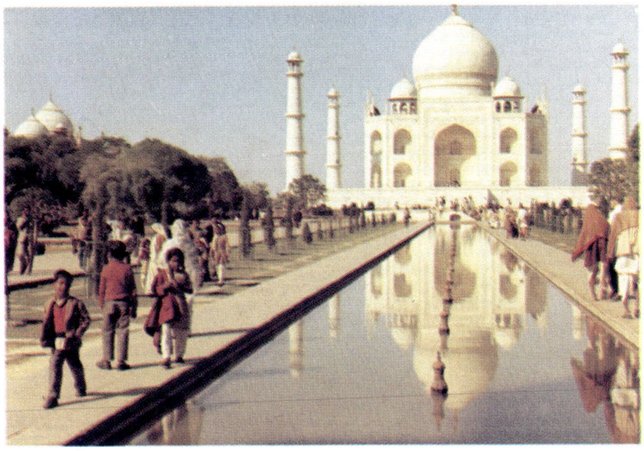

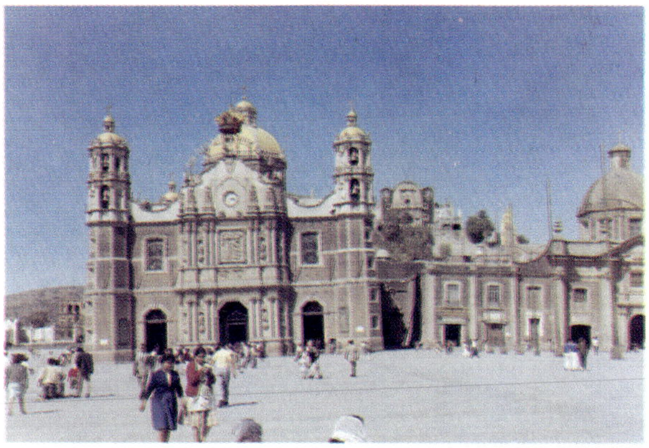

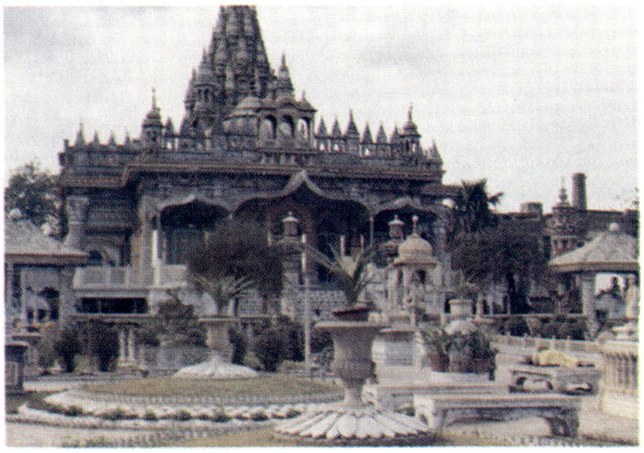

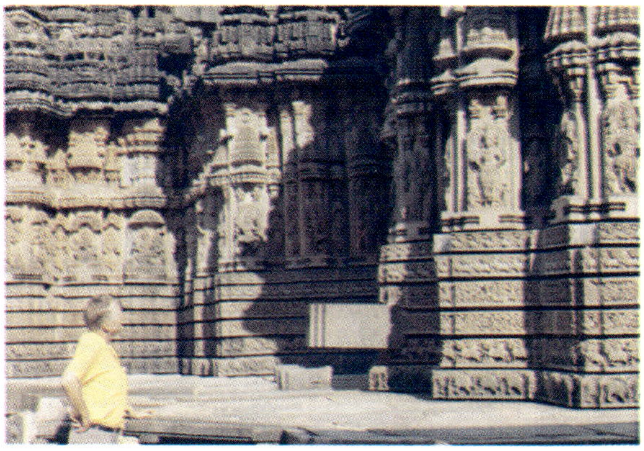

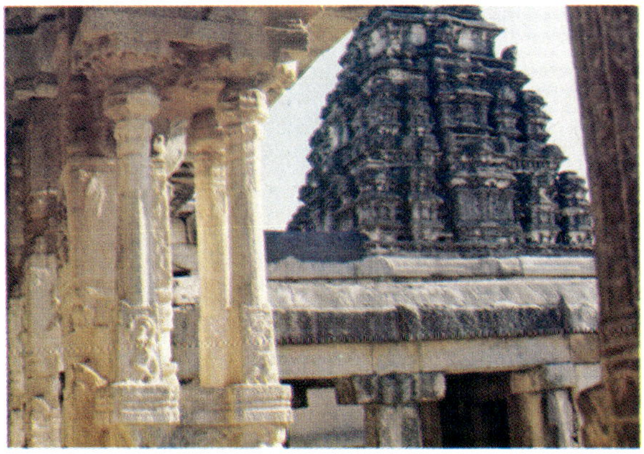

Beautiful temples throughout the world inspired us to ponder what man's mind is made of. Everything that is created originally comes from man's mind, but when we see destructive things created from man, it is well we look back and see what it is possible to build in a world of beauty.

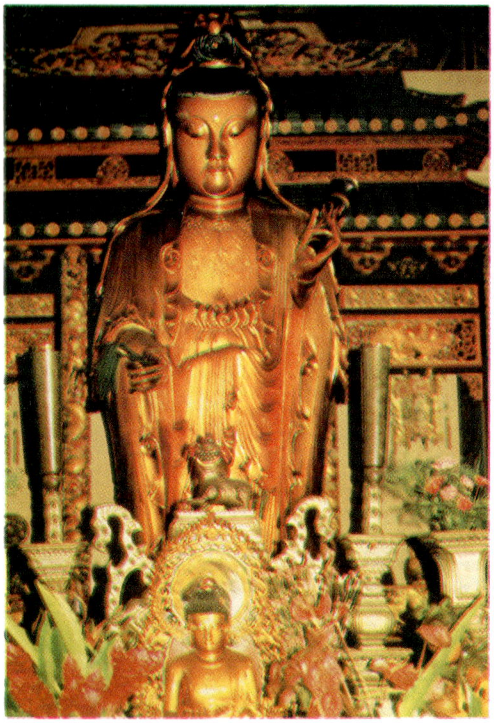
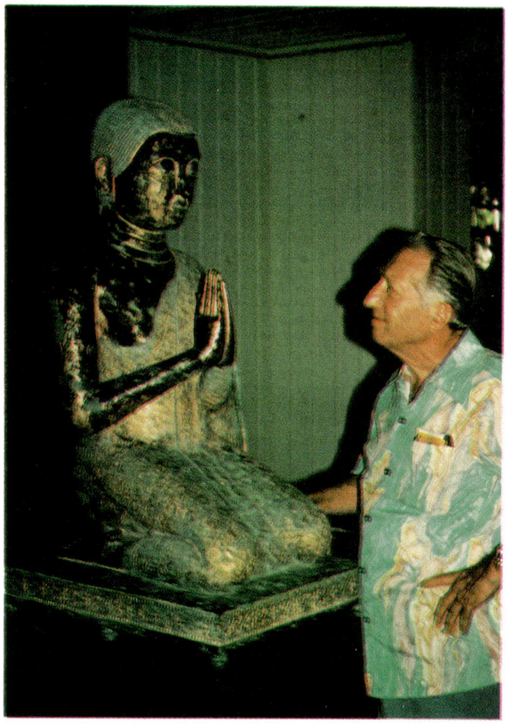
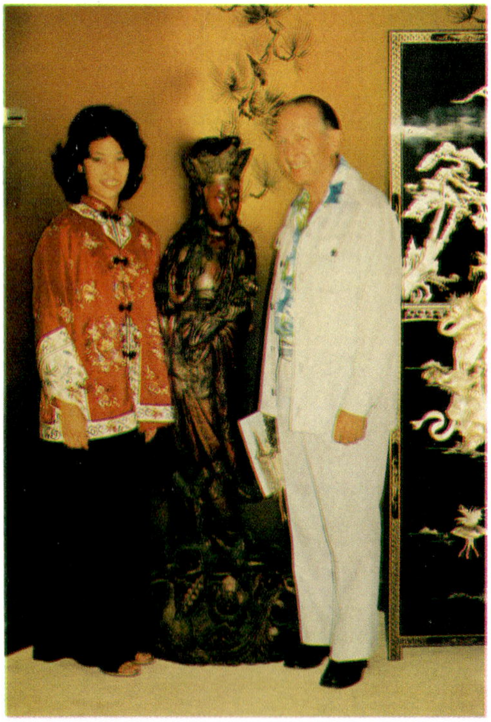
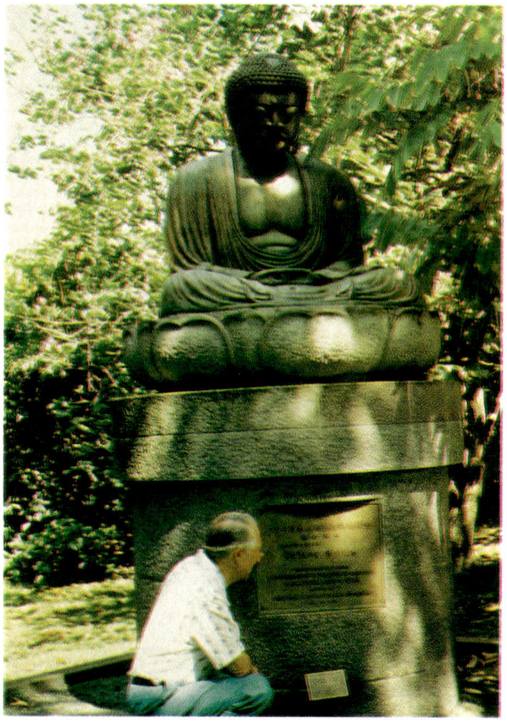

In the Far East, we find many representations of Buddha which fall in the category of sacred art and as a reminder of the truth and enlightenment he brought. Every culture has its ways of seeking spiritual truth, and religion has had a great impact on the art and architecture of many nations, East and West.

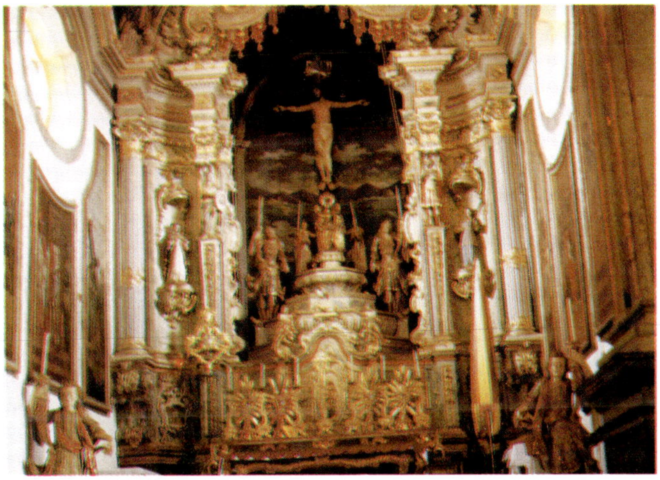

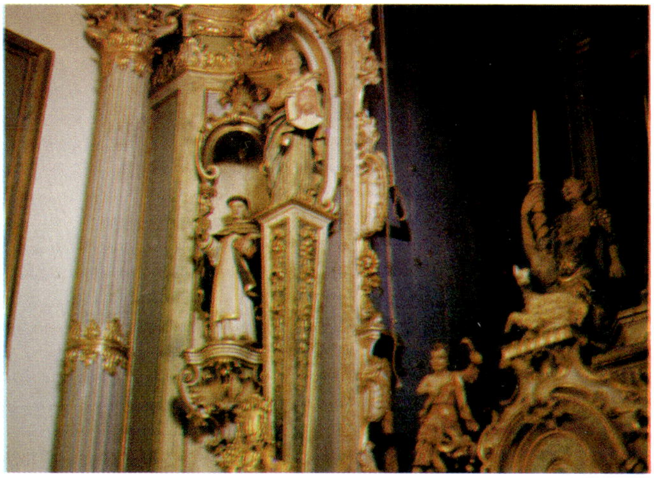

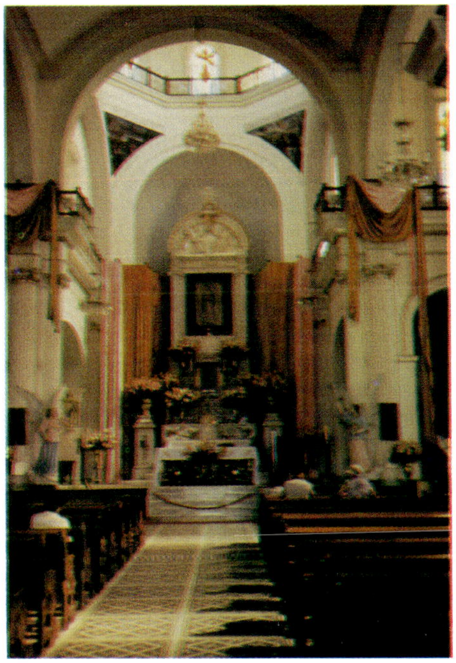

I have visited many beautiful churches in South America where the interiors were calming and breathtakingly beautiful. There was a feeling of peace, harmony and goodwill, qualities that bring healing to body, soul and spirit. It is a lovely experience to see these churches, yet if we do not bring the real church inside us when we attend church, they are only empty buildings.

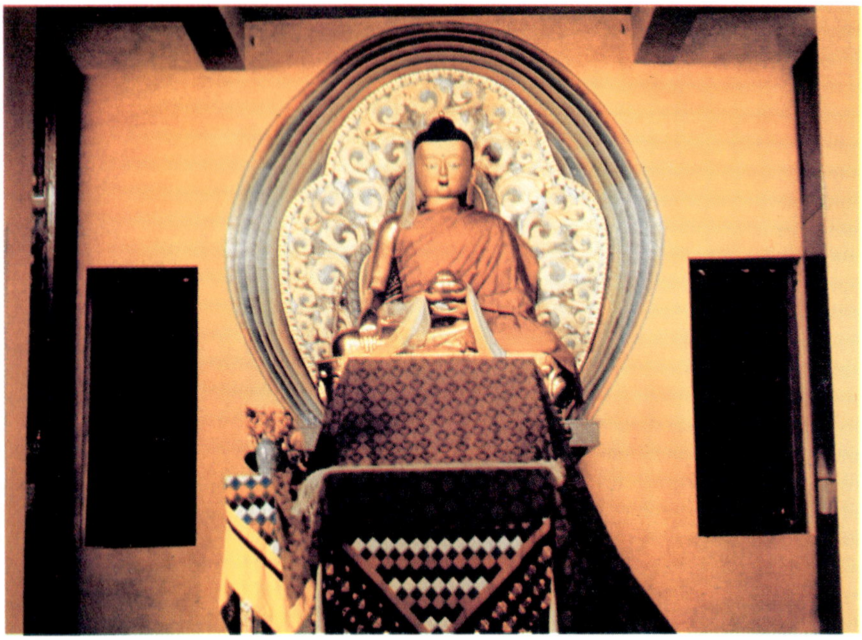

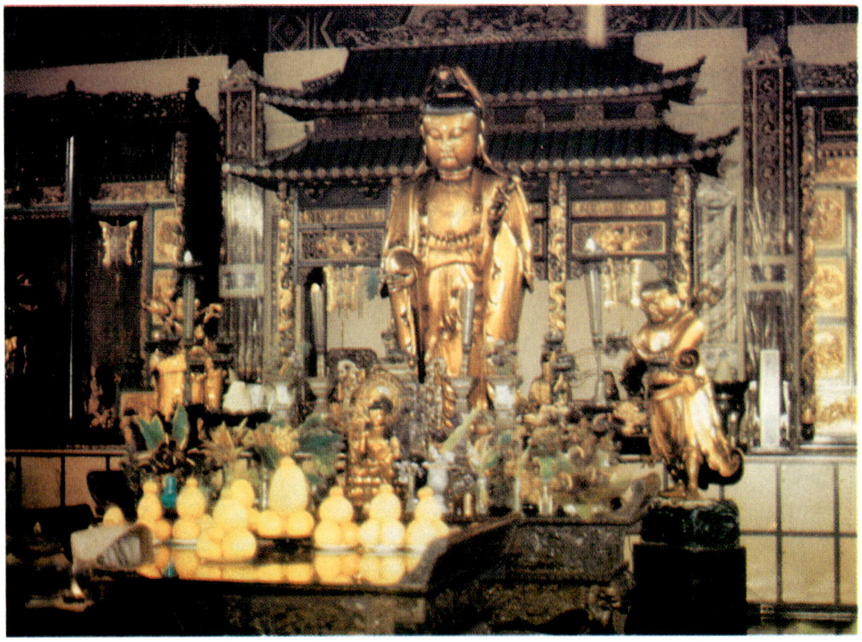

Top: This was the private shrine of the Dalai Lama of Tibet, in exile since the communists took over his country. Bottom: The female deity Quai Lin in this Chinese temple presides over food left for the spirits of the dead.

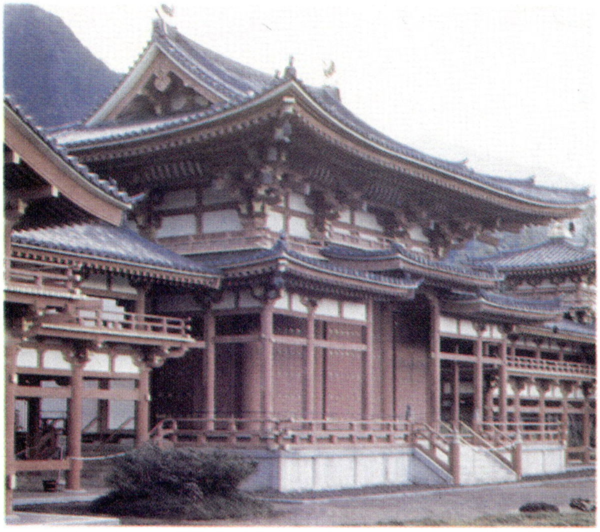

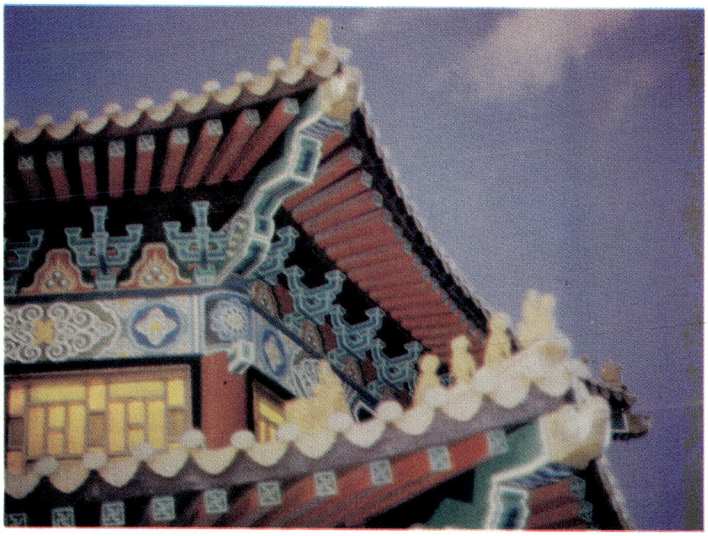

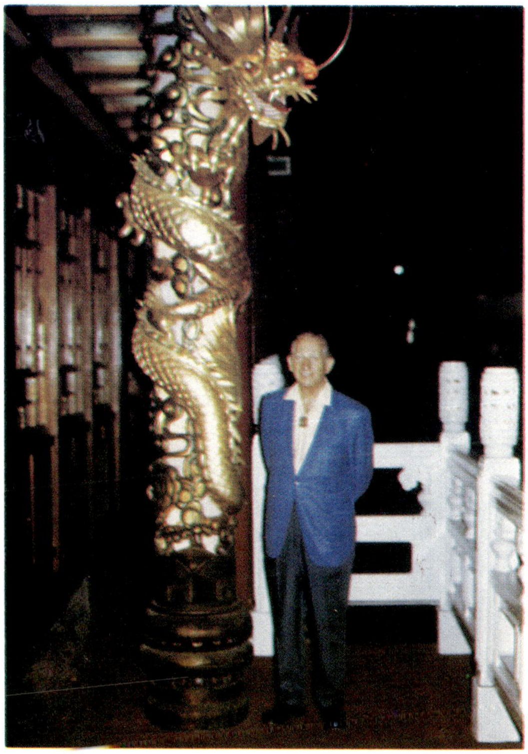

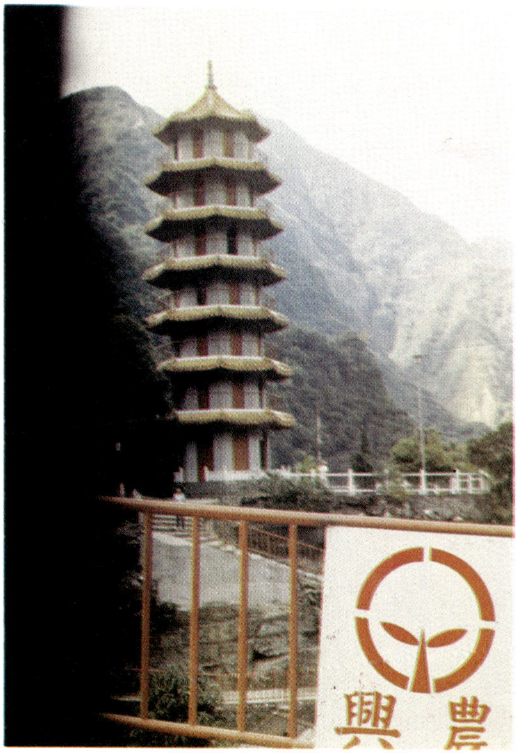

Upper Left: A Japanese temple gives a feeling of serenity in a busy, crowded country. Upper Right: Here is a detailed portion of a Chinese temple. Lower Left: :The dragon as represented in Chinese religious art is not a symbol of fear, but of benevolent protection. Lower Right: While we traveled through a part of South China, we saw this pagoda, lovely against the setting of mountains.

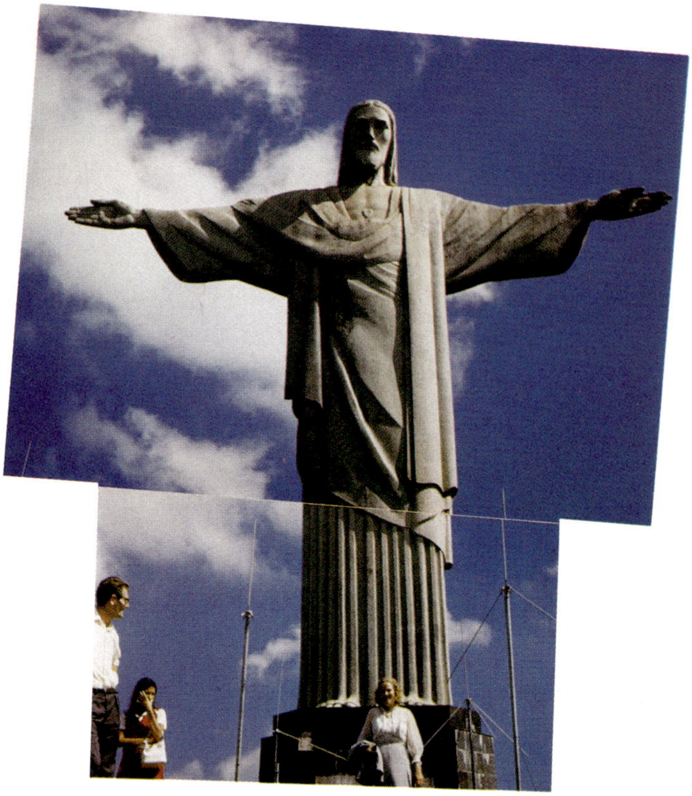

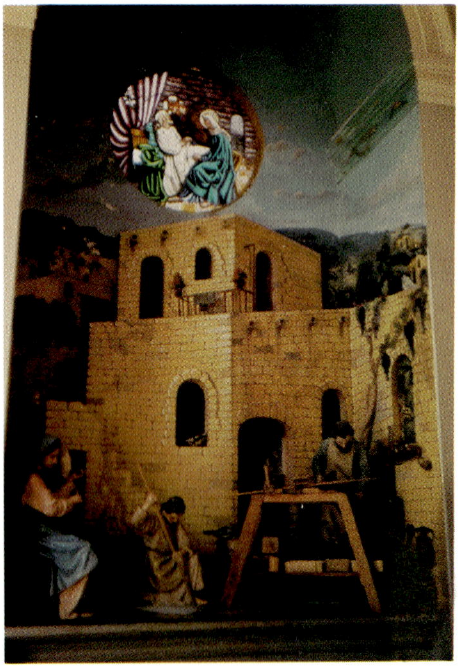

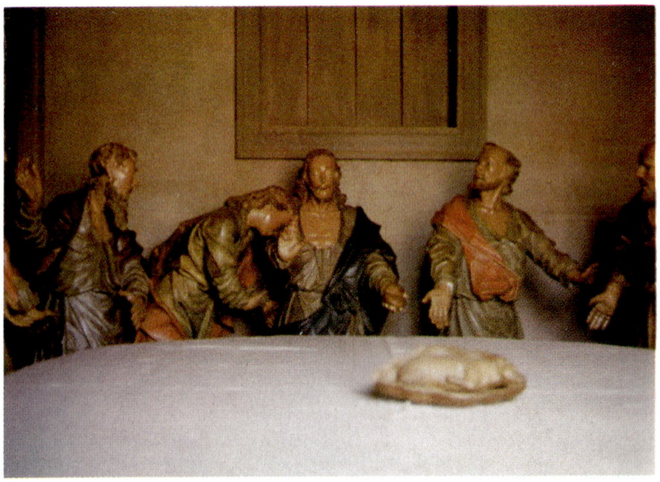

Top: On a mountaintop above the harbor at Rio de Janeiro, Brazil, a towering statue of the Christ is outlined against a lovely blue sky dotted with puffy white clouds. Lower Left: At Congonhas de Campo, Brazil, we visited this lifelike scene of a carpenter's shop as it would have appeared in the time of Jesus, who was trained as a carpenter by Joseph. Lower Right: These sculptured figures of Jesus and His disciples represent one of the stations of the cross. While we were moving past this scene with other sightseers, a man pulled a gun and shot the figure of Judas.

ing what uplifts people, the good words. You find that if you keep practicing, just like you would practice playing the notes on a piano, soon there won't be any sour notes. Soon you will play well. Many people will love to hear you play."

Life is an instrument we play, but we must realize that sometimes we have to play through inspiration. We have to do it because we are living the higher and the better life. As I explained to this person, "We live a life of creating things. You can so twist this body with distorted thinking that you will hardly know what is going on."

Many years ago Leonardo da Vinci painted the famous picture of Christ and the Last Supper. He spent seven years getting all the portraits for the people who went into this beautiful painting. He found his model for the Christ in a church choir. He went out into the streets and he found "Matthew" and painted him into his picture. Then he found and painted the others, one at a time. Finally, he had Jesus and all the disciples but one. It was very difficult for him to find the exact face he wanted on the street. Who do you suppose that was? Judas. In the end da Vinci had to go into a prison to find "Judas." While da Vinci was working on this last portrait, the prisoner modeling for him asked, "Do you know who I am?" The great artist looked at him carefully and replied, "No, I've never met you before." The prisoner said, "Yes, you have. I am the Christ that you painted seven years ago." It is hard to believe how people can change.

No One Is 100 Per Cent Materialistic

I don't think a person can live a material life entirely. To get married because of physical attraction alone, for example, would be a terrible mistake. You marry a person for love and beauty and happiness, harmony and sharing. Look at all the wonderful things that we really marry a person for. They say that true marriage comes from heaven. Well, heaven is made of these things.

In a way I am married to each one of my patients. We are brought together, aren't we? For a time we give and we share kindness, happiness, peacefulness. We are giving to one another. This is the heaven we must have in the healing art. This is the heaven we have to seek in order to have a good body.

A good marriage can help bring a good body. It is good to be married if, through marriage, we find love, beauty, happiness, harmony and sharing. But there are some people who shouldn't be married. I don't believe in divorce, but I will tell you this: If you aren't married for all the higher and better things, you aren't really married. You're living in slavery. You are not living at all. You are trying to make life out of something that is dead. I bring this up only to encourage you to seek the finer things in your marriage.

This healing business is dependent on an interior activity in our bodies. It is very difficult to describe to you just how that works, but the Good Book tells it nicely when it says, in effect, that the spiritual becomes active when you shine, when you move, when you rise.

Now, this physical world is faulty. It is limited and ever-changing. But when you go into spiritual avenues you often find very reliable material — guidelines, rules, laws that we can use in our lives. These may approach the reliability of scientific fact. For instance, whatever you are seeking in life is also seeking you. Yes, that's true. And to change what is in the world, we must first make the change in our minds. We are going to have slums in our cities as long as we have slums in our minds, for example. Slums begin in the mind. So to change physical things we must change our minds.

It is our concept that we have to change. We control our muscles, all our physical functions, our food and drink, our vices and other behavior. Why shouldn't we develop a way to have dominion over some of the mental thoughts that come to disturb us?

How about all these inferior ideas that come to us? A lot of people apparently believe that one bad turn deserves another. They believe in vengeance. Do we have to live that way? No. Vengeance is by choice. Vengeance harms the user and drains his energy.

We have to learn to use our energy properly. You don't crack open an egg with a pick-axe, do you? No, you tap it lightly. We have to know when to use the feather and when to use the sledge-hammer. We use the lighter method as often as we can.

As one man told me, "Take it easy, doc, and relax." Let's take it easy, mentally. Is there any reason why we can't have this attitude toward life? We have to get rid of our grievances. We have to rearrange our lives. We have to reorganize our recreation and our leisure time. We should refresh our lives. Sometimes we have to take a vacation from ourselves and the things we dislike doing. We have to make life worthwhile.

Someone once told me, "We live on the external and we live on the internal — but we also live on the eternal." Mother told me, "You don't have to worry about dying. We are living in eternity right now. When you die you simply go on from where you left off."

Wise men are made, not born. Each day you become wiser and wiser. A wise dominion will come to you. This wise dominion, which is yours only, comes from experience, and by changing your life to a higher one and a better one.

Your countenance shows what is within. Why don't you give your face an expression of all the lovely thoughts you know? This is what I mean when I say, "It walks, it talks and it will finally get to your face."

We have what we call a God nature. If I could see this God nature working through a person, it would so relieve the nervous system that I wouldn't have to worry about his high blood pressure or tensions. He wouldn't need tranquilizers. He wouldn't need all this regulated relaxation. He wouldn't have to worry about sleeping. He would relax and let go.

Let God Take Over

The moment you do this, you will find yourself walking in youthfulness. Illness will disappear and fifty per cent of your troubles will leave you right now. I cannot discount the fact that we don't eat right physically and we don't drink right. Any human being can become sick. Doctors and nurses become sick when they don't use the proper foods and get the right amount of rest and relaxation.

There is an old Chinese proverb that tells us there is no possible rearrangement of bad eggs that can ever make a good omelette. We must start with the good things, otherwise we are going to have disharmony in the body.

Someone sent me this shopping list from Milwaukee, Wisconsin.

A Lady's Shopping List

One of these days I must go shopping.
I am completely out of self-respect.
I want to exchange the self-righteousness I picked up the other day for some humility, which they say is less expensive and wears better.
I want to look at some tolerance, which is being used for wraps this season.
Someone showed me some pretty samples of peace.
We are a little low on this, and one can never have too much of it.
And by the way, I must try to match some patience that my neighbor wears. It is very becoming on her, and I think it might look equally well on me.
I must try on that little garment of long-suffering that they are displaying. I never thought I wanted to wear it, but I feel I'm coming to it.
And I mustn't forget to have my sense of humor mended, and look for some inexpensive, everyday goodness.
It's surprising how quickly one's stock of goods is depleted.

We are all seekers. So now let us seek the teacher. Those who teach have usually gone through problems and troubles. They have an understanding that you can use. So let us seek the teachings — let us learn. There is an obligation we have as a student, and that is to open the door. Then we will meet some of the great things that are in store for us.

You should insist on peace of mind, health and happiness. This is what God wills for you, but you have to insist on it. You have to set a time for it and put everything else aside to let it come in. Two thoughts cannot occupy the same mental space at the same time. It is either one or the other. You can't think peace and war at the same time. You can't think health and disease at the same time. You've never seen anyone walking down the street discouraged and depressed singing, "Happy Days Are Here Again." It just doesn't happen.

We find that we are single-minded beings. We walk that path of single-mindedness. Poise is the key to happiness. Don't make lecture prayers. Don't neglect being thankful or blessing other people.

You Can Control Your Mind

So this mind of yours is to be used as it was meant to be used, and you have the privilege, from the inside, of working out a real self, a self that many people may never know. The real goodness is on the inside; that is what we should seek on the spiritual path.

The inside is where ugliness, misery, injustice, poverty and painful situations begin, but happiness also begins there, as well as joy, goodness, beauty and righteousness. All these things come from the heart. As a man thinketh in his heart, so he is — and he reveals it to others. As a man thinketh in his heart, he automatically affects every cell in his body. As a man thinketh in his heart, he makes his own future. As he thinks in his heart, he touches other people. Let us be kind and good to other people.

It is not what you have in life, it is what you enjoy in life that counts. Some people can be poor and happy. Some people can be rich and miserable. This should be brought to our attention many times.

There are many levels in life. They claim that we live on as many as 120 different levels in life. We have to recognize that there is a right way of thinking. Thinking has to be perfected. If you use the spiritual avenue, the mind will always work better.

We have to be wise enough to take care of ourselves. We can't be victims of life; we have to be masters of life. Learn how to think good thoughts and let them pour forth, because we live on what we give out. We have to be aglow, and this is something that emanates from within ourselves. We have to give of ourselves.

If we would realize the consequences of our thinking, we would realize that as we put these laws into effect, these words into effect, these principles into effect, certain things come back to us. That is why I believe the Lord when He says, "Vengeance is mine." The Lord is the Law. Events will boomerang back upon us if we try to get even with other people.

Constantly work to advance. Build a life for yourself. Seek out God's immensity. Just think about that for a moment. The immense truth in life is that when we have peace and harmony within ourselves, our bodies follow it. The body is a servant to the mind and reacts according to the way you think.

There are reactions in the body that will change black hair to gray in a period of hours or even minutes. I have seen people get congestion, stomach problems and blocked bowels. I have seen high blood pressure in countless individuals. I've witnessed patients coming in with that awful mental attitude and I've watched them walk out after they have changed that attitude. We can all find a life that is worth living.

We turn to God, the living Law. He calls us his beloved. God is love, and that love is for us. With a living Father, we can certainly ask Him for all that is good. He is the teacher of all good and the giver of all good. This is where our inheritance comes from. Let us turn within ourselves where God lives, and we will find out who we really are.

It is here that we can find our happiness, our joys; and it is here that illness will begin to depart. It dissipates, breaks us and begins to leave. You can see that there is something in spirit that every living person needs. It is not a matter of going to extremes on the spiritual side. It is not a matter of seeking the spiritual, day and night.

We Must Do Our Part

I remember a man hospitalized with big leg ulcers who prayed unceasingly for thirty days with a *Bible* in his hand. Yet, he was eating fried pork chops, pickles and ice cream. God isn't just in the *Bible* or up in the sky somewhere where prayers go. He is with and within us. How can a God of consequences bring us a good life if we don't do our part in balancing the physical, mental and spiritual?

We must balance our lives. We must learn what to do as mental beings, learn what to do as physical beings, and realize that we get good direction when we turn to God.

You will never be lost if you do that because God will never let you down. As we look upward and outward, let us not forget to look inward. As we look to the Father, we look for that wisdom and guidance. As long as our hand is in the Father's hand, all will be well.

We may not have bread, but we will be provided for. We recognize God as the great one, the powerful one, the all-intelligent, the all-creative, for good, for harmony and for peace.

To recognize that we must be the kind of people who deserve the kind of food that makes us well — that is the beginning of the good life. We must recognize that within ourselves, where we make our lives, our behavior begins, changes begin — and it is here we find freedom from worry, freedom from envy, freedom from destruction and freedom from disease.

So we start with today and we start within the Father, and we come out living the good life, the spiritual life. To be a good servant to the spiritual gifts is necesssary. We must have compassion on those who know the least and those who have yet to learn their lessons. We must remember that we were there one time. Through our growth and through the Father's guidance, we can bless them.

We are thankful that we are finished with lying, cheating, stealing and taking advantage of others. We are thankful that we live on the higher way. We are thankful for the Father's guidance. We go forth insisting that by doing all the good we possibly can, good comes forth.

We are looking to our true inheritance, knowing that we have a loving Father who has given us a wonderful life to live. All we ask is that we be awakened to this, for the awakened one is the one who truly lives. We ask for that life as we walk in obedience to God. Walking in obedience is walking in the light, and then all will be well. When all is well, sickness slips away. Health and harmony come in. We are thankful for that thought. Let us walk in obedience to God's will. We have really been blessed.

From the Doctor's Pen . . .

NATURE'S FIRST STEP

I lived as a seed in the world of God,
Green as the grass growing upward.
Tho' I lived in a spot that seemed so small,
I used what I had and became all inclusive.

Color itself was first noticed in a rose,
And I leaned forward to grasp the feeling of smell.
Within myself that which made a rose all I wanted,
Grew till my whole insides glowed colors of God.

Nature seemed strange when I picked up some earth,
And I saw black mud lay motionless to my unseeing eye.
But when, after the heaven dropped her hand of rain,
Heaven and earth came together and made a blade of grass.

I saw my first lesson, how one needs the other,
How growth is the God-power waiting for mixture.
The song of a bird as it comes from a warbling throat,
Is motionless mud and the power of God doing their work together.

So your today is here on the wing or in song,
But know this within—that all can begin
Where heaven and earth get together looking up or down;
They look to each, their vision seeing none other.

So it is a need in the world to be greater than one,
To lift to the heights those that are motionless clay,
To reach down with the power that's invested in you,
Sealing with cement of growth all separation.

As you walk, these two are one working together;
Your feeling at home needs plaster and maker.
As you look at yourself, you're these two in one—
All Power, walking, as motions of heaven and mud of earth.

Chapter 16

I Will Dwell In The House

Go through life
elevating people.

Most of us are looking for the finer things in life. Sometimes we think these things just "happen" for us. We have all met people who believe that success and failure are only a matter of luck — good luck or bad luck. But the truth is, we have to *make* the finer things happen. I am not talking about the "nose-to-the-grindstone" approach to life, for we have already shown how detrimental to life and to health that approach is. What we are talking about here is change. We have to change ourselves to bring what is best for us into our lives.

In other words, there is always a "good" morning inside what seems to be a "bad" morning. We often measure life according to the mind and how it experiences the storms and winds of the world. Now, our physical bodies are of the same creation as the winds and storms, and a miniature hurricane could be howling right now inside you. Perhaps you have been throwing sticks and stones. You've been doing many things to that wonderfully created body of yours that you are going to have to stop.

We have begun to understand that the physical body is not as physical as we once thought it was. We once believed that this body was made of the dust of the earth — intricate combinations of atoms and molecules. But then we read about Christ dying on the cross, commending His spirit into the hands of the One who gave it to Him. We have within us that which is much more than the dust of the earth.

Some of us live as though we were just 150 pounds or so of dust. Some of us think that life is just the pumping of the heart, the breathing of the lungs. That boils down to a kind of "vegetable" existence when you look at it closely, doesn't it? We have to reach out for something higher and bigger to make sense of this life. So we begin to think about that spirit spoken of by Christ. We begin to wonder what goes on in that spiritual realm where God interacts with us through spirit. We begin to understand that the physical realm is very much affected by what goes on in the spiritual realm, down to the "marrow of our bones" and our state of health.

As far as our health is concerned, I feel we do not "tabernacle" with God enough. We do not "church" with God enough. Attending a one-hour church service on Sunday isn't going to do you much good unless you practice what you learn. You don't just learn truth, you practice it and grow in it. You have to learn and practice love. Are we born with love as a natural thing inside us? I've watched my children quarrel and fight and I don't know where they learned to do that. They didn't learn it from me. You have to teach them to love and encourage them to practice it. It doesn't come easy.

Some "kids" are past the age of forty and still don't know how to love. They are still quarrelsome and violent, still caught up in that "I'll-get-even-with-him" stage of childhood. These are the attitudes that get us into trouble with other people and into trouble with our own health.

From a health standpoint I have observed that we display a very unspiritual attitude both in our eating habits and other aspects of everyday living. Being a Christian isn't just a matter of correct belief in certain spiritual values. It isn't just a matter of thinking the right thoughts. It comes right down to daily living, down to the minute-by-minute experience and behavior of our lives. All spiritual values have physical implications. We were not created by the Father in heaven to be loving and good inside our minds but abusive, cruel and hateful toward our bodies. Can you see the conflict in this?

The laboratory of life is in the mind. We believe we deserve the best. The real challenge, then, is bringing those wonderful spiritual principles and mental beliefs into action at the physical level. I believe that the same principles apply at the spiritual, mental and physical levels. It's that simple. There is a Christian attitude toward physical life as well as spiritual and mental life.

The Mental And The Spiritual Control The Body

There is a state of continuity to the spiritual life. We can go forward or backward. We can progress for a while, then fall back. But the idea is to go forward. There is no beginning and no end on the spiritual path. Can you see that the spiritual and mental flow into the physical body at the level of action? They most certainly do, and it is vitally important that we see this.

Memory belongs to the mental path, but memories can affect us at both the spiritual and physical levels. When we bring back a hateful memory, we are both violating a spiritual principle and introducing a disturbance into the body. This is why we teach you to get rid of the old and take on the new experiences as we journey through life. If we don't let go of these negative memories they will impede us on both the spiritual and physical paths.

We know that mind interacts with the body to produce physical changes. Anxiety can even affect the growth rate of a man's beard. Now, we can work toward a cure for an ailment at the physical level, but it does little good unless we have the mind working with us and not against us. When the mind is hindering a healing, we bring the spiritual values in and "clean house." We get rid of the litter and trash, the anxiety and resentment, that are hindering the healing at the physical level. Then the physical body, which is the servant of the mind and the spirit, responds and adjusts itself.

The body is given a bad time often in this life. I know of a woman who was given a series of penicillin shots to heal a certain problem. It worked, but she promptly developed arthritis. She began taking a common brand-name pain reliever for her arthritis. Again, the drug helped, but while she was taking it iron became depleted in her body and she became anemic. The iron she took to get rid of the anemia caused a constipation problem, for which she had to take a laxative. This is the way it goes. One problem so often leads to another, with the powerful modern drugs and their typical undesirable side effects complicating the situation. Disease is one disharmony after another, that's all. But to get rid of it, we have to get to the root cause.

Thy Will Be Done

When we have fully integrated the spiritual values into our lives, we will bring the kingdom of heaven into our minds and bodies. Heaven to me means the Divine Presence working physically, mentally and spiritually with complete harmony at all levels. There is a line in *The Lord's Prayer* that goes, "Thy will be done, on earth as it is in heaven." If you really took this seriously, you would work toward having a perfect body and perfect health. When I examine the people who come to me for help and see the state of their bodies, the state of their minds, the state they have been living in, then I am left with an overwhelming conviction: We need to change. You need to change. We can have heaven on earth. We can have wonderful lives. Change is the key.

One of the most interesting aspects of truth is that it doesn't change. Facts change. Truth does not. Every truth that has been taught since the dawn of the human race is still with us today. Who makes truth come alive? You do. The only time that is really worthwhile is when the Divine power is flowing through us. Some of you may understand where disease comes from, some of you may not. There are some very simple solutions to some problems. Is cholesterol complicating your life? The solution is not to cut down on fried foods. The solution is to get rid of them entirely. The solution is to toss your frying pan into the garbage can.

Back To Eden

Let's take a journey, in our imaginations, back to the Garden of Eden for the moment. Can you see the lush green trees in your mind's eye? Can you see the sparkling clear rivers and streams and hear their melodious sounds? Look over there at those plump, deep purple wild grapes, clusters and clusters of them! Look at those fruit trees, their limbs heavy with ripe, delicious fruits of all kinds. And, my goodness, have you ever seen so many nuts and berries in your life? Don't they just make your mouth water to look at them? Now, take a good careful look around — make a complete circle. Do you see any hamburger stands? Donut shops? Soda fountains? Candy stores? Coffee shops? Liquor stores? Drug stores? You can't? Well, to tell the truth, I can't either. Now, here come Adam and Eve, but I don't see her carrying a can opener, do you? And television won't be invented for thousands of years yet, so it doesn't stand to reason that they have any frozen TV dinners around. And do you know what else is missing here? Think about it. Think hard. That's right! There's not a single hospital or doctor's office in the whole garden!

I think you get the picture. We want to be healthy, don't we? Then we are going to have to live closer to the farmer than the can opener. We have to live closer to the orchard than the frozen food packing plant. We have to live closer to God than the doctor's office, drugstore and the hospital!

We Are What We Eat

Not long ago I was browsing through a shop at an airport and I noticed a sign that said, "Have an in-between snack while you are waiting for the plane." Below the sign was a rack displaying rows of plastic bags of what are called "cracklings." So I read the label on one of those bags, and what do you suppose they do to prepare this nice snack for you? They take the skin of pigs, bake it to a crisp in an oven and salt it to taste. Imagine that as an in-between snack!

You can eat three healthy and nutritious meals a day, but you can also foul them up completely by what you do between meals.

It isn't simply what we eat that makes a good body, although the proper foods are very important. You have to have good digestion before the body can properly utilize the foods you eat. What would prevent us from having good digestion? The person who sits down to a meal bringing his worries, fears, and troubles with him will not digest his food right. The child who is harshly scolded or disciplined at the dinner table will not digest his food right, nor will the parent who scolds or disciplines him. Good digestion results from having a peaceful mind and thinking good thoughts.

I suspect that God had a wonderful time putting the beautiful colors in fruits and vegetables and in giving us eyes to see them with. I suspect that God had a marvelous time placing the delicious tastes and aromas in peaches, apricots, melons and other foods, then giving us the senses of smell and taste to enjoy them with. Beautiful, nice-smelling foods really stimulate the appetite, don't they? When we eat with a hearty appetite we enjoy our food and digest it well. God has been very kind and good to us.

This body gets kicked around. It can only respond to the situations we put it into. When we go out in the cold, it shivers. When we go out in the heat, it perspires. When we put it in an embarrassing situation, the face blushes. That is why we have to be good to it. We want the body not only to feel good, we want it to feel wonderful.

If you tell someone you are sick, you are claiming something that doesn't belong to you. You are putting a thought into the nerves and the brain that doesn't belong there. Sickness is not our inheritance, and when we claim it we are not acting like the children or our loving Father. You must rise above it. We must become better for any experience that comes our way. "Rise" is a spiritually powerful word. Use it often, as often as you need it. Say, "I am rising above this." Then you will be bringing the spiritual, mental and physical levels into harmony.

There is more to the physical body than meets the eye. Our bodies are made up of gases, liquids and solids. Chemical changes are going on constantly, assisted by the vitamins and minerals. A delicate acid-alkaline balance is being constantly maintained, and the body temperature is kept at a certain level that is just right for all these processes to balance out. Fine electrical currents flow through the nerves as the brain regulates the organ functions, as we receive sensory information through the sense organs, as our muscles obey our every command to move. Glands secrete, releasing hormones into the system that shift the body chemistry. Old cells die and are eliminated as new ones are born to replace them. Our bodies are wonderfully made.

Some people are wearing their bodies out faster than they are able to rebuild them. Vitamins are used up faster than they are replaced. If you take vitamin B to stop the nervous system from breaking down, you'll find yourself taking it continuously. You could repair the nervous system "in the twinkling of an eye" if you could see the need to change. You have to turn. You have to look again. See life a little differently.

Let us learn to recognize the changes we need to make in our lives, realizing that "it is the spirit that quickeneth; the flesh profiteth nothing." Let the living spirit flow into and throughout the temple you live in.

Condition Your Mind

I feel that you are going to discover some wonderful ways to help yourself as you realize that you must give attention to the spirit and mind before the body. First things first, as they say.

A man came to me once and said, "I need to lose some weight." So I put him on a reducing diet. When he came back the following week, he hadn't lost a pound. I knew the diet was sound. Why wasn't he losing weight? I had treated one lady who lost 176 pounds, but this man hadn't lost a single solitary pound.

I asked the man to sit down and I began to inquire about his life habits. We soon got down to the heart of the matter — or the stomach of the matter in this case.

"Well, doctor," he began. "I've always had this terrible fear that other people will get more food than I do. I'm afraid that I just won't get enough to eat. So at the end of the day, before I go to bed, I eat a whole chicken."

I began to work with this man, realizing that we had to do some changing in the mind before we could make progress with the diet and the weight reduction he needed. I had to take care of fear, of selfish desire, of craving. But these aren't in the stomach. They are in the mind, where the control center is. This is where the action starts.

There is an old folk saying that goes, "The way to a man's heart is through his stomach." To the extent that there is any truth at all to this, you ladies out there should realize that "the way to a man's stomach is through his mind."

For a while there was some controversy over the legal aspects of human heart transplants, but I am much more interested in the human brain. When the brain goes, it doesn't matter a great deal what you do to the rest of the body. When the brain goes, your physical body is dead. The brain is the most important part of the body.

If the legal questions can ever be resolved and if medical science can find a way, the transplanting of human brains would force us to change all our understandings. Imagine a person looking his doctor straight in the eye and saying, "I'd like to have a brain that doesn't have any hatred or violence in it."

The heart is often said to be the center of our spiritual being, but this is only a figure of speech. It isn't the heart activity but the mental activity that determines what kind of person we are and whether we are alive or not.

We Have To Go To The Top

Suppose you had a stomach ulcer and wanted to grow new tissue there to heal it. We know that in order for the ulcer to appear in the first place, there had to be something of a war going on in the mind and body. And we know that by taking in the right foods we can get rid of the ulcer. But we must also realize that we can treat this condition by getting rid of the ulcerous thoughts, the warlike thoughts in the mind. How? We replace them with good thoughts. Get into a harmonious way of thinking.

Replacement therapy can be carried out mentally and spiritually just as it is physically, and this is what I am showing you how to bring about. Lift yourself up to your true heritage. You are a child of God. You belong to God. Godly ways are above man's ways, which is why we must learn the lifting process. First, you learn to lift yourself, then you begin to lift others. I must lift you to a higher level of thinking. You must lift me. We help one another.

We must seek illumination. Illumination broadens the understanding, and this is an inside job. No teacher can give you understanding. Even the Christ could not give it to you if you weren't ready for it. If you were sick, you could sit in the lap of the Christ and not be healed — unless you had faith, unless you could tune into that consciousness. You have to lift yourself to the truth that He taught.

Truth Or Consequences

The student of truth deserves the finest there is. He deserves a good body — and you can't keep the good body away from him. The person standing in a Las Vegas casino with a bet in one hand and a drink in the other is gambling with his life. His consciousness doesn't tell him he is going to have a good body.

As you live on the physical plane, so you live on the mental plane. But I must tell you that the mental is between the spiritual level and the physical level. We improve our physical fitness by what we draw from our heavenly Father. Many people don't draw enough on Him to make a good physical body. Too many are caught up in fears, not thinking as they should. What you fear will come upon you. If you live in fear constantly, that is all you will see.

We may be praying amiss. So many of you ask God for help with your problems. You give those problems to Him, but ten minutes later you take them back again. You don't know how to leave them with Him. You don't know how to go on to new experiences thankful for what has passed, thankful for what is yet to come.

This society we live in will never be any better until God flows through man enough and through enough men to lift up society. As it is now society drags man down. We live under the law, not above the law, and not close enough to God.

Is Your Thinking Groundless?

People have to be reached in different ways, but we must have some kind of common ground. The best way to approach these new ideas is to stand on Holy Ground. You will hear people say, "That fellow doesn't have any ground for what he believes." You have to have a base to stand on. You have to have a basis for looking at things. Otherwise you are groundless. You have to stand on Holy Ground, you have to stand in a solid place to recognize truth in what is presented to you.

We can't say, for example, that "the majority is always right." Truth is not determined by how many people believe this or that. What's right is right. What is right is grounded in God. To be right you have to be standing on the path that makes it right.

Many were brought to Christ to be healed, and all were healed. Some had to be reached in different ways. There are people around who are not going to have a healing for quite a while yet. There are people around who are not going to live long enough to get a healing because they refuse to change their attitudes in the way necessary to get to a better way of living.

You have to put a little effort into this thing. We must realize that this physical body is a garment woven from what we think, what we believe, what we feel. In a way of speaking, you "wear" your friendships. You wear your attitude in the stance of your body, in the countenance of your face. This comes from within. Some of you should notify your faces that there are many lovely things inside you.

Before he became a Christian, the Apostle Paul had been a persecutor of Christians. On the road to Damascus he was blinded when Christ appeared to him. Christ's countenance was so bright, so powerful and shining, that it blinded the man. What an experience it would be to be blinded with joy, with happiness! How wonderful it would be to be blinded that way! Of course, Paul received his sight back later.

I know of a lady in New York who prayed

that she would never see her husband again. God answered her prayer in a way that caught her by surprise. She became blind. When she realized what had happened, it took a whole year to get her sight back again. Doctors would call this a psychosomatic illness.

Today, psychiatrists are trying to find the answers to these mental phenomena. But they are looking for a physical solution, not a godly solution. They are looking for a solution in ways that can be seen, heard and touched. Often we refuse to accept that there are ways "ye know not of," perhaps in dimensions we haven't touched upon yet.

Once on a cold winter's day a wealthy lady was driving down Broadway in New York City. She saw a thinly-clad barefoot boy wistfully staring through a shop window. Pulling her car over to the curb, she parked it and approached the boy. "What are you doing?" she asked him.

"I was just asking God to give me a pair of shoes like those in the window," he said, shivering as he spoke. The lady led him into the shop where she asked for a bowl of water and a towel. After washing the boy's numb dirty feet, she asked the clerk to bring her half a dozen pairs of warm stockings. Putting a pair on him, she selected a good pair of shoes, fitted them to his feet and said, "Now I think you'll feel better." With tears in his eyes the little fellow grabbed her hand and exclaimed, "Are you God's wife?"

Are We In The Right Place?

Isn't it interesting how God will sometimes put us in exactly the right place at exactly the right time either to help someone or to be helped by someone? This is not something you can touch. This is not something the psychiatrists can explain. We are all God's children, aren't we? Hand in hand, we could really accomplish great things! If, as His children, we would do the will of the Father of all creation, wonderful changes would take place in this world! How do we get started with this? We must start with ourselves.

We have to prepare ourselves to take care of this physical body and we must first approach this mentally. I always start with the mental way. We must start with good feelings.

The body always needs preparation. You have to prepare it when you get up in the morning. You have to prepare it when you go to bed. You have to prepare. We have a saying: "Prepare to meet your Maker." We should do that every day.

Abraham Lincoln said, "I will study and I will prepare myself. My time will come." That is what we have to do. If you wish to get well, prepare yourself and your time will come.

Update Your Thinking

A married couple came to our Ranch with a serious problem. The wife said, "All he talks about is going back to his home village outside of Boston, so he can sit and talk to his old cronies. I hear this in the morning when he wakes up. I hear it all day long. I'm tired of hearing it!"

"How long has this been going on?" I asked.

"Twenty years," she sighed. "It's all he talks about."

"Why don't you send him back there?"

"Well," she admitted, "I'm afraid of losing him."

"Do you really think there is something back there to hold him?" I asked gently. "Do you want to just go on living the way you are now?"

After thinking over our conversation this lady decided to tell her husband that he could go back. She decided to take the risk. She told him she wouldn't stand in his way.

So, with a good deal of excited anticipation, he returned to his home village. But it had changed. The old swimming hole had been filled in. All the streets were paved. The old base burner in a store now owned by an old pal of his had been removed. When he walked into the store, the man he used to pal around with was too busy to talk to him. He wanted to sit down and talk to his old friends, but they had forgotten who he was. They had changed — and so had he, he finally realized. He couldn't wait to get back home to his wife. She was delighted, and now they are a happy family.

A lot of us are living in a world of memories of who we were or what we did twenty years ago. You must let these things go. Come back to the here and now. Update your thinking and learn to enjoy the present. The Creator isn't just a God of the past, He is present in each moment of each day.

Too often we put God away on reserve. We don't keep Him on "active duty." We just call on Him for emergencies. But He is around all the time! We could receive His guidance a great deal more if we would only open to it.

This is why religion is often so sterile today. We view our God as distant from ourselves and ourselves as distant from Him. Then when we hit difficulties, we have to make a "long distance" call to Him. We only tend to use God for our own convenience.

There is a lovely poem by Leigh Hunt that I'd like to share with you.

Abou Ben Adhem

Abou Ben Adhem, (may his tribe increase!)
Awoke one night from a deep dream of peace
And saw within the moonlight in his room,
Making it rich, and like a lily in bloom,
An Angel, writing in a book of gold;
Exceeding peace had made Ben Adhem bold,
And to the presence in the room he said,
"What writest thou?" — The vision raised its head,
And with a look made of all sweet accord,
Answer'd, "The names of those who love the Lord."
"And is mine one?" said Abou. "Nay, not so,"
Replied the angel. Abou spoke more low,
But cheerily still and said, "I pray thee, then,
Write me as one who loves his fellowmen."
The angel wrote and vanish'd. The next night
It came again with a great wakening light.
And show'd the names of those whom love of God had bless'd,
And lo! Ben Adhem's name led all the rest!

It is our thinking that we have to work out in order to get our healing. With the right attitude healing will come automatically.

Experiences come and go. Don't hold onto them. I've had people at the Ranch, who, if they could have let go of the experiences of twenty years ago, would be well today. They are still living in the past, still living in that place from which their physical problems came. People say, "How can there be a God if this terrible thing happened to me in the past?" Their attitude is destroying their lives. We have to rise above all that. We have to go beyond it.

It says in the Good Book, "In my Father's house are many mansions." Get out of the mansion you are now in. There are many rooms to explore. Don't be afraid to go into the next one. You are preparing yourself for the upper room.

Don't Let Your Mind Get In Your Way

So many of you are stuck in one track, one experience, that it has taken over your whole life. You are in a rut if you stay there. What is a rut? A rut is a grave with the ends kicked out. And you know what graves are for.

We must realize that we have to make a move in life. A man lay paralyzed near the pool of Bethesda at Jerusalem for thirty-eight years; mentally he had not moved. Then he heard that voice. It comes to a person once in a while. It came to Moses. It came to Elijah. It came to Job. And to that paralytic the voice said, "Rise and walk." He heard it and obeyed.

But, you see, most people would say, "I can't walk! I've been paralyzed for thirty-eight years!" Do you understand what they are doing to themselves? They have made the decision to remain exactly where they have been for thirty-eight years. They aren't going to move.

When this paralyzed man heard the voice, his mind didn't get in the way. What did he do? Without thinking it over, he got up, picked up his bed and left. He moved!

We have to die constantly to the old experiences. That is what Paul meant when he said, "I die daily." The cells of the body die and are replaced by new ones. This body is in a state of flux. Leave the old, come to the new. Don't be like Lot's wife. She looked back. She looked back to her old experiences, and what happened? She turned to a pillar of salt. You don't heal salt or earth or physical substance. You heal the mind. The mind is what makes the salt. You must keep this body limber, pliable, open to new experiences.

Many people are prisoners in their own minds, prisoners to their thoughts. I think that it is time we are released from these thoughts. Paul said for us to "Prove all things," to test them, to try them out to see if they are right. You can't "prove" an experience without putting one foot in front of the other to move into it.

You see, I've never been able to get a person to quit smoking until he decided he was finished. Not until he was ready to go on to something else. You can never go on to the next experience until you are finished with the last one.

What did Christ tell the little Samaritan lady who came to the well to fill her vessel? He offered her "living water," the water of everlasting life. Isn't that a lovely gift? And she was wise enough not to hesitate. She accepted that gift.

People come to me and say, "I've tried this. There is no way out." Well, I can't help those people. No one can. There is no room in them for the good things because their vessels are filled with old, stale memories. You have to pour out the old. You have to come empty. Then you will find that something very lovely will happen.

I have mentioned that nature and society are vessels for our use. But today they are not being used for good purposes. The vessel of society could be filled in a very wonderful way if we would start out with God. But we are all fighting instead because we haven't been able to find a common denominator, a Holy Ground to stand on and listen. We haven't opened our ears to the real wisdom, and that is why we are in trouble today.

At one time my teacher, a Scotsman named Murdo MacDonald Bayne gave me a poem I will never forget. He had been a captain in the British army and he gave me this poem before he passed away:

Spring blew trumpets of color,
Her green ran in my brain;
I saw a blind man groping
Tap, tap with his cane.

I pitied him in his blindness
But, can I boast I see?
Perhaps there walks a spirit
Close by who pities me.

A spirit who sees me tapping
The fine sense cane of my mind
Amid such unseen glories—
I may be worse than blind.

What gracious gifts are all around us, if only we'd open our eyes!

One of the greatest experiences we can have in life is to learn from our bodies. Our bodies will teach us a lesson. There is never anything that happens to you in the form of war, aches, pains, ills or disharmony that has its existence in the body. If you look for and accept God's harmony, in most cases these pains or other things will leave. How do I know? I know. I know from experience. It has been done many times here at the Ranch. So many times.

Stop Blaming Your Body

Many of us resent out bodies. We blame our bodies for our ailments. People bring their bodies to me and say, "Take this body away from me. I don't like it. I can't stand it. It isn't what I want. It's too ugly." They actually resent their bodies. But their bodies still belong to them, even if they'd rather leave them on my doorstep. It is on *their* doorstep, and they have to take care of it. All I can do for you is to awaken you. Did you know that? I can't do anything else for you but awaken you.

Since the body follows the mind, resentment comes about as a result of the mind's errors, not the body's. There is no place in the *Bible* that tells us to despise, to punish or to get rid of the body. The body is the temple of the living soul, the temple beautiful. It is not created by human hands but by God, the Creator.

King David said, "I am fearfully and wonderfully made." We are all "fearfully and wonderfully made" — and why shouldn't we be? We are made in the image of the living God! What a wonderful thing this body is! We must take good care of our body and mind.

We learn that the body is *two* — the flesh is the willing servant to the spirit. That is why spirit must come first. Not mind, spirit.

Do Unto Others

One night at the Ranch we showed pictures of the various masters and their healings in various parts of the world. I have traveled to many of the shrines and have studied many of the healing arts. I want to know all of the healing arts. Not many years ago the Episcopal Church in England, in an unexpected departure from its usual practice, allowed a priest to lay his hands upon a person for healing. They realized that possibly a person has to be touched for some things to be healed. What touches you? What do you feel? This is very important, you know. Let me tell you about a few of the experiences I've had in this area.

I knew a lady who had been taken to a mental institution. That night I said a prayer for her. Previously I had been suffering with a cough for about six months. After I prayed for this woman, the cough was gone! I wondered what had happened — after all, I hadn't prayed for myself. I only wanted this little lady to be taken care of. Although I didn't realize what had happened at the time, it would later come to make a great deal of sense.

Well, I didn't think much further about this instance, but one day I was driving along the highway with my wife beside me when I developed a terrific headache. I seldom get headaches, but this one was just blinding. I had to pull over to the side of the road. I couldn't drive anymore, as I explained to my wife.

Now, when I feel sick I just want to be left alone in a corner. I don't want anyone to touch me; this is the kind of person I am. As my wife reached over to touch the back of my neck I was just about to tell her not to do that when I thought, "What is she reaching for? She is trying to bless me, trying to make a change." You know, we sometimes tend to close the doors on the nicest things in life. Just as I was ready to close that door, I let it open again. She hardly touched my neck — and the headache left! It was gone! To this day I am not certain what happened, but I do know her touch blessed me.

Lourdes, France, is famous for its healings. We once visited there hoping to see a healing — and we indeed saw one. But first we were shown into the doctor's library by a priest, who was kind enough to locate for us the medical reports on fifty-two people who had been healed by faith alone.

Now, Alexis Carrel, the Nobel prize winning scientist, once sent extensive questionnaires to these fifty-two people who had been completely healed. He wanted to know what they were thinking of, what was on their minds while they were at Lourdes hoping to be healed.

Carrel asked them questions like, "How did you pray? What did you ask for? What did you say in your prayer?" He asked many questions, but the answers were different on all of them — except one. There was only one question in response to which every one of the fifty-two people answered exactly alike: "When I prayed, I didn't pray for myself but I prayed for somebody else to get well." They were praying for *somebody else* when they were healed!

Now, perhaps, you will understand what Christ referred to when he said, "What you do unto the least of these, you do unto me also."

Do you think I can be happy when my patients are unhappy? Do you think I can be happy that people come to me with disease and disharmony? No, this is a difficult thing. But I am happy when they get well. I am happy as I see the healing begin to take place. Can you see your obligation to lift other people? This is something that has to be done in life. You must lift others to lift yourself. It is a *must* in life. Now we will get back to what happened in Lourdes because we sometimes find that people are lifted into a healing under very surprising circumstances.

Anatomy Of A Double Miracle

After I had examined the medical records of those who had been healed in Lourdes by faith alone, I went out to take some photographs with my camera and found myself talking to a tall, good-looking man from Russia. When he said he was a Communist, I said, "I understand that Communists don't believe in God." He replied curtly, "I don't." So I asked, "Then what are you doing here?"

"Well, " he answered, "I just came here to see what all these crazy people were doing. If there is a God, this seven-year-old boy standing next to us would get his sight back."

And the boy *did* get his sight back — that very day!

I witnessed a healing — in fact, two healings! Because when the Russian saw the boy healed, he said, "Now, I believe." Yes, I had seen two healings in one day!

What I want you to see is the working of the law in this. The Russian wasn't interested in himself — even as an atheist, he only wanted that boy to be well, and *that* is a prayer. That prayer did not go amiss if you know what I mean!

You don't have to love what people do but you have to love people. You have to help them find the right attitude. You have to put them in the right frame of mind. You have to be good to them, and that is all you owe anybody.

On the other hand, many of you are so dependent upon others, so tied down to them that if they are not happy you can't be happy. You can't get your happiness from other people. You can't live on other people. Find something within yourself to live on and develop that glorious nature that is yours and yours alone! Overcome evil with good. We do this by going from within outward. We change from the lower level of life to the higher level. Go directly to God to straighten out your problems. You don't need a go-between.

Wouldn't anyone be happy to be healed of some supposedly incurable disease? The reward I really value in my work is to see how thankful and grateful a person is for a healing. That repays me over and over, much more than any money. It is almost unbelievable! I look for that blessing. I would like to see all of you well!

Now, as we stand before God, we stand on Holy Ground. We stand one with Him, hand in hand, and we recognize that all good is right here and now.

We recognize that there is no sickness in spirit. We recognize that all good has been given to us. It is the pleasure of our heavenly Father to give us His kingdom. It is for us to see, to turn, to look again. It is for us to rise and shine, to come and to go. These are the activities of spirit. May we realize that. May we be good to one another.

Let us lift up other people. As we live with these friends of ours, this life is our home. As we live in Him, in our environment, His creation is our home. Let us recognize that our prayer is always heard. It is not the church on the hill, in the valley or in the city that recognizes what is good, it is the church within. Without that church within we could never recognize the church on the outside. Let us learn to prepare ourselves. May He guide us in that direction.

We will patiently wait and know that our experiences will bring us to that day when all ill health will leave, when sickness will vanish and all of these troubles and problems will pass away.

We are in a new day, a new land. Let us stand on Holy Ground. Let us remodel our house. Let us go into this temple and recognize that we must place it upon a new foundation, a foundation of rock.

If we want a better home to live in, there must be windows to let the sunshine in. We must have good circulation. There must be fuel and there must be heat. There must be warmth to share with our friends. We must build a fence of faith to enclose all of these things.

Let us keep an open door so even strangers may come in and know that they come to a house that welcomes them as well as friends. Let us not see them as strangers. Let us not see men as men but as children of God. Let us transform our sight to such purity of vision that we may not see the iniquity of man. Let us recognize that as we rebuild the body with physical foods and the mind with knowledge, we will not perish. We have life not only of an internal self that is good, not only of an external self that will become better, but as an Eternal Self that will live forever.

Let us remember that when we put this house together we want the finest wood. We want the finest materials to make this house over, and we look to Thee, Father, for these fine materials. We look to all Thou hast given us, for we know what we have inherited. It is our heritage to have the finest things. For we, as your loving children, know we have been promised all this.

I know that God will never let you down if you will live in this house, because this house is the temple beautiful in which God dwells.

Be active in silence,
Strong in peace,
Keep thy strength in gentleness,
Rest with the song of wings about thee,
Fill the inner reaches with love,
Bathe in the Spirit
For it is sweetness to thy bones,
flesh and health.
Keep in this Holy Estate and, listening, obey!
— *Anonymous*

"You are created for joy."

Chapter 17

The Vibrations of Health

Health is not everything,
but without health,
everything is nothing.

Most people go through life never realizing that the body is the servant of the mind. The body does anything we demand of it. Recognizing this truth will quicken your life. You must know that you are ultimately responsible for what happens in your life. The buck stops with you. You are the one who leads yourself either into problems and troubles or into the good things of life. You decide, and those decisions take place at the level of mind, of thought.

I used to wonder when I heard people say, "Thoughts are things." To me a thing was solid, something you could see, hear and feel. But then I began to understand. A thought is a vibration. A thought can certainly be felt, can't it? And thoughts can have very real consequences in this world.

What is this deep thing we call our feeling? Now and then I wonder about these feelings of ours and what they do to the body. I wonder why these feelings come as vibrations. Do you know what a hate vibration can do? Do you know that a hate vibration can actually crush you?

Have you ever watched the faces of people change when they have been called insulting names? When you are happy, your face looks entirely different. Thoughts *are* things, and thoughts actually change our bodies. And these changes can be dramatic, cumulative and more destructive than we realize.

What a shock it is to discover that thoughts can destroy the body! Since this is so, don't you think you ought to turn away from negative thoughts? Almost casually, we permit destructive thoughts to enter our minds every day. It's such a habit, we "don't give it a second thought," as they say. Well, it's time to give it a "second thought." We are the decision makers. We decide what thoughts we will have. We must know that there is absolutely no wisdom or good to be found in a negative thought.

When we turn back to the real wisdom in life, we change our bodies. If more people did that we wouldn't need all the doctors we have today. We have psychiatrists and psychologists who make a living from the poor life habits that lead people into unhappiness. We have chiropractors who make a living from people's accidents, many of them resulting from carelessness. Of course, some things you can help and some things you can't.

But you *can* help by thinking kinder thoughts, uplifting thoughts, peaceful thoughts. Some people believe that peace can come from a pill or capsule. But it can't. Peace is a state of mind. Peace is a state of being. It isn't something we buy at the drug store.

Choose The Road You Travel

Many people just let things happen to them. Many people just allow any old thought to wander into their mind. You must choose your thoughts. Our vocabulary, the words people use in everyday conversation and thinking, has been examined and analyzed, and one-third of our vocabulary in this country has been found to be destructive to the human body. These words just slip right into our thoughts and mouths along with the others — when we let them. Just as you choose the road you travel, you can choose the words you use. It takes practice, but you can do it.

We were not created to live in the constant shadow of death. We were not created to live in constant fear of the end. You must learn to be as discriminating about what thoughts enter the door of your mind as you are about who enters the door of your house.

We have been promised life, life more abundant, and that is wonderfully uplifting. Let us claim that promise. It is hopeful. It is good. Every thought of this kind is life-giving, and as it flows through us it helps the body to create a better cell structure. If you can't live in thoughts that are creating a good body, you are destroying yourself. You break yourself down. We need to find out what kind of thinking is beneficial, what kind of vibrations are good for us to live in.

Years ago when I first began to look into this, I wondered how thoughts could have a physical impact on the human body. We hear people say, "When I heard the news about my son, it hit me like a ton of bricks." "It hurts me to have to tell you this." "She was gripped by fear." What gripped her? Certainly not a person. Then, what was it? It was the thought itself. Thoughts can touch, wound, hit or hurt — and the body responds.

I never realized the full power of thinking to affect the body until one time when I visited England. A special and somewhat peculiar coffin was being built for a man who was about to die. This fellow was so crippled and bent over that the coffin had to be constructed in an odd, curved shape to fit his body. Yet, just after he died, his body straightened out! What had been keeping him crooked? It was in his thoughts!

As I studied people, I became aware that often they are weary. Worry makes us weary. Worry wears us out. Worry chokes us. Where do worries come from? They are thoughts, aren't they?

I'd like to shout, "Let's get revitalized!" Surely we are intelligent enough to know that we can't be revitalized if we continue to walk the weary way, the worry way, aren't we? If you are wearing yourself out mentally, I can't revitalize you physically. We'd be working at cross-purposes. It wouldn't do any good. Revitalization comes when there is an enthusiasm for life, when there is joy and happiness! This creates a new vital energy that will flow through you and recharge every cell in the body. But the person who is tired of life, tired of people, tired of his job, tired of financial problems — this person can't hold his shoulders up and walk as the "upright man" does.

The walk of the upright man gives a different perspective to me. He is a person who has his head in a different consciousness. He is a person who holds his head up because he is thinking the higher thoughts. On many occasions I have written inscriptions that say, "Take the upper road in life" in the books I have authored. Try to think in terms of the upper thoughts, the upper road. That will lift your head up. Let's do some good thinking about our thinking and see what it does for us.

Scripture tells us that first we must seek. If you will seek, you will find. If you want good health, if you want the good life, you must start by seeking it. You have to make the first move for anything that you want in life, and that includes good health. Don't expect a doctor to take care of that for you. Don't expect anyone to help you. Get started doing something for yourself — and be cheerful about it!

If we really want to have an untroubled mind, we have to leave behind the old ways that gave us the troubled mind in the first place. We can't be like the fellow who walked into the health food store and said, "I'd like to buy some whole wheat cigars." It isn't just a matter of finding a better substitute for something bad.

The Cream Puff Consciousness

People look for coffee substitutes and meat substitutes. They look for low calorie soda pop and imitation ice cream. Why don't we find out what is good for us, what is real?

I recall a man who came to my former sanitarium with very high blood pressure. I worked hard with that man but I couldn't make any change in that blood pressure. It was mystifying because I was used to seeing the blood pressure go down after the right treatments. I changed his diet. I did everything I could think of, but the man left with a 240 blood pressure just the same as when he came in.

Not long after that, I was walking past the local bakery when a lady came running out the door and stopped me. "You owe me a bill," she said, "and I want to get paid for it."

"But I 've never bought anything in your bakery!" I protested.

"Well, one of your patients certainly did," she said. "He bought three dozen cream puffs — on credit — before he stopped coming in."

Three dozen cream puffs! There I had been, trying everything possible to bring that man's blood pressure down, and he was gobbling up cream puffs every single day! No wonder I hadn't been able to get anywhere!

Many of us have a cream puff consciousness. We want the health problem to go away but we don't want to give up our cream puffs. And we truly can't "kick the cream puff habit" until we get rid of the cream puffs in our heads first. If we are going to change our habits, we have to start by changing our minds, transforming our minds, lifting our minds to higher ways.

When I first began reading the *Bible* I often wondered about the passage that began, "In the beginning was the Word, and the Word was with God, and Word was God." What could this "Word" be? After much thought and study, I realized that it was nothing less than Truth, the fundamental vibration of God's Truth. When we are not in harmony with this Word, this vibration, our lives go poorly. This is the vibration that can transform our consciousness, our lives — if we let it.

Scientists tell us that heat, light and sound are all made up of waves, of vibrations. We hear by vibrations. We see by vibrations. We are warmed by vibrations. The scientists that study quantum physics tell us that when you get down to the things atoms are made of, the subatomic particles, the smallest things there are, these too are made up of vibrations. What that means is that even our sense of touch, the basic sense that tells us that something is solid and "real," depends on vibrations. This may seem strange to you, but everything we can sense or know or experience is made of vibrations.

Keep Your Life At The Higher Level

We live, then, in a spectrum of vibrations. We are surrounded by them all the time. If truth is the only right kind of vibration, then what does a lie do to us? That's something to think about, isn't it?

Every word in every language in the world has its own special vibration. When we speak of love, the vibration is peace and harmony. We feel these vibrations when they come to us. They affect our bodies. Good vibrations are what we owe the other person. The Golden Rule tells us, "Do unto others as you would have them do unto you."

People who don't know any better give out the worst vibrations, the lowest kind. Some people don't know what it is to give out good feelings to other people, and because their bodies are affected by what they are giving forth, they reflect that disharmony at the physical level in themselves. They are harming themselves. They say that ignorance is bliss, but is it? The question is, what are we going to do when we meet such people? Are we going to let ourselves be dragged down because they give out bad feelings? We don't have to let that happen, but most of us do.

This is why I say that we must be careful when we ask somebody how they feel. They may tell you, "Oh, I have a terrible headache," or "My ulcers are acting up again." They tell you how this or that awful thing happened in their family, and then you start feeling sorry for them, so sorry that you get stuck in their rut of thinking. Then you start talking about your headache. You start talking about your problems and troubles. And between the two of you, you have two sets of troubles playing teeter-totter with one another. Each of you leaves the other feeling worse than before you began talking.

Get away from this low vibratory state of living. Avoid low vibratory words and tones of voice. As we have said before, one-third of our vocabulary is too dangerous for safe human consumption. One-third of the words people commonly use are destructive to the nervous system and to the human body. So we must pick out a good vocabulary — and use it. We want to get our lives to the higher level and keep them there.

To be aglow with the spirit is to be expressing a vibratory rate that raises us constantly. In order to do that, we have to live in an environment where it is possible to express the higher vibrations. We must pick out friends who are good for us, friends in whose company we feel good.

Low vibrations don't belong in our sphere. This is what spiritual teachers mean when they talk about levels of consciousness. When we have been in a low level of consciousness and we rise above it, we get into a higher vibratory rate, a higher level of consciousness. When we get into the higher vibratory rate, our body follows. As the body follows, a smile starts to come from within, and the face changes wonderfully.

We are surrounded by words. We hear, "He was deeply hurt." Yes, we understand that words can be painful. "She took it to heart." "It weighs heavily on him." "Her conscience disturbs her." These are nothing but words, nothing but vibrations. They are nothing but feelings — yet their vibrations interact with the vibrations of the body, lifting it up or dragging it down. The same is true of thoughts. All negative thoughts disturb and distort our nervous system. "My goodness, you look absolutely wonderful today!" Isn't that a better way to go?

The Secret Of Happiness

Have you ever heard a bird sing an unhappy song? Well, neither have I. All day long they have to forage for their food, but they always seem to find time to sing a little pleasant song now and then. Maybe we can learn something from them.

I hear people say, "I want this. I want that. I ought to have this and have that." These people have their minds so set on the things they want that they don't stop to appreciate and enjoy what they have. I don't know if people like this ever notice the birds singing outside, but if they could stop and listen, they might learn something.

We have to get away from wanting. We have to enjoy what we already have. This is one of the little secrets of life. If we don't have this attitude we are too hard on ourselves. We are too hard on our nervous systems. Learn to enjoy the things you have as much as possible. He who ceases to be thankful may be living, but he's asleep on his feet!

Eventually worry worms its way into the deeper self, the innermost vibration. That is where it can really wreak havoc. There at the core of our being it tears down body and soul. What a man is deepest, he really is. Hate destroys. If hate reaches the innermost being, it becomes a terrible thing. Clean it out! Clean house as quickly as you can!

We have to fix up these bodies by cleaning up our minds. Some people are very negative about what they do, and they do that negative thing very powerfully.

A mother was listening to her son worry over an examination coming up at school. "I just know I'm going to fail!" he asserted miserably. His mother replied kindly but firmly, "And I just know you are going to pass!" We must be positive about what we are going to do, and we must teach that attitude to those around us.

We can go through life positively expressing the negative. We can hate with vengeance. We can aggravate the negative in life. We must learn to use thought lightly "as a feather." We don't want to use thought like a hammer, hitting people over the head with it.

When the harsh thoughts are carried to the body, the nervous system suffers. And who makes a living on this? Yes, the doctors.

It is time to get into the higher vibrations. Vibrations organize matter. Now, if we put a magnet under a piece of paper and sprinkle iron filings on top of the paper, the filings will all fall into a beautiful pattern showing the magnetic lines of force. These magnetic lines of force are vibrations, invisible to the eye, but very real nevertheless. All vibrations organize matter.

If I had a little spigot that I could attach to the foot of the person who comes to me with health problems, and just drain the resentment out of him, I know that person could get well. The *Bible* says, "Resist not evil." It is this resisting and resenting that maims and kills, not the evil itself. Evil can't attack the nervous system — but resentment can. We have to learn to live without resentment.

In all his work man is limited by what he focuses his eyes upon, what he turns his ears to hear, what he reaches out with his hands to grasp. Money comes and goes. Time comes and goes. Those who don't tune their awareness to the godly life miss it.

As we begin to lift ourselves to the higher level, we realize that our time is an aspect of "foreverness" when we live with a God of Life — and foreverness has no end. As we rise to this truth, we rise to life. There is no pleasure in dying. You must live and express that livingness. Plant the seed of livingness in your mind. Don't be like the lady who was just "dying to get well." You have to *live* to get well!

Your Life Is From God

What have we inherited? If you think only in terms of the genetic inheritance from your mother and father, there's a possibility that you will only live the proverbial three-score-and-ten years. We have to recognize what our true inheritance is. If you seek your inheritance from the heavenly Father who promised, "that whosoever believeth in him should not perish, but have eternal life," you can have a different kind of life. You don't look at death. You don't look for the end.

Then you can walk differently. By living a godly life you will be able to change the whole vibration of the body. Life within you can change entirely. Then your physical body will serve you in a wonderful new way. You won't have that tired, worn-out, weary body any more. It will be revitalized.

Do You Work For Ulcers, Inc?

The man who works for "Ulcers, Incorporated" doesn't have a job; the job has him. He is not master of the situation, but its victim. He is the victim of his own attitudes. "It kills me to be around that boss of mine — I can't stand it," he says. Perhaps he even runs away from that job and finds another one. But he will only run right into that same problem again unless he turns to a new kind of life.

We have to turn to a new kind of life. That is the point of what I am talking about. We have to present a new idea of life to the body's cell structure. Your physical body doesn't know what to do. It takes in everything you give it. It takes coffee and donuts, pickles and ice cream. It makes the best body it can out of those ingredients. But you can't expect it to do much with caffeine, sugar and acid.

In a similar way your nervous system has to be presented with a better life idea. All the messages that constantly pour into and throughout the nervous system must be uplifted by your attitude toward life. If you are not building up the nervous system, you are tearing it down. We have to go the spiritual way.

In all spiritual ways, throughout His life and teachings, Christ showed Himself as the Son of Life. He didn't speak about death in anything. He is the Son of Life. "I am the resurrection and the life." When He was dying on the cross He told the thief beside Him, "Today shalt thou be with me in paradise." He spoke always about life.

"Father, into thy hands I commend my spirit," He said on the cross. Christ is living in that spirit. He never spoke about death. Death is man's idea. We must associate with life. Otherwise we are constantly breaking down the physical body.

Be conscious of good because our consciousness is what we live in. It is what we are aware of. Many people don't like to go inside themselves because they have guilt in there — stored in the closet, so to speak. They have a guilt consciousness. Or they are not aware of good when they look within. You must clean up the ideas inside your mind. Give it a good house cleaning and sweep out those dusty old closets. Live according to your higher consciousness, according to your higher beliefs, your higher understanding. There are good ways inside you.

So go inside and clean house. If you can clean the inside and then come out, every cell in your body is going to feel it. The cell structure of your body will respond to the vibration of the new thoughts you give out.

Let's Learn How To Live

George Bernard Shaw once said we die because we don't know how to live. We kill ourselves by our lethal habits. Low moods come upon us when we are tired and fatigued. They can be hard on us and hard on those around us. We must not be afraid of trying new ways. We must not be afraid of the desire to take up new ways. We have to change our lives if things aren't right. We can't just sit and watch life go by.

Work with the idea that everything is for your good. We need that exuberant enthusiasm that young people have. They just want to jump into life with both feet and live. We have to drive into this river of life and start swimming. "Come on in, the water's fine," we hear the young people say. And it's true! The water of life *is* fine! Don't ever sit around in a rocking chair and let life slip by. I don't believe in retiring. The mind never gets old. You can think your whole life long. Your thinking may slow down a bit, but the extra knowledge and extra wisdom you have developed make up for it.

You will have more appreciation at the end of your life than ever. You will appreciate beauty more. You will know the value of music more. So old age should be composed of wise days. They should be beautiful days. They should be wonderful days. You can appreciate life more fully than at any other time of your life.

Don't be afraid to change your attitude. Don't be afraid to look inward and let wisdom unfold — to develop new thoughts and to replenish your mind with better thinking.

Let go of old fears. Fear is a terrible thing. As President Franklin D. Roosevelt once said, "We have nothing to fear but fear itself." Fear is a condition of the mind. One person can fear one way, and another can fear another way. Some don't fear at all. Those people who don't fear usually have a consciousness filled with other things. There simply isn't room for fear.

The Mind Must Be Free Of Fear

To have an untroubled mind we must get away from fear. I can't help but think of that famous radio and television personality Arthur Godfrey when he left the hospital following a long bout with cancer. After such long suffering he said, "There are many things to think about. Life is a privilege. It is granted to those who live a life." When he was asked what he meant by "living a life" he said, "There are three things. We have to strive for personal excellence. We have to leave this world a little better for our passage through it. And we have to try to learn how to live without fear."

These are great statements to think about. We cannot live with fear. We may not have bread but we will be provided for. We must have faith. We cannot allow ourselves to have a fear of people, fear of traffic, fear of a job, fear of time, fear of lightning, fear of the Russians, fear of darkness, fear of airplanes, fear of sin, fear of not being accepted socially. When we think of all the fears a person can develop, it is no wonder that the body becomes exhausted. It becomes weary from carrying these thoughts.

I have been taught that if we believe in God, we draw from God. If we believe in life, we draw from life. But if we believe in fear, we draw death, and this I know is true. That is why so many people today are only half alive. To be fully alive, to have an untroubled mind, we must have peace of mind. We can find it within ourselves.

Everybody is looking for a Shangri-La. I remember a time when I had many troubles and problems. All I wanted to do was to go to the South Seas, sit on an island under a coconut tree and let the coconuts fall into my hands. I thought the ideal life would be to live that way. But you don't have to run after some Shangri-La. It is right here. It is this moment. If you start chasing a Shangri-La, you may be chasing it the rest of your life.

We can end our negative thinking. When anxiety and fear dominate us, it is foolish to think we can find peace of mind. It is an impossibility. When we live in our physical losses, our energies leave us. Vitality comes only when peaceful thoughts are in our minds. Then peace flows into our cell structures.

We dissipate life by our words and by worrying about our relationships. I mention this because I have repeatedly emphasized that we have to carefully pick our friends in life. People who are hard on us, people who are difficult to understand, people we can't get along with — these are the kind of people who dissipate our energies. They dilute the quality of our life.

Peaceful feelings toward the self and others

are extremely important. Peace means harmony. It means right thinking. It means justice. It also implies a code of ethics by which to live. If we want to have peace, we must live in such a way that we are not encumbered by guilt or shame or hostility. When we are at peace we have no hostility within us.

Hostility destroys our vital energy, and we will never harvest anything from hostility but destruction to the body, mind and soul.

On the other hand, love knows no boundaries to its endurance, no end to its truth, no fading of its hope. Love outlasts anything. It stands when all else falls. Love can revitalize us. We must have love within us. I have mentioned many times that love is to be passed along to others, not only because they need it, but because we need to give it for our own good, for our own body's good.

Love Rejuvenates The Body

When you love, you enter a new dimension. Your body takes on a new vibration. You make your life important not only to yourself but also to others.

The bank teller can feel rich when he handles money. But is he? You are truly rich only when you feel good inside. I stress this because feeling good is a state of vibration. It is a state of consciousness. If you can reach this state of consciousness you will change your body because, as we have pointed out many times, the body follows the mind.

A well-known proverb says, "As a man thinketh in his heart, so he is." Walk the higher road. Take the good thoughts into your heart. Then the body will change. Raise your sights. The finer things will come to you.

Let there be peace on earth. Let there be peace in the hearts of men. How can this happen? Let peace begin with you. Let peace begin with me. Then it will happen.

We know the way. We are glad when we are told to go into the House of the Lord, the House of the Law. The House of the Law is a house of justice. It is a house of peace and harmony. As we go into this house, we know we have something wonderful to live for, something that we make worthwhile simply by living the higher way.

As each of us brings into harmony what is within, it is good to know that God is one with us, that we are one as we walk and talk in this kingdom. When we live in this kingdom we realize we are heaven bound, that our body is the temple of the living soul — we are not earthbound. We are on our way to a higher place, a place that has been prepared for us.

We are thankful we can change to better ways, that we can accept those ways from on high for our body's good. To accept the spiritual lessons being taught us is to understand that all heaven and all earth have been vested in man. We have the privilege of experiencing that heaven here on earth through right thinking.

Our bodies respond to those peaceful moments we share with God. What a special privilege it is to live in the higher realm. I know it is good to follow Him, to be touched by the Spirit, to know that the feeling we have extends far beyond the boundaries of the skin. It is by living in this spiritual life that we touch Him and feel Him.

Prayer Is Thanksgiving

We are thankful for all the things that are given to us in heaven and earth. We are looking only for what is good here — in heaven and earth. All good that we accept will be expressed though our bodies.

One of the great admonitions is, "Abhor that which is evil; cleave to that which is good." Let us learn to see as God sees: purity of heart, purity of mind, purity in each other. Today we enthusiastically act upon this wisdom: there is all good in everything we touch, everything we feel, everything we see.

When we see good in everything we turn our eyes upon, we are truly blessed. You are a good person in my eyes. You are a blessed one in my heart. I pray that these words may be a great blessing to you this day.

"Age is opportunity no less
Than youth itself, though in another dress,
And as the evening twilight fades away
The sky is filled with stars, invisible by day."

—Longfellow

Chapter 18

Be Alive With The Mental and Spiritual

Knowledge is so proud
that it thinks it knows so much,
while wisdom is so humble
that it knows so little.

We should all be interested in improving our bodies. Each day I look for ways to improve my body and to upgrade the Ranch. I like to see things getting a little bit better each day. If I buy a car I want it to be a little better than the one I had before. Strolling through the grounds at the Ranch, I look for ways to make them more beautiful than they were before. In other words, we would all like to think of the world as being just a little bit better for what we have done here.

Everybody needs to think this way. Some people are satisfied in drifting along with their everyday ways, not realizing that they are not doing the best they could do. Of course, it is possible to drift through life thinking you are perfectly happy this way. This is like the worm in the horseradish. He thinks it is the finest place in the world because he has never been anywhere else. How can he tell? He has nothing to compare it with. He has never touched some of the finer things.

Let's take this idea to the mental and spiritual levels to see how it affects the body and how we can apply it to find a better way to live. Now to be upgraded means this: I want you to be closer to *kingship* and *queenship*. I want you to move closer to *kingship* and *queenship* than ever before. What do the words "king" and "queen" mean to you?

A long time ago in England, three men were being interviewed for the position of driving the king's coach. Each one was asked how close to the edge he would take the carriage if he drove through the mountains. The first man said, "I am so skilled at handling horses and a carriage that I could drive within three inches of the edge of a mountain cliff, and the king's coach would be perfectly all right." The second man said, "I would stay a foot away from the edge if I were driving the coach." The third man said, "If I were driving the king's coach, I would drive it as far away from the edge as possible." The third man got the job.

You are driving the king's coach, and there is a king inside of you. This is the kind of kingship I am talking about. If you are responsible for the kingdom of life you live in, that king's domain within you, then there must be a king inside, taking care of it. The most wonderful thing you can do with your life is to take good care of this king within yourself.

Some of us don't have many ideals. We don't step up to the higher road in life. We may think we are perfectly satisfied. We may live in physical comfort. But we don't live in mental and spiritual contentment. I spoke about the king and the carriage and then I mentioned the kingdom, the king's domain. It is an entirely different *king* I am talking about.

Comfort comes to us at times with the physical things of life. We can buy that kind of comfort. We can have comfortable clothes and comfortable houses or apartments. We have comfort around us. But did you ever sit with somebody and feel uncomfortable? Have you ever had dinner with someone when you just didn't feel comfortable? There is such a thing as mental comfort as well as physical comfort. We have to learn to distinguish between these two areas of our lives.

Life Has Many Facets

Most depend on the physical things, the material things, as the only aspect of life they can really hold onto. We must realize that there are other ways. The reason we become discouraged is often because we think our physical possessions are the most important values in life. But there are other values, other facets to life. Those qualities of character which take care of us in times of discouragement, depression, trouble, stress and war are very important. What qualities do you find in yourself? You have to stop and think about this.

If you have never studied, if you have never reached for the higher values in life, how do you expect to be strong enough to take care of weaknesses? If you are as weak as the weaknesses you are handling, they will overcome you. If we find ourselves thinking evil when we meet with evil, then evil will stay with us. If we want good, we have to think about good. We have to manifest good. Then good will stay with us. I mention this because if we want good health, we have to live in what brings good health. We have to saturate our bodies with peace and harmony. Let evil be overcome with what is peaceful and harmonious within you.

If you can't realize that all is well with you no matter what experiences you are going through, the experiences will tear you apart. Don't let your experiences get the best of you. A lady, sixty-eight years of age, told me she was working out some kind of social security when someone told her, "At seventy you will be finished." You can't listen to people like that. Don't look ahead to seventy and think you will be finished. There are places where you can get a job if you want one. Some people have been told they can't expect to get a job after forty, and of course that is true only if you let yourself be fooled by that kind of negative thinking. So, don't let yourself be deceived.

People say to me, "Doctor, I'm afraid I will never get well." Don't tell me you are finished! This is a finishing thought, and it doesn't belong in your body. Whenever someone says, "I am nervous; I am sick, ill and discouraged; I am through," then they are claiming thoughts that become part of them. Those thoughts saturate every nerve and cell in the body.

A happy person is generally a wise person. The happy person has accepted the experiences that have come to him, and he knows that they have come simply because they were on his path. We can accept our problems and turn them into wisdom.

When we learn to see obstacles properly, we will use them as stepping stones to the higher and better life. When we reach the higher and better life, we will greet those obstacles with pure joy because we have learned that we can use them for our own progress. We have to do this to get out of sickness and ailments. We have these physical problems today because of what we have believed in the past and may still believe. We have to go farther in our beliefs. We have to expand our understanding. We live in our understanding. Cultivate the better thoughts. Wonderful joys lie beyond what we can see!

This morning a lady said, "Now, I see. Really, I have been dead to all this, haven't I?" Of course she had! If you're not living, you're dead. You have to wake up and see. You are only living when you know that good thinking and good spiritual ideas make a good body.

You could change your ideas now. You could accept and reach for the finer avenues in life and you would have the secret of good living. You must reach out. If you never have a dream, you will never have a dream come true.

The Person — Not The Disease — Must Be Cured

I have seen every disease cured but I haven't seen every patient cured. My problem is the patient, not the disease. I am giving you professional advice. If you don't have a desire to go someplace, you are not going to get anywhere. As comedian Jack Benny once said, "Well, I'm not giving all my money away to charity and to this, that and the other thing." And someone said, "What are you going to do? You can't take it with you." Then Benny said, "Well, then, I'm not going!" Some of you people out there aren't going either. You aren't going any place. You are stuck right there with the physical values you believe in.

Personally, I believe many people like their sickness. They don't know where else to go or what else to do. Some people don't know what door to knock on to seek help.

Sometimes we let people have their problems because they need that experience to grow. The people who evolve out of their problems and their sicknesses should be happy that they are living a better life and going another way.

One of our California governors said, "I think it's nice to pray, but when you get off your knees you have to start rowing for shore."

Let's go back to the physical question and let's take care of it. Let's not just get up on cloud seven and stay there. Then we are no good any more from a physical standpoint. We have to do something for each other. There are many people who become completely involved in the spiritual side of life and become hermits. They don't want to have anything to do with people. You know — the air is polluted, the food is devitalized, everything is going downhill — and the first thing you know, they go off by themselves and live alone because they want perfection. We are never going to find perfection in this material world, least of all by running away from its imperfections. I would like to tell you that perfection sits right next to you. You can go through all these worldly things, and they will not affect you. You are affected materially only if you are materially minded. This might sound strange to you, but your viewpoint can change only if you make up your mind to change it.

Some time ago, a man told me there was only one statement in the *Bible* that he believed: "It came to pass." Everything in our experience has come to pass. You have to believe something as you go through life. I make a living on people who have poor beliefs. I know that if you believe a lie, you live a lie. There are many people whose minds I just have to change before they can be healed.

"Doctor, will I get well?" Of course you will. "Do you think I can make the change?" I know you're going to make a change.

People tell me you can't build new cartilage, you can't build new brain cells. I ask them, "Who have you been listening to?" Another person told me she only had six months to live. "Who told you this?" I asked her. "Do you believe it?" And, what did she do? She believed it. She reached for death, and it found her. She died.

We Use The Law Rightly Or Wrongly

The point is, what you reach for, you can have. Many people are walking around today who had once been given up to die. They didn't believe the crazy ideas that were handed to them. Some doctors tell patients they are going to die when they have an extremely serious medical problem simply because the doctors themselves don't know of any further ways to treat that condition, beyond what has already been done. That is, what the doctor is really saying is that *he* has given up. Now the patient doesn't have to go along with this. You have to be very careful what you believe. The doctor's limitations aren't yours, you know.

When you are working with this physical body, it is the end result that you must keep in mind. This physical body had to be produced in mind, in thought, before it became word and deed. It was created according to law, with each cell, organ, bone and limb precisely designed, located and developed where and when it was supposed to be. The fingers were put there because of the law. The nose is on the front of your face and nowhere else because of the law. It had to be right — and it is, because of the law. When a physical problem arises, then we go back to the law that created the body. We go within to the law and we trust the law to correct the problem. We do this at the level of mind.

Now, the development of the fingers had to be directed. The development of the nose had to be directed. But have you ever stopped to think that this mind is directed, too? It has some ninety faculties that I know of, such as the critical and the analytical faculties. It has a "reaching" faculty. Otherwise, how could we reach for hope? How could we reach for love? How could we stretch forth and get some of the lovely things we have in our lives?

We must go on from where we have left off. Leave the old quickly. The more quickly you leave the old, the better your future is going to be.

When you were in the third grade in school, did you know what was being taught in the eighth grade? Could you conceive of it? No, you couldn't understand what was yet to come. Most of us still can't. Christ said, "I am the way, the truth and the life." I wonder what ways He had. I would really like to know what ways He had. Wouldn't it be wonderful to possess some of this wisdom?

There is a special place in our minds from which we can experience life as wonderfully as it really is, but I can't show it to you. You have to go inside and find it for yourself. Now, there are people who consider themselves so practical that they won't believe two plus two equals four until they see it on paper. They won't believe they are going to get paid until they see the money in front of them. They want perfect health *before* they will believe that a certain treatment or approach to healing works. They want the demonstration or proof to come first. Well, I have news for them. They are putting the cart in front of the horse.

The demonstration comes *after* you believe. "You show God to me, then I'll believe," people say. Believe first, then you'll find God. That is the way it works.

Some time ago a resident at the Ranch handed me a slip of paper. On it were the words, "The Laws of Nature are the habits of God. The Created Universe is His Body." Some of you may have the idea that God is a stern but kindly old man with white whiskers. I think He is everything — personal, impersonal, physical, mental — I think He is everywhere. I don't believe you can find a place where He is not. We find that the real power in this world is not in material possessions, but in the power and life that we ourselves possess. This is where our strength lies.

Asking for strength doesn't guarantee it will come to you. You earn it. You work for it. When you change the consciousness of your thinking mind so that you realize where all power is, you will have all the strength you will ever need. Most of you wear yourselves out looking for a source of strength, trying to find a source of strength, before you learn it is inside you. It is already there.

One lady told me, "I think I'll try you." I said, "You aren't going to try me. I'm all right." This idea of trying is misleading — you can wear yourself out trying. You are going to find a direction to go one of these days, and when you find it you will stop trying. You will be "doing" instead of "trying to do." Then you will have something wonderful.

I read one time, "An educational book is understood in proportion to the growth of the reader's mind." When you read a book, you will get something entirely different from it than the next person will. You will understand what you are ready to understand, no more and no less. We go through life understanding it only from the level of where we are. When we get to a higher level, we will understand more. This is brought out in a dedication to "The Memory of Perpetual Youth":

The babe in the cradle feels;
The child in his teens thinks;
The youth in his 30s has an idea;
The man in his 40s invests and creates.
The middle-aged man constructs and
reconstructs;
The man of 70 to 90 reflects and rejuvenates;
The man of 100 rests and takes a vacation;
The man of 150 is surely an advanced thinker.

You don't find the advanced thinker at the age of twenty, do you? But I believe you should advance your thinking as quickly as possible because there is really no age in the mind and in the spirit. We tack age on to these ideas. Time is here to stay. We come and go.

Many of you are looking for better times to come. The better times are here. The sooner you see that better times are here, the better for you.

For advice and sympathy, go to your friends. For money and books, borrow from strangers. For little or nothing, go to your relatives. For thought, power, wealth and joy, go within. Lastly, learn to be self-reliant and discriminating. Separate and discard thoughts that do not belong to you.

People come to the Ranch and ask, "What kind of resort is this? You know, doctor, I would like to get well." Do you know that to recondition yourself, you have to recondition the mind as well as the body? If we recondition our mind, the body will follow. The shoulders droop when we are depressed. When you are discouraged, you can't sing, "Happy Days Are Here Again." It doesn't work that way. You have to find the uplifted way.

When I speak of upgrading, I mean to rejuvenate. You want to rejuventate the tissue from day to day with good foods. Wouldn't it be nice to upgrade the mind? This gives the nervous system a good time, and it certainly needs a good time after what most people put it through. When I say it needs a good time, I mean we should have a beneficial current running through our nerves. Good thoughts generate this current. The best way to do this is to consider what is natural, what is good, what is right, what is best for you.

We Arise By Lifting Others

In India they say a good man is one who works like water under the ground to feed the roots so plants will grow. Real love allows you to grow, nourishes you, gives you the water you need, the sunshine you need, the nice thoughts you need. Love helps you put yourself in order. No one has ever become well until he put himself in order by way of others.

You don't really get well until you start helping others get well. This is a law. This is a hard lesson to learn. But, from experience I know you'll never be happy until you start lifting other people. And, to be healthy, you have to be happy. Beggars aren't happy. You have to be on top of life to be happy. When you lift other people, you lift yourself. You bless them, and they bless you. They need to be blessed. You need to be blessed. Live so that you are blessed. Don't go through life seeing how much you can get, how much you can rob, cheat and lie yourself into. Stop all that and evolve. Start clean and fresh and from this very moment.

You can give your body a good life. When you give your body a good life, many physical problems disappear that were caused by tension. I take care of physical symptoms. Not everything is mental or spiritual, but if we start there, it is easy to get the physical body well. To repair tissue is the easiest task. But it isn't easy to get you to change your mind. It isn't easy to get you to stop the harsh thoughts that you think about others. This is the most difficult task in the world.

It Is Your Mind That Must Change

I don't think I am letting any cats out of the bag when I say that people have difficulty changing their mental habits. We constantly hear complaints like, "If he only understood me" or "Everytime I am around him, something wells up in my throat." We can't always change other people but we *can* always change ourselves. It may be difficult, but we can. At the same time, we have to realize that we may be around others who *don't want us well.* We can defend ourselves against this by right thinking, but it is necessary to spend as much time as possible with people who love us, who want us to be well and who uplift us. Often we can change the situation by uplifting ourselves and by doing good to those who do not wish us well. In that kind of atmosphere, we often find that they will change. We don't *try* to change them, we simply go about our business and let them change themselves. If this does not bring about the necessary change, then you will have to leave that situation for the sake of your health.

People have not been trained to be good to one another. We don't know we are supposed to be good to one another. We don't stop to think that people and relationships are more important than possessions. When we don't accept an opportunity to lift someone up, to build someone up, to care for someone, we lose a blessing for ourselves. We lose. There is also a reciprocal law here. When you are good to others, they are good to you. When you are good to others, you make yourself wanted and needed. You need me, and I need you. We have never been taught this, but it is true. How many people can sit down together and warmly reason out the solution to a problem and make a decision on it? We need to work together on ideas. We separate ourselves from one another — and from God. We think that God separates Himself from us just as we separate ourselves from one another! We even divide

Him! We have to come back together. We have to reason together and share ideas together. We are all God's children and we must change our minds to think in this way.

With God we have everything. The Good Book says, "All that I have, son, is thine." If you get right with God, you don't even have to know the commandments. Now, there are some people who are at a level where they live under the law. They only understand when they are told, "Don't do this, don't do that." They have to have somebody standing at their elbow reminding them, "Don't spit, don't swear, don't chew, don't grab." I encounter people at my lectures who constantly ask me, "Doctor, is smoking okay? Is drinking okay? Is coffee okay?" People always ask me about their bad habits. I wish they would ask me about some of the good habits! When we know we have everything, we don't have to follow the "thou-shalt-nots." If we believe in God and follow God's will, we will be following the "thou-shalts" instead.

You don't need to worry about your body. Leave that body alone and straighten out your mental direction. If you toil without a direction, without a destination in mind, you will get worn out and get nowhere. An airplane pilot was asked by a passenger how things were going. The pilot replied, "We're lost but we're making good time!" Know your destination. Then put your feet on the path that leads to it.

We are going places but sometimes we are not accomplishing anything. I see a man going along day by day. He gets older but he never gets anyplace. Some people haven't reached the age of eighteen when they die at eighty. Wouldn't it be wonderful for everyone to be as Christ was by the age of thirty-two?

There is never enough for greedy people but there is plenty for those in need. To have no bread and yet know that we are going to be taken care of is to feel well inside. This works very well from the standpoint of the nervous system.

Once I spoke to Dr. Robert A. Millikan, the scientist at the California Institute of Technology who was awarded the Nobel Prize for measuring the electrical charge on the electron. At the time he was investigating cosmic radiation. I said to him, "You have broken down molecules into atoms and you are even making measurements on subatomic particles. You are doing these experiments with cosmic radiation. Is there anything beyond that?" He answered, "That's where man ends and God begins."

Most people have never gone beyond their own bodies or the immediate circumstances of their daily lives. There is another world, the *real* world. If I put a pen on my desk, it has no power of its own. The real power comes when I put it to work. You will find that the real power comes into our lives when we let God use us for His purposes.

If we could harness this power and put this body in good order, we would have the most wonderful servant in the world. Our body was designed to serve us. This servant has over a million nerve fibers leading from each eye back to the brain so we can see light, colors, shapes and textures. You are an instrument of over two million strings, and you don't yet know how to appreciate it. You don't know how to play it properly. To play this body properly you have to learn the mental and spiritual notes.

Wouldn't it be wonderful to change your life so much that when you went home your dog would bark at you because he couldn't recognize you? Wouldn't it be nice to change your life so that people would say, "Goodness, he's a changed man!" Or, "Look at her, she is simply transformed!" Wouldn't it be good to walk that way?

Unless we start walking that way mentally and spiritually, our body has nothing to follow, and in the absence of direction it may follow hate and the other negative things. So we start from within and work outward. Then you will have something to radiate. As we radiate life, harmony, peace and goodness, the whole body feels it, and the nervous system works beautifully. I treat people ill from abuse, not ill from ordinary work. I treat people for overuse of the body or sometimes underuse. If you don't use this body you lose it. Our body is meant to be used. Find out how to use it.

What are Thoughts?

We say that "thoughts are things," but then Albert Einstein showed that matter and energy are equivalent, didn't he? Thoughts are energy, energy that travels as vibrations. Thoughts have a certain rate of vibration. We find that when the lower thoughts bombard our nervous system, it starts to act and react. We hear someone say, "You said this to me last week, and I don't like it. I'm going to get back at you." I can tell you that by holding that kind of grudge, you place your nervous system under great tension, and the first thing you know, you will find yourself in a doctor's office or hospital. It is claimed that hospital patients average taking fifty-two pills a day. Why? For control of the physical condition, they say. But, then we are out of control. We are controlled by the pills!

Usually we don't judge people rightly. We judge by the physical appearance. You have to judge people by their inner selves. You must look for the good within. We sometimes hear people say "He brings out the worst in me." Try to bring out the best in others. You can do that only by bringing the best out in yourself. And when you bring out the best in yourself, you are healing yourself.

If you spent every day healing yourself by positive thinking, you would win. We become wrecks by beating other people down. Leave people alone. Don't depend on people for your happiness. Let people go! The one idea you should be interested in is elevating yourself. The next step up in life is never to take a job that will harm another person.

How far does judgment reach? It goes right on to heaven. Where is heaven? Within us. That is why we must lead good lives. "Behold, I stand at the door and knock: if any man hear my voice and open the door, I will come in to him and will sup with him and he with me." This knocking at the door requires an open consciousness to allow the best aspects of life to enter.

The Christ said, "My sheep hear my voice." I am wondering if you know what this Voice is. We should all study enough to discover that Voice. We will hear it even if we are deaf. We will see even if we are blind. Maybe the blind man sees more. We may be worse than blind because we do not see the right things. I wonder if you see the difference between the physical, the mental and the spiritual. We have to get away from the idea of human power to let that godly power bring health and enlightenment to our nervous systems and minds.

So many peole are looking for a demonstration. In the time of Christ many people were hungry, and He showed His disciples how they could feed 5,000 men and several thousand women and children with five loaves of bread and two fish. After the Christ fed those people, they gathered up twelve baskets of leftovers. The next day Christ told them, "Ye seek me, not because ye saw the miracles, but because ye did eat of the loaves and were filled." He had shown them the secret of everlasting life, but they didn't see it. They only remembered what they had put in their stomachs.

Something called Infinite Substance exists. There is such a thing as "practicing the Presence." There is an opportunity to "Lift up your eyes and look on the fields, for they are white already to harvest." These are understandings we have to grasp in order to see. Many wait for it. Try it. All we have to do is claim it. We have been told many times, "All that I have is thine."

People who have the idea that they are going to get to heaven by violence are mistaken. We cannot do as President Franklin Roosevelt once said: "We're going to have peace even if we have to fight for it!" You cannot storm the ramparts of heaven. You may only get there by the heavenly way, the way of the innocent child who hasn't learned negative ideas. A child hasn't yet developed the vocabulary and knowledge of the negative ideas.

Today, many people live in constant fear — fear of the devil, fear of mankind, even fear of going out at night — all terrible fears. Lecturing around the country, I once had 2,000 to 3,000 people attending my talks. In Chicago one time, about 1,000 came. Many told me, "We're afraid to go out at night. We're afraid to go out in this district any more." What is man coming to?

We should live, not in fear but in the love of our fellow man. What a terrible thing to have to go through life afraid of people and violence. Violence and lawbreaking are making attorneys rich — and we have more attorneys than ever. You can read in the newspaper about court cases where each side employs several attorneys!

The same thing is happening in our health care system. In some cases people are examined by several specialists before they begin to treat you. Specialists are even watching other specialists. We aren't looking at the whole problem. We have to learn how to ask. Some have the idea that God gives more to one person than to another. They say, "You are just lucky. God has been good to you." I don't think God picks out one person and says, "I'm not going to give as much good to you as to the others."

How Much Good Can You Use?

Life is like a fountain. You can go to that fountain with your vessel and fill it up. How much can you take? If you want much, bring an empty vessel. But if you bring one alreadly half-full of greed and problems, you are in trouble. If you return again and again with an empty vessel, you will find something good each time. I hope you will try it.

This fountain flows forth with that Infinite Material which goes before us to make straight our path. Some of you may already be on this good path, and you must realize that the more you have, the more is expected of you. Every level of consciousness brings certain responsibilities.

We have to stop saying "mine and thine." This can become an obsession. Life is glorious, and all things are here for everybody. You can have everything you reach for, but you have to reach for it.

Very few people reach for more than the material things, but you can reach for faith to change this physical body. You can reach to the law of acting and believing you have received it, that you already have the things you have hoped for. There isn't anything you could ever hope for which doesn't already exist. Do you want to go beyond the physical?

It gives the Father great pleasure to offer you His kingdom. We must recognize that. To reach, one must stretch out one's arms. Why can't we reach out with the mind? We can! Sometimes I think we need a mind-stretcher to help us attain our goal. We have to be equal to the goal we reach out for. This is most important. Some of us may have a long way to go, but, you see, these thoughts can be given to us in a very short time, and our reach is then extended.

We have heard of people "stretching the truth," but what we want to do is stretch our minds to get some of the eternal truth. It is right here for us. "Heaven and earth shall pass away, but my words shall not pass away," it says in the Good Book.

Can you touch substance now that you can depend on? Can you find anything at all you can depend on in this world? Can you always depend on your employer, your friends, your relatives? It is difficult, isn't it?

No real discouragement exists in this world. There is no depression. There is an overabundance of wheat, corn and all the things we need. The concept of depression came upon us because of man's limited consciousness in trying to do things his own way. We have the land, the soil, the seed and everything to meet the needs of everybody, but depression came to us because of negative thinking. The person who can raise his consciousness to the level where he doesn't live in depression is ready for the new life!

As we go forth and reach out and attain all we should have, the complete abundance that has been promised us, I am sure the body will follow. When we say, "First seek that kingdom, the King's Domain, and all things shall be added unto you," we find that we leave behind the negative things: discouragement, depression, tension, resentment — all the things that bring us dis-ease. We change it now to radiate Thy Light.

As we radiate that godliness, we recognize peace and harmony working within us — not peace at any price — but love at all costs. We change our ideas to the higher laws, to that love which passeth all understanding, which gives us complete harmony within. And as we reach and touch one another, we uplift and take care of one another, knowing that, "What we have done unto one of the least of these," we have done unto Thee also.

I know that as we are for one another, we are going to be cared for, because this is the living bread, this is the staff of life. As we go forward now, let's live. Let's love without thought of compensation, anticipation, anxiousness, the things which finally become flesh. We find that as we live in this perfect harmony, we will be cared for because we believe in God. We know as we follow the godly way, He will never forsake us.

Prayer

Let us meditate silently for a moment on what I have said.

We are going to change our thinking, Father, because we realize everything is within us, that it is the Father within who does the work, and as I gain faith within, the works become rewarding.

Faith without works is dead. That which I believe will finally touch my physical body, the kingdom and the world in which I live.

Chapter 19

Anxiety

What you are seeking is also seeking you.

We can have anything we seek — but not unless we reach for it. Now, this raises several questions. How can we reach for the better things? How can we raise our lives to a higher level and make our expression of life a better one? How can we have a better handshake, a better walk, a better talk?

The times we live in have been called the "Age of Anxiety." Unless you have something of a higher nature to draw on in time of need or trouble, you are going to face serious problems. There will be times when you will struggle with greed. There will be times when you will be faced with such difficult situations that you will think "fight or flight" are the only possible solutions. There will be times when that ogre we call depression will try to drag you down. You must have something at all times to draw on.

To get out of our troubles and onto the higher path, we must learn to draw on the Higher Self. When we are in tune with and drawing upon the Higher Self, we need never feel lost, lonely or lacking in anything. We have an unlimited resource in the Higher Self.

The story was once told to me of a saint in India who, while walking along a path to a river, saw a scorpion drowning in the water. He reached in the water in an attempt to rescue it, but the scorpion stung his hand, and he dropped it. A second time he reached into the river. The scorpion stung him again, and he pulled his hand away. As the saint prepared for his third try at rescuing the scorpion, a man who had been watching said, "Don't you know that it is the scorpion's nature to sting?" The saint replied, "Yes — but it is my nature to forgive."

What is your nature? Are you like the scorpion, ready to start a fight if someone touches your life? Do you let the things of this world discourage you? Do you open yourself to receive hurt or harm from your experiences or from the words that are spoken to you? If you do, emotional symptoms will develop within your mind that will ultimately take their toll on your physical body. It will affect the cell structure of the body, and that is when you come to me and ask for help.

Where Do Troubles Start?

I believe that if I closely examined all of the actual causes of physical problems, I would find that as many as eighty percent of them start in the mind.

People have the idea that if they rest the body, the nerves will improve. This is true but only partly so. If you rest the mind, the body will This is getting back to basics. If people who experience tiredness, fatigue or exhaustion could set their minds at rest, their bodies would follow. What comes from the mind produces physiological activity within the body.

Why are so many people in the United States taking tranquilizers? I am convinced that it is because in time of need they feel they have nothing else to draw on. They haven't given their inner resources the slightest consideration.

Our attitude, our emotional state, even affects our breathing. The person who lives in fear does not breathe correctly. Since the body needs a certain amount of oxygen to funtion normally, alterations in breathing rate, together with shifts in body chemistry such as those caused by the release of adrenaline, can cause severe problems over a period of time. Only the person who has a reserve within, who lives in joy and appreciation, can let the chest go and be free to receive the right amount of oxygen.

Nearly all the people who come to me are middle-aged to elderly. The young people are getting by so far, but most of the elderly lack sufficient oxygen. Without sufficient oxygen you can't burn up the body's waste materials. Without sufficient oxygen you can't generate heat in the body. But happiness and good feelings can give the elderly a good open chest, enabling them to bring in the necessary oxygen. Of course, it always helps to go to the country where the sweet-scented evergreens, flowers and grasses make every breath such a pleasure. Then you will breathe correctly.

If you are down on the world, you won't breathe corrrectly. You really don't want to breathe. I've heard people say, "I wish I were dead." Many people who come to the Ranch say that at first. This attitude complicates and worsens any physical problems the person has, making things much more difficult.

Treat The Whole Person — Not The Disease

The day is coming when doctors are going to treat the whole person rather than the disease. Doctors will be looking at the family environment, the childhood background, anticipations, anxieties, food habits, all of these things together. We need to know what our patients have done in the past and what their hopes are for the future. It is enormously difficult to treat a person who comes in and says, "You're the ninth doctor I've seen. What do you think you can do for me?" My usual reply is, "Just what do *you* think I can do for you?"

We have to learn to develop and constantly unfold a Great Within for the sake of our own health. We must have elevated thoughts for the good of our cell structure. You may think you are only "buttering up" other people when you express positive thoughts to keep in their good graces — but you are doing *more* good for yourself, whether intentional or not. You need to express good for your own good. It isn't a matter of expressing it for the sake of others. When you can change any idea that comes to you for the better, then you are evolving and making that Inner Self a better self. This is what you have to do.

The American Indians were very resourceful in matters of health. They had their medicines, but the Medicine Man was busy, too. Dressed in his ceremonial robe and horrible mask, his job was to frighten away the evil spirits. The Medicine Man would dance around his patient and make terrible noises to scare away the evil spirits that were causing his patient's problem, and in a day or two the patient would recover. The main job of the witch doctor or medicine man was to turn his patients' minds toward recovery. As for the patient, he had no negative ideas to deal with because he left those to the doctor. He just naturally recovered.

Your work can become pleasant the moment you get rid of aggravations. I know you can actually get well if you will relieve your nervous system of problems and troubles, because they are responsible for "clogging up" these vital communication channels in the body. Once you clear the nerves of these obstacles, then peace and harmony can begin to flow through, telling the cells and organs to rejuvenate. This is the lesson, the healing lesson, that all religions teach: Rest! Christ said, "Come unto me all ye that labor and are heavy laden, and I will give you rest."

Most people need rest. Something has to happen within you before rest can come to the physical body. You must go to the mind first. I'm telling you how to give your mind a good rest.

If you will just let go of your aggravations, even those that come from any sickness you may now have, you will stop the cycle that produces and sustains physical problems. The person who talks about sickness produces acids that hinder healing, acids that the body has to take care of. The body has enough to do. Why give it more work, more problems, more acids, more mental disturbances?

Learn To Walk In Peace

To break that cycle right this minute, still your mind for the moment and know that everything is all right. When you can walk in this world — and it is a mess these days — quietly, reservedly, with joy and happiness, knowing that you are one with God, knowing that all is well as long as you are on His side, then nothing will disturb you. You will be able to walk through anything with a peaceful mind. The vibrations of your body will reach a level where all that is experienced is good.

Health, harmony, peace and beauty all come from the thoughts, beliefs and attitudes that influence you and from how you use them to influence others. They come from what you are trying to accomplish.

As we have previously mentioned, one of the keys to life is correct breathing. I want to emphasize this because we find that in nature the fast-breathing animals die early, and in my experience this applies to human beings as well. The person who lives in fear breathes very quickly, and fear takes a devastating toll on the body.

A person who is happy, joyful and satisfied breathes sixteen times a minute. A person who lives in anxiety with feelings of depression has to breathe eighteen to twenty-six times a minute. You breathe according to your mental attitude. You wear yourself out by using up excessive mental and nervous energy.

A cynical person is likely to develop lung troubles. People simply cannot breathe properly when they live the pessimistic, cynical, antagonistic way of life. The frequent interference with the normal breathing pattern in these kinds of people contributes to the development of lung disturbances. On the other hand, a person who learns to sing brings joy to the heart — and the lungs. They develop an entirely different lung structure than they had previously. No one can go through life condemning, distorting and disturbing other people without affecting his own lungs.

You have your problems. Mostly likely they are "people" problems. There are people you should leave alone in life. There are people you should set aside in life. You have conditions in your life that you have to put aside. You have to divorce yourself from these circumstances and you have to do it in a nice way. Learn how to handle your problems from a spiritual standpoint.

Are You Emotionally Fatigued?

Most of the physical problems I see today result from what we can call emotional fatigue. Fatigue starts in the emotions, in the mind. When a person is highly emotional, he has a lot working on his nervous system. He is going to wear that nervous system ragged unless he gets "off it." The first thing you know, there is a conversion of this emotional symptom into a physical symptom in the body. This is what doctors are treating so many people for today.

Anxiety is a kind of low-level fear, and, like fear, it connects with what scientists call the "fight or flight syndrome." People often want to get away from something developing within themselves that bothers them. But you can't run away from yourself. When an internal problem develops, you become anxious about it. You build up mental frustration.

You want to fight or run, but there is no place to go, nothing to fight. The enemy is on the inside, not the outside. The constant nagging urge to fight or run from this invisible enemy is emotionally exhausting and nerve wracking. Most people wear themselves out with this kind of anxiety.

To get rid of it we must start with the mind. If you don't have a naturally spirited body that wants to walk and work these difficulties out, your shoulders will slump, gas will build up in the stomach, and the heart will suffer more pressure. But when we live on the joyous side of life we lift our arms, we stretch them, we reach for the good

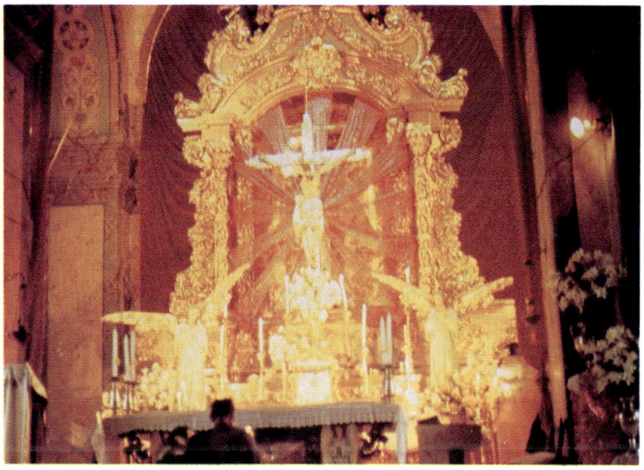

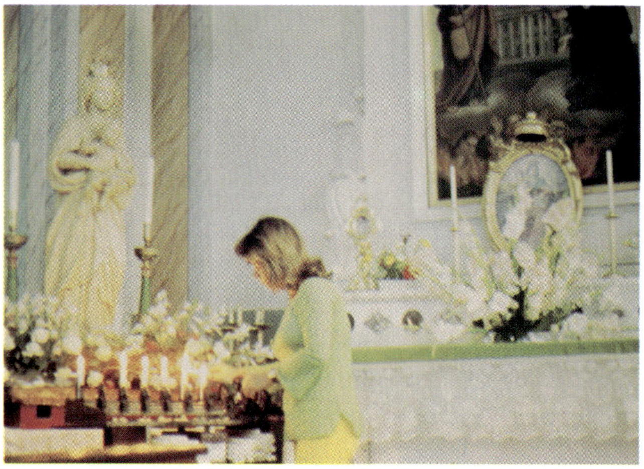

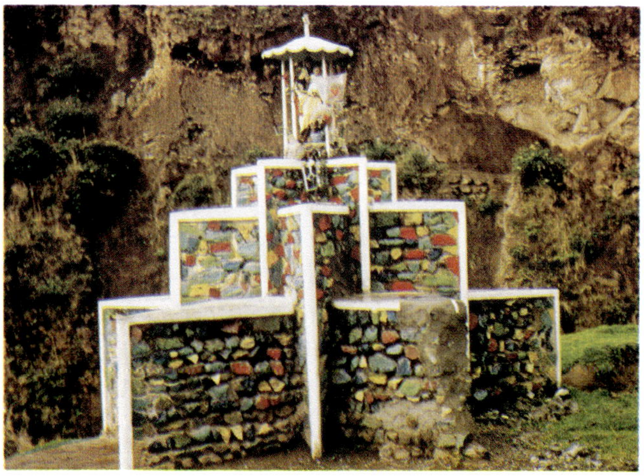

Upper: The gold altar in this South American church seemed almost to glow with its own golden light, reminding those who have eyes to see that the real treasure is inside us. Center: Candles are lighted in this church along with prayers of intercession or thanksgiving or prayers for special favors. Below: This roadside shrine was made so people would stop and pray here. Built at the edge of a dangerous curve in the road, it also served as a reminder that several people had died there in automobile accidents.

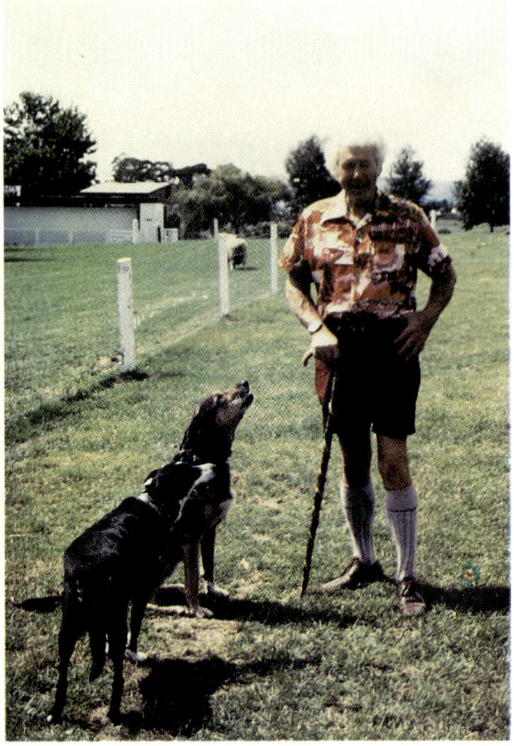

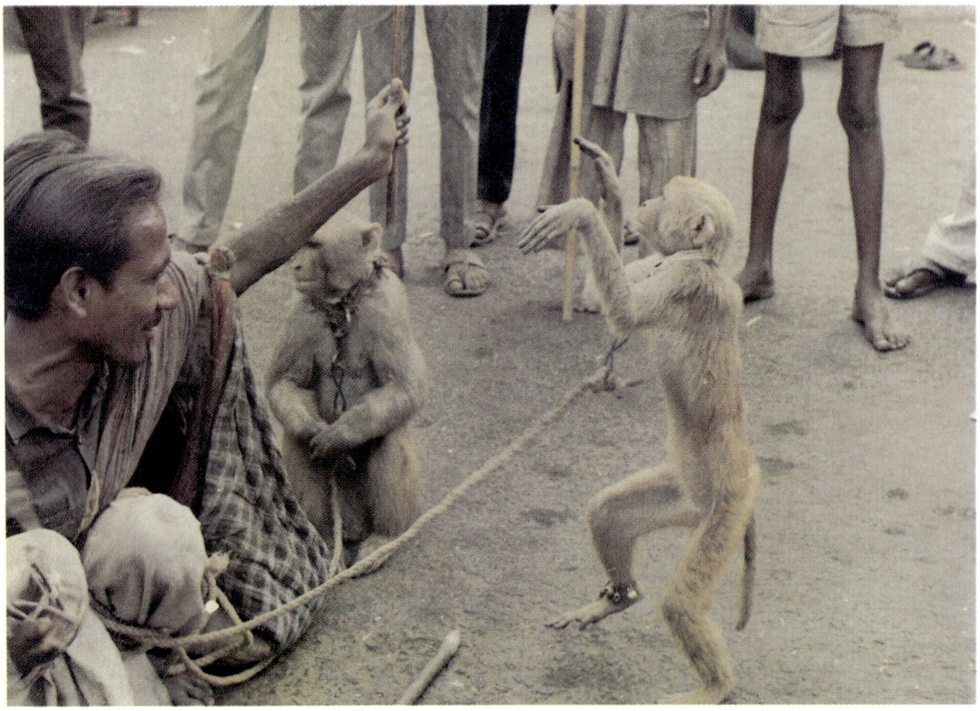

A smile goes a long way in spite of language—the language of the inner self is always contacted between both animals and humans—and I hear between flowers.

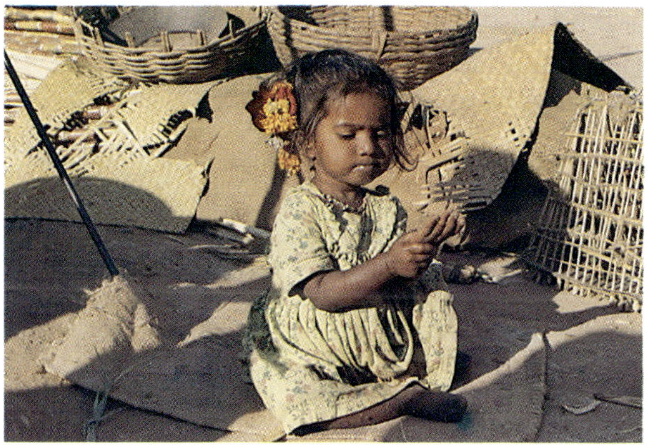

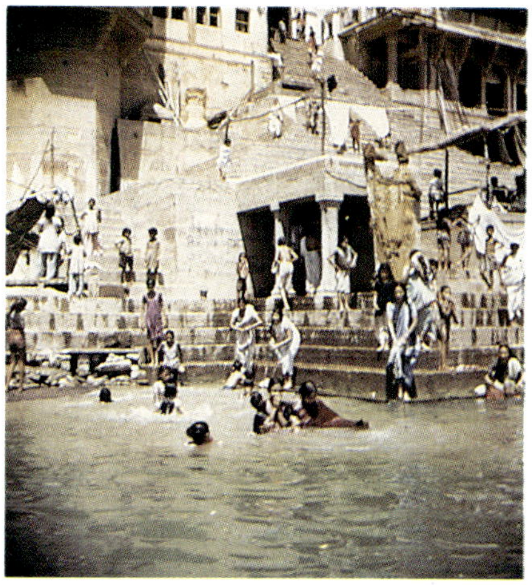

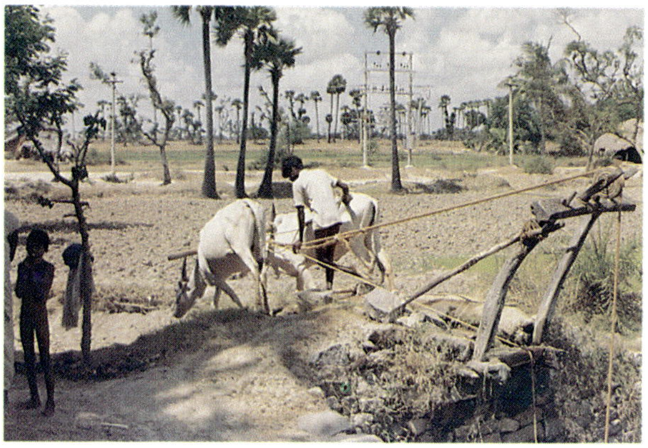

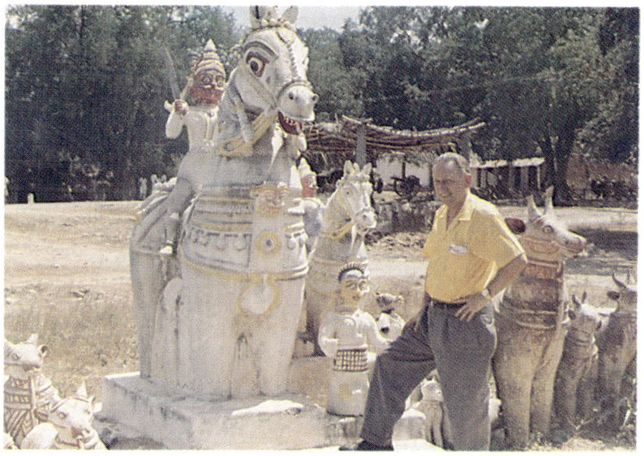

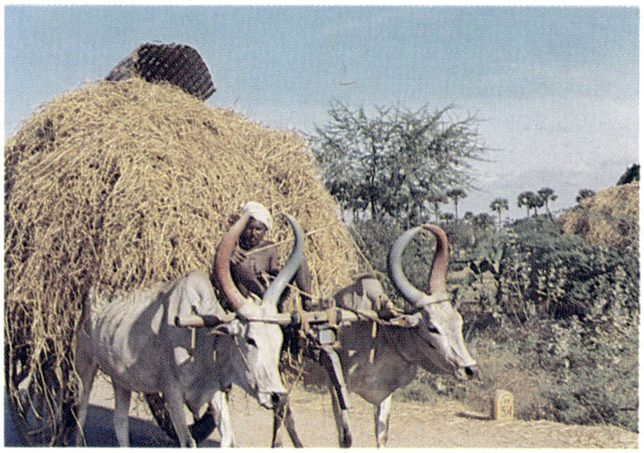

1. A lovely little child of India. 2. The healing waters of the River Ganges have touched many people, giving them new hope and, in many cases, even health. 3. Here is a water hole where the oxen bring up water to irrigate the surrounding land for growing foods. 4. In India, cattle are considered sacred. They are used as beasts of burden, but they claim it is God's chosen animal to be used by the human race. Great care is taken in their grooming as you can see by the color on their horns. 5. In India, much energy and attention are given to the spirits that protect, care and help.

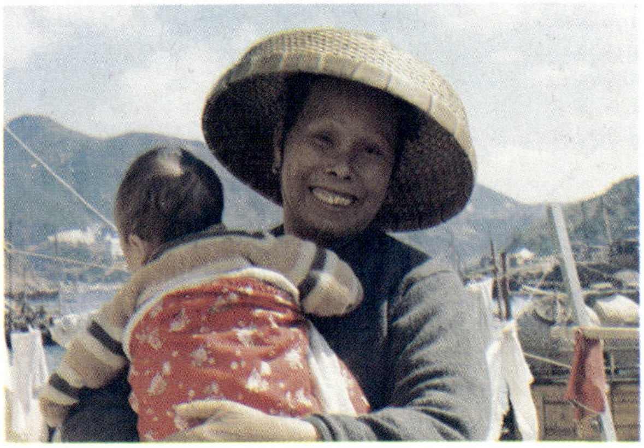

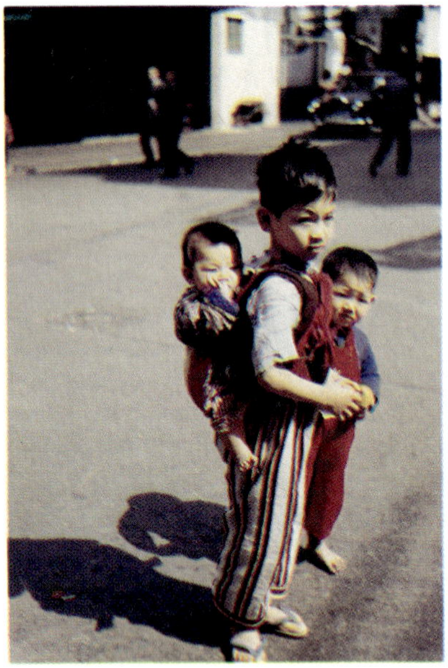

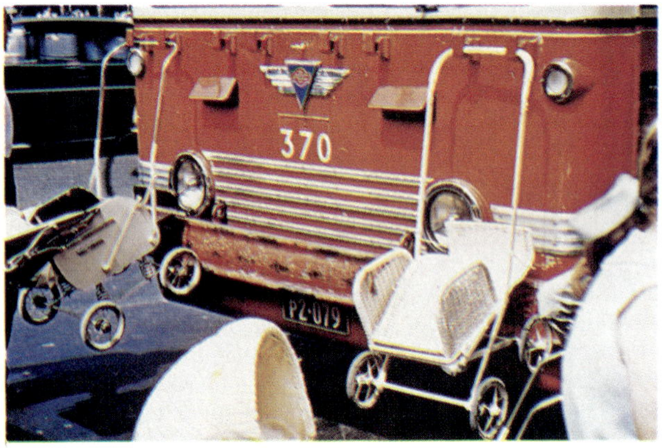

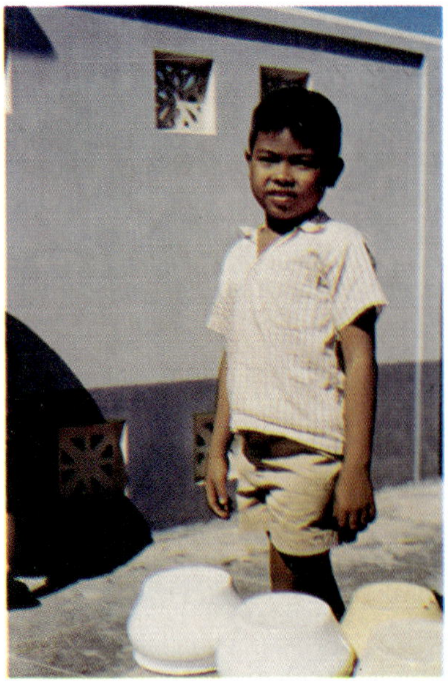

Hong Kong. 1. In spite of having so little, the people show much love as can be seen in the wonderful smile on this mother's face. 2. This is the front of a bus in one of the southern cities of New Zealand where those who take their baby buggies along hang them on the outside of the bus. This is certainly a great help to the mother who doesn't want to carry her child. 3. The young carry the very young, but we find these people are taught to care for their siblings at a very early age. 4. Children are taught to work early, keeping their hands and minds busy.

things, we are alive with life. When we are living like this we keep our minds and bodies in better condition. When you are living in fear or anxiety, the worst thing you can do is to sit alone in your house or apartment, dwelling on these things. First, tell yourself, "I'm going to leave these things behind." Then get active. Do something physical like cleaning house, even if you don't feel like it.

If you want to get rid of depression, nervousness, gas in the stomach and pressure against the heart, get outside and take a morning walk. A wonderful variation on this is to take a very early morning "grass walk" without shoes. Believe me, you can't stand still barefoot on that cold, dewy grass! You have to move! Focus your mind on the fresh coldness and texture of the grass as you walk. As you let this experience take your mind off all the negative things, begin to fill it back up with better thoughts. Look at the sky, the trees, the sun, and count your blessings. There is much that is good about your life. All you have to do is open your eyes to it.

Maybe You Need A Worry Stone

While visiting the Virgin Islands I heard about an unusual thing that the people there call a "worry stone." A worry stone is a small smooth green stone with a hole in it. People hold this stone in their hands and "get rid of their worries" by rubbing them into this stone with their fingers. Whatever the worries are, the Virgin Islanders just concentrate on letting them pass into the stone instead of holding onto them. When I was young, I did something like that. I woke up with a terrible toothache one Sunday morning, and of course no dentists' offices are open on Sunday. So my dad put a clothespin on one of my fingers. My finger hurt so much I couldn't feel the toothache.

Of all the people who come to the Ranch, more of them have problems caused by worries than anything else. If you could get rid of your worries by rubbing a worry stone, wouldn't that be wonderful? But I think many people would just use that stone as a reminder to keep on worrying. You can't really cure yourself with a worry stone. The worry is really inside the head, which puts it out of the worry stone. I think it is time that you toss worry and anxiety out of your head and your life once and for all. They don't belong there. This is the real lesson I have for you.

One way to make a new beginning is to develop noble sentiments. We are here to live a noble life with a noble purpose. We are here to see and bring out the nobleness in each person. To live a noble life is to go through life living the higher consciousness. If you don't have a higher law within to draw from, the physical condition deteriorates. You have to rise above things. You have to rise above by constantly elevating your life through noble thinking, noble words, noble ideas.

Perfect your ideas so you bring the best thoughts to yourself. Whenever your mind is not occupied with higher thoughts it is open to lower thoughts, and lower thoughts bring on dis-ease. Disease comes from disharmony. Chaos brings destruction. Harmony brings good health. We must realize that good health evolves though self-discipline, through making sure your mind is tuned into the higher path.

Practice self-exaltation. Rise above negativity. We must have direction from the Higher Self in order to have our bodies express good health. We have to reach the higher levels of life and we have to lead other people to higher levels. Then everything else will follow.

Prayer

As we go through life, we are thankful, Heavenly Father, that Thou hast given us breath, because we realize that this breath is the Secret of Life. We recognize that spirit and breath go together. We realize as we take this breath of life, we have become one with Thee, and Thou hast given us all the loving thoughts, the privilege of feeling well, of looking for the good, of living the Higher Life, of knowing that all ways can be well with Thee, that our troubles will cease and we can have rest in Thee.

The Law of Life tells us all is well for those who live the good life and follow the path of righteousness. We need Thee and we need Thee every hour. As we walk and talk, let us recognize that the Spirit we walk with and talk with will guide us to the right physical activities for our bodies.

Chapter 20

Establish A Ground To Stand On

You can have everything you want in life; but you have to take everything that goes with it.

One of the great laws is that nothing can disturb you unless you give it your consent. You are in complete control of everything that happens inside you. We hear people say, "You lost your temper." Do you think someone can force you to lose your temper? Oh, no! You lose it all by yourself. We never hear the expression, "He lost my temper," do we? Nothing can get inside unless you allow it to happen.

You might say that we live in permissive times. In other words, we allow too many things to happen to us. We allow sickness to come upon us. We allow problems to come upon us that make us nervous wrecks. We allow mediocrity and failure to come upon us, preventing us from being everything we want to be in life.

We are powerful beings but we abuse that power. We say, "He made me miserable." Or, "She makes me sick." In cases like these we have put our power into lies and then we live those lies. No one can *make* you sick or miserable. They do something, and then you choose how you respond. *You choose.* Yes, you can choose to be sick or miserable. But it is not true that someone can *make* you sick or miserable. We are a law unto ourselves.

This is quite a power, isn't it? To be able to make ourselves sick? To be able to make ourselves miserable? Once we realize that we have such a power, we only need to turn it around to bring what is good into our lives.

Good things are available to everyone. If you want courage, just claim it. If you want peace, just claim it. It is yours. No one else can give it to you or take it from you. You and you alone have the power to make it happen. You are a channel for the life that flows through you. You can either dam it up as it comes to you and repress it or you can let it loose and live it.

To make the right choices in life, we must establish some kind of ground to stand on. You need to establish a firm foundation for the home you live in. Where is your home? You may say, "Home is where I am happiest." Is that necessarily at 274 - 7th Street? No. Happiness is a state of mind. Happiness is a quality you can take anywhere on earth. You are carrying your home with you. How can you find a proper foundation for it, a proper ground?

The ground you choose for your home is found only when you are absolutely quiet, unconcerned with everything outside your body.

This is the real you. This is where you really are. This is your domain.

This is what you build on when you build within yourself. We don't build on the shifting sands of the emotions. We don't build on the uncertain swampland of the intellect. We build on the solid rock at the center of the inner silence. Then what we create will be strong and permanent, capable of withstanding the storms and winds of life.

Can a wise man become sick? Previously, we have read how the youth in his 30's has an idea. The man in his 40's invests and creates. The man of 70 to 90 reflects, beginning to see how life can be changed. And, the man of 150 is very wise. He has to be wise to have reached that age!

When you are wise you will not be sick. When you are wise you will have grown out of your problems and troubles. So, seek wisdom. Wisdom comes as we learn to overcome. I don't want to wish sickness or trouble on anyone, so I will wish you many "awakening" experiences. There are actually no terrible experiences once we have learned to draw wisdom from what comes before us. Experiences are all helpful when we meet them with the right attitude.

Why do you say, "I'm miserable," when it might simply be that you are going through a period of adjustment? Look again. See what you can learn from the situation. A prolonged period of mourning for the loss of a loved one is inappropriate and unhealthy. A period of mourning should be heartfelt but brief. The shortest sentence in the *Bible* is, "Jesus wept." Why did he weep? He wept for His friend Lazarus who had died. Then He stopped and brought Lazarus back to life. Get into those problems, solve them and get back out again. Take your stand on that strong inner ground and come back to it when you need to. We should use this ground our whole life long.

The sickness that may have taken over your body, mind and spirit is consuming the valuable time of your life. You brought in this sickness. You can't blame anyone else. There may be some difficulties you can't control, but you can control how you respond to them.

We are talking about the establishment of a king's domain, the kingdom within. All my life I have been seeking the spiritual values, not so I could become skilled at preaching sermons, but because of what the truth of the higher path brings into my life. Aren't you looking for something? Aren't we all seekers?

I believe that my life flows forth from the kingdom within me. My beliefs are "grounded" in that kingdom. No matter what is around me — violence, death or hell itself — I'm going to conquer because my foundation is built upon rock. I have been practicing and learning for a long time. I have spent my share of time in hell. I discovered that I had created that hell myself, and hell held me captive only until I realized that I had to overcome. For the first time in my life, I realized what the Christ meant when He said, "I am in this world but I am not of this world."

Is it necessary for anyone to be bad? Does anyone have to lie, to steal or to cheat? Do you think you have to? My mother often said, "You can have anything you want but you have to take everything that goes with it." What goes with lying? What goes with cheating? What goes with stealing?

I know people who have become so sick of being sick that they are no longer sick. They have discovered that the word becomes flesh. They learned to change the word. We react to thoughts. When someone calls you a name, what do you do? How do you react? When someone tells you that you are wonderful, that you are lovely or handsome, what do you do? You put yourself in agreement with that and become lovely or handsome. Who doesn't want beauty? Who doesn't want to be desired?

Walk In Beauty To See Beauty

Do you know how to see beauty? I mean, really *see* it? You have to be well inside. You have to be able to walk in beauty to see beauty, to attract beauty to yourself. Beauty starts from within and works its way outward. You are never going to improve the outside until you change within. So, you begin by appropriating beauty within. Then, as Christ said, "He that hath, to him shall be given."

The person who is pure cannot 'see' the bad; he looks and his sight is too pure to see anything but good. It is too pure to see the negative within a person. The moment you become too pure to see the bad, that which is not good in others, you know you have reached the level of complete forgiveness. It is a form of blessedness. But the moment that you dwell on wrong and say, "What a terrible person," that thought reflects back inside you, and you sink to that poor level. Sickness is a result of negative thinking.

Sickness doesn't come from tension alone but also from wrong words, wrong thinking. Of course, tension wears you out. Restrictions in the circulatory system reduce the flow of blood to many parts of the body. Eventually, high blood pressure may result. It is hard to predict what particular kind of sickness will result from negative thoughts.

Thoughts become matter. Your thinking is flesh "in the making." You must realize that your mind is bombarded by thoughts all day long, and these thoughts will have an effect on you. You must establish a ground to stand on so that you are not tossed to and fro by these things.

Make up your mind to be positive. Start an epidemic of good feelings among those around you. If someone doesn't want to be good, that's his choice, his business. But do you know what my business is, my choice? My choice is to be good. I'm going to be good to my nervous system. I'm going to be good to my mind. I'm going to be good to my body. I'm going to be well whether you are or not. Now, you have to have that attitude.

One Sunday morning I was down in the garden when they were planting. You know, growth takes place on Sunday just as it does on the other days of the week. Plants have no awareness of time. They only know sunshine and water and the glorious good air and all God's good. As long as plants have these, they grow. They don't pay attention to Monday or Tuesday or two o'clock in the afternoon. They grow because all good has been given to them.

To express love toward other people is to make sure they have what they need to grow. Make sure others grow. Feed them love. What feeds the other person will also feed you. That's why we start with ourselves. As you nourish others, you nourish yourself; as you condemn others, you condemn yourself.

Why do I say this? Eventually, as a result of wrong thinking, you get to the point of a disturbed nervous system. Can a person who hates be well? Can a person who resents avoid being crippled by his thinking? To be a mental cripple is one of the most disabling afflictions I know.

I would like to be able to give all of you an untroubled mind. Wouldn't that be a wonderful gift? But I can't do it for you. The state of your mind is in your hands. But I'm going to walk with an untroubled mind today. How about you?

You are the king of your inner domain. You rule it. It is your responsibility. Do you want hate in it? Do you want violence in it? No one ever fired a gun unless the signal came from his mind first.

Peace And Health Go Together

Unless we become peaceful, nonviolent and nonresistant, we cannot be well. Mahatma Gandhi announced, "This is it. This is the law of life, the godly way to go." And he moved the entire country of India. All of Great Britain's army couldn't prevail against Gandhi and his message. They threw him in jail, but he simply said, "I'm going to do the right thing. I'm going to sit in jail as long as they want to keep me here and I'm going to do it nicely."

We have to decide what we want to look at and what we want to see. How do you shake hands? If the other man won't shake your hand, you should shake the dust from your heels and move on. It is his loss. You still have the Christ consciousness working within. You are still one with the God working within. Stay within that realm, and sickness will never touch you. The mind controls the body. The body is a servant to the mind.

When I point my finger at you, my mind is pointed at you. When I ask you to stand up, it is the spirit that quickens your mind before you can do it. The flesh didn't know what to do. It just followed you. You respond mentally and spiritually. So it is the power within, the power flowing in your body that makes you move.

I want you to see something you can rise to. Three spiritual words have great power: "*Arise* and *come* and *shine*." You can't shine misery. Let the spirit shine through the face. Let your face display all the lovely things inside, the godly ideals. Your face *can* change if you change from within. What you are deepest, you really are. That is the ground you stand on.

Do you know there are tranquilizing thoughts? Have you ever heard the slang expressions, "cool it" or "don't get shook"? What do you think they refer to?

Here is a fascinating article I found a few years ago:

GRANDMOTHER'S DUTIES

In addition to the duties listed, Grandmother read her Bible and had family prayers, which was the main reason she didn't need tranquilizers. Grandmother, on a winter's day, milked the cows, slopped the hogs, saddled the mule, got the children off to school, did a washing, mopped the floors, washed the windows and did some chores. She cooked a dish of home-grown fruit and pressed her husband's Sunday suit. She swept the parlor and made the beds and baked a dozen loaves of bread.

She split some firewood and lugged it in, enough to fill the kitchen bin. She cleaned the lamps and put in oil. She stewed some apples she thought might spoil, churned the butter, baked a cake, then exclaimed, "For goodness sake! Calves have got out of the pen." And went and chased them in again.

Gathered the eggs and closed the stable, back to the house and set the table. Cooked a supper that was delicious and afterward washed up all the dishes. Fed the cat and sprinkled the clothes, mended a basketful of hose; then opened the organ and began to play, "When You Come to the End of a Perfect Day."

I think that if Grandmother had let herself get aggravated, she would have let the calves wander. I think that if Grandmother had hate in her heart, she couldn't have played "When You Come to the End of a Perfect Day." It isn't work that kills, it's the aggravation that can go along with it. I'm positive that the mind can kill. I'm positive that the mind can destroy. The mind is capable of producing tension, disturbances and resistance. The mind plots the destructive deeds, and the body carries them out.

Before you can stand on "untroubled ground," you have to move away from "troubled ground." There are many troubles around. Some of you are married. Some of you are wealthy. Don't think these can't be aggravating. Even troubles can cause trouble. Gossip about troubles can trouble you. Grandma used to say, "I used to teil my troubles to everyone I knew; and the more I told my troubles, the more my troubles grew."

What do you want to grow in the garden of your mind? What do you want to nourish in your mind? Ideas, like plants, must be nourished. Plant beautiful bright flowers and healthy, satisfying vegetables and fruit trees in your garden. Then nourish them. Living should not be a process of decay. Uplift it.

This is the way to get well physically. We can't have a good physical body until we change what is in the mind. We have to go to the "top" to change the body. We will never be well if we are living down below, if we are wishing, hoping, begging, pleading for something bad to happen. When we are on top we are giving out all the good vibrations; we are lifting other people. Nobody can lift another person unless that person has first lifted himself. Rise up and start to help others. Through others you help yourself. Start doing good for others.

Then you will get rid of your sickness, your troubles. As the mind goes, so goes the body. When you are down below saying, "I'm poor, I'm sick, I'm miserable," then that is the kingdom you are claiming. If that is the sand you are walking on, it is going to slip from under your feet. You will cry out, "Everything is terrible! Please, help me!" But people will avoid you because they want to be free of that kind of distress.

Now, I want to help people free themselves by awakening them. You can't give people freedom. To give them freedom, to give them good food and then leave them in the same old state of consciousness is not helping them. It has been said that if all the money were taken away from the wealthy in this country and given to everyone in equal shares, in five years thc original wealthy minority would have their fortunes again. Some people are "money-minded." Some people are "love-minded." You can be rich but if you don't have love in your heart you won't be well. Sickness goes along with a strict money-minded attitude.

When you view the world around you, it is very much like an unruly youngster. It's like a badly behaved child — and it's being treated like one. The world is taking a terrific beating these days — a spanking, a licking, a whipping. Why can't we seem to get out of this? Aren't we out of kindergarten yet? When are we going to learn? Isn't it time to graduate?

The Wise Man Has A Master's Degree

The best decision you can make is to grow as fast as possible, to graduate from the grade you are in, from the experiences you've had, from the life you've lived 'till now, from the kind of person you've been. The wise man always graduates. The wise man gets the master's degree. Be perfect as your Father in heaven is perfect. That is the master's degree. When Christ said, "It is the Father in me that doeth the work," Thomas responded, "Lord, show us the Father." Then Christ said, "When you have seen me, you have seen the Father."

When you look at a person, do you look for faults or virtues? What do you think a person is supposed to be?

Every fence has two sides. Everybody thinks the grass on the other side of the fence is greener. More often than not, the grass on your side is just as green as the grass on the other side, but by one of those curious quirks of human nature we seem to put greater value upon what is on the other side. Now there are two sides to everything. Virtually everything in life is double. The American Indian talks about the "forked-tongue," the person who says one thing but means another, a hypocrite who is as dangerous as a rattlesnake. We have heard of the "two-faced" person and the "double-entendre," the latter referring to an expression with two possible meanings, a frequent "punch line" in jokes.

Every Thought Has Two Levels

Very few people go through the Bible and see the double meanings. Christ talks about these in "The Sermon on the Mount." Before, there was the law: Thou shalt not kill — thou shalt not do this or that. But, you know, that is for those in kindergarten. Once you find that the goal is being perfect as the Father in heaven is perfect, you don't have to say, "Don't do this, don't do that" anymore. If you want the perfect way, you establish the laws of love and harmony in mind, and then you are finished with the old law. It is automatically included in the new.

You have to set your sight on what you are going to do and what you are going to be. You do this mentally. Then the body follows. We are double — we are mental and physical. But the physical follows the mental.

We are sometimes double in another way. A glum-faced man went in to see a psychiatrist and spent half an hour telling the doctor his troubles. The psychiatrist responded, "You need to break out of this depression. Take a day off and go to the circus on the edge of town. Have a few good laughs. The clown over there has everyone rolling in the aisles."

"I am the clown from that circus," the man replied.

We are capable of laughing on the outside while we are crying on the inside. This is disharmony, and of course sickness comes from this kind of doubleness. Seek harmony.

The kinds and varieties of doubleness that we find in man are almost unbelievable. One psychiatrist took a scissors and cut two photos of his face in half, right down the middle. One of the photos was reversed so that he could put the two left sides together and the two right sides together. When he did this, the composite photographs appeared almost to be of two different men. The two left sides together made him look narrow-faced. The two right sides together made him look broad-faced. On this man — and most of us as well — the two sides of the face do not match.

The left side of the human body is different from the right side. One shoulder is higher than the other. One leg is longer than the other, and the feet are different sizes. You buy shoes to fit the larger foot, the wider foot. Many women have to have their dresses form-fitted. A lady who recently came to me couldn't understand why she had all the symptoms of thyroid trouble, yet her lab tests showed nothing abnormal. But there are two lobes to the thyroid gland, and one side turned out to be over-active while the other was under-active.

We also have to take care of that which doesn't fit in our society and our family as well as in ourselves. We must find our weaknesses and overcome them. We each embody both weakness and strength, and it is wise to increase our strength. If your weakness is hate, get rid of it. If your weakness is fear, get rid of it. Develop your strengths.

What you put your attention to grows. You have to learn to accept everything. Fighting things only makes them worse.

Some of you must learn to accept your wives or husbands. You may think you have a half empty glass of water, but let's put it another way. You have a half full glass of water.

Good Advice Is Good Medicine

You understand that when I say, "I don't care," I really do care. Otherwise, I wouldn't be trying to help you. You have to take that forward step yourself. I want you to realize that when you bring that body of yours and its problems in to see me, I know that your body has been at the mercy of your mind. Your mind may have been giving your body a terrific beating. If so, you need a lesson. Sickness is that lesson. But lessons are useless unless you learn from them.

I wish more doctors would sit and talk with their patients. So many give you a prescription and send you off to the drug store. You come into the doctor's office with your "coffee-and-donut" habits and you leave with the same consciousness. There is no uplifting. There is no learning. Because nothing has changed, you will be sick again.

Those who come to see me have to pay just as with any other doctor. The difference is that when they leave, they take with them a blessing that will last the rest of their lives. You can't measure this in dollars and cents. People walk differently when they leave here.

Once again I want to remind you of what happened with my little five-year-old girl when I came to the door and asked, "Who's beautiful in here?" She exclaimed, "Me!" You have to claim the best in yourself. You are what you are because of what you claim. Stake your claim and start plowing your "ten acres." Plant wonderful things in that ground. "As you sow, so shall you reap." You haven't really practiced this, have you?

I think Christianity is the most wonderful philosophy I have found, but I see so little of it practiced. I have never really seen Christianity practiced. It couldn't be, or we wouldn't have so many different churches, for one thing. There is only one God — why is there so much separation? Your God is my God. There is no *real* division.

We are all the children of God. We are all in the same kingdom. All this separation and division represents an underlying disharmony that is causing much of the strife today.

There is a better existence, and we can discover it. I believe that the only reason disease is on the upswing is that we have forsaken many of the godly axioms. I don't mean to make a fetish out of so-called "godly" ways — we can be mean and appear godly, too — as in the case of religious fanatics who abuse those who don't believe as they do.

You can have a wonderful business if you open your eyes to these things. A man came to me one day and said, "I had a great furniture business going, and do you know what happened? A man opened a competing furniture store across the street from me. What am I going to do?"

"Pray for him to succeed," I suggested.

"You want me to pray for him?" he almost shouted. "He's taking my business away! He's taking the food from my children's mouths!"

"Pray for him," I repeated. "Hope that he has everything good. The more people who come to his place, the more who will see your store. If you keep doing right, people will come to you."

He left my office, and in three months his business was booming so well that he had to move to a larger location on the other side of town. He had taken my advice, and it worked.

If we could only see how these prayers work we would be more faithful and expectant in our praying. By wishing good for the other person, we are always happier and better off.

Surprising Answers To Prayer

Not long ago I received a very surprising and delightful answer to prayer. I was wondering how to decorate my color room, what we call the Oriental room. The only change I could envision was to have a mural for the background, a lovely visual decoration for people to look at and enjoy. I wanted this room to be so beautiful that it would attract people to come and meditate there and feel uplifted. A friend of mine from New Zealand said, "Everything you do here creates a nice atmosphere, good vibrations. That's a wonderful feeling!" I wanted that room to be consistent with what my friend said.

So I went to a Japanese store and to many other places looking for murals, but none seemed right. Some looked good at night but not in the daytime. So I said, "Wally, go ahead and do this one." Just then a lady came into my office needing advice.

After I had taken care of her, she said, "This makes me very happy, and I'd like to do something for you. I have a Japanese mural that is four feet by seven feet. (Wally was putting in one that was four feet by six feet — my prayer was only off by a foot!) This lady had thought about giving her mural to a museum because it was so beautiful. But she said, "Doctor, I think the most wonderful place to put it would be in your Oriental room." I couldn't believe my ears! I had sent out a prayer, and half an hour later it was answered.

Of course, prayer is a two-way street. A woman came in and said, "I'd like to get married. I've lived so much in poverty that I want to marry a rich man." She started praying for a rich man and soon she met him. She came running into my office saying, "You know, my prayers have come true — but the man weighs 380 pounds! I don't want a fat man!"

"Why didn't you pray for a thin rich man?" I asked.

She didn't marry him. As it happened, he died two weeks later. She could have had all his money, but chances are, she still wouldn't have been happy. Can you see how foolish such a prayer can be?

I think prayer is nothing more than putting your wishes, your complete desires, your undivided attention, in one direction so that something really can happen. There is no such thing as a "vacuum" in nature or in life. Something has to fill it. Prayer creates a kind of vacuum toward which whatever is prayed for begins to move. Prayer is an attracting power.

If you don't want a fat man in answer to your prayer, you will have to be more specific when you pray. But I think sometimes it is better to say, "Thy will be done, not mine," so that whatever we are doing. we are working on a godly path, and whatever moment comes to us is the moment we are supposed to have. The moment you accept your experience and realize it is for a lesson, then you are ready to move on.

The Inner Self Is A Powerful Self

Do you understand how the physical and the mental sides work together? These are the two ways I am speaking of. If we get this inner world straightened out, the outer world around us will change. We will find we are working with something entirely different. Sometimes you may be working with disease. Sometimes you may be working with prevention. "An ounce of prevention is worth a pound of cure," as the saying goes. I find it difficult to work with people coming to me all burned out. It isn't really the right time to repair the barn door after the horse has run away. We need to fix that door ahead of time. Why can't we do right to prevent disease?

Prevention is necessary. Once when I was traveling with my friend Wally through the mountains on the South Island of New Zealand, I asked him to go to the local airport and reserve a plane for me so I could take some aerial photographs. He reserved the smallest plane they had. Those people at the airport removed the wall panels from that little airplane so I could just lean over the side with my camera and take photos. As I strapped myself into the passenger seat, I couldn't help but think how small that plane was in comparison to those enormous mountain peaks we would be flying between.

We took off and were soon flying over those mountains. As I leaned over the side with my camera, I thought, "I've never seen mountain peaks this close — or this jagged." I began to wonder about the safety of this tiny plane as the pilot maneuvered around those huge dangerous peaks. "What if something happens?" I asked the pilot. He smiled and answered, "Before we left, I made sure nothing would happen."

That's prevention.

On another occasion a man took off in his light plane from Lake Wohlford in Southern California without checking his gas gauge, not realizing that the night before some kids had stolen most of his fuel. He was about 500 feet up when the engine coughed and died, and his plane crashed into the mountains. We need to look ahead.

Peace Of Mind Comes When We Plan Ahead

Once you have taken care in preparing for a certain situation, relax and enjoy it. Worrying about all the little things that could go wrong can cause you to "crack up" mentally. So, accept your lot and go along with the plan — after adding the proverbial ounce of prevention.

Now, there are people who refuse to listen to advice about prevention. We must not condemn them — or anyone else, for that matter. If we can't help a person, we must not hinder him. We shouldn't hinder a man in his progress. It isn't what we have, it's what we enjoy that counts. Can you see the two sides of this idea?

Many people fear what is yet to come. They look for things to fear. They look for signs that their fearfulness is justified. Then what they fear comes upon them. They attract what they fear, and if you are a fearful sort of person, I want you to learn that you can release fear completely from your life.

What is it that casts out fear? LOVE. Look again: "Perfect love casteth out fear," it says in Scripture. When you are filled with love, there is no room left for fear. Can you find the other side now?

If we can change the negative approach we have been using to one that is positive instead, then we have won. I think James Allen put it very well when he said, "As you think, you travel." Isn't that a wonderful idea? And as you love, you attract love. You are today where your thoughts have brought you. Tomorrow you will be where your thoughts have taken you. You cannot escape the results of your thoughts. But you can endure and learn, accept and be glad.

You will always gravitate toward that which you secretly love most. You will realize that vision. Into your hands will be placed the exact results of your thoughts. Whatever your present environment may be, you will fall, remain or rise with your thoughts, your vision, your ideals. You will then become as small as your controlling desire or as great as your dominant aspirations.

So, we are going to recognize that God is the Universal Mind, the Universal Path. We are going to treat people as we want to be treated. We are going to treat people right whether they like it or not. We don't have to love what they do, but we have to love people because we know they are on the path, too. They are seeking whether they know it or not. They are human. They are the children of a loving God. They must have a chance to make good just as we have the chance to make good.

Let Us Help People To Grow

I can't say I have never lied but I am glad I don't lie anymore. And because I have lied, I have to give others a chance. They are growing just like I grew. "I have cheated," they say, "but now I am finished with cheating. I am glad now that I can see how thoughts can disturb and destroy. Now that I know, I can do something about it. I was sick of the kingdom I was once in. So, I moved and I found that by sowing different thoughts, different ideals, different actions, different words, my life has changed. I never could have had a ranch with thirty-five people working for me when I was only eighteen years old. Can you understand that? I have attracted power to myself for my time. Some of you may say, "Thank God, I don't have his responsibilities." I thank God that I don't have your problems — but I also thank Him that I am able to help you with them.

Work to advance. Unfold the Great Within, the godly potential within you which can grow bigger and better than anything you have ever realized. You will never know what a beautiful life this is until you get out of kindergarten, until you stop squabbling and start growing. Take care of your "ten acres" as you would a sacred, Holy Ground. It belongs to you in the sense that it has been loaned to you. It is here for your use. Ask for the direction and the guidance you need to properly care for it. As you attract positive ideals to yourself, they will eventually affect your cell structure, bowels, kidneys, heart and eyes.

It is hard to believe such a wonderful path is ahead. Let us not strain — let us reach. Let us not force — let us shine. Let us not strive to get up — let us arise beautifully, without effort, because we find that in the Law of God everything works peacefully, harmoniously. Let us go through life quietly, beautifully, seeking the best of other people and giving forth the higher vibrations and thoughts which should be coming from us. Try this path and you will find a better life ahead.

Be Renewed By The Transforming Of Your Mind

The better life comes when we have transformed our mind. "Be ye therefore perfect even as your Father in heaven is perfect." We can be hell bound. We can have hell right here. The Garden of Eden is here, too, but man has put a chef, a stove and a can opener in it. Man has corrupted the Garden of Eden.

We have to return to the path to higher consciousness. We have been going our own way too long, and it hasn't worked. We must return to nature. We must return to God. We have tried the way of this world, and it has swallowed us up. It has given us disease and unhappiness. It has given us resistance and disturbances. It has given us people problems and food problems. Realize that in coming back to nature's path, God's path, asking to be admitted to God's kingdom which is within us, you establish the ground you should stand on. It should be Holy Ground.

Say to yourself, "This is me. This is my ground, and no one can disturb it because it is mine alone." I can tell you that when you walk, you will not walk the way someone else thinks you should walk. Nor will you copy the walk of someone else. You will walk as though the Father and you are one. You will find there will be no sickness because there is no sickness in spirit. There is no disturbance in spirit. There is only harmony and peace. There is only goodness and joy.

Assume that everything is all right, and all will be well. All is well. You have the privilege of choosing. You have free will. Think it over. All power is yours. You have the power of heaven and earth to move your life up, move your thoughts up. It is within your grasp.

When I say that all is well, realize that you must practice this concept. Start using it now. Everything is all right. You have been blessed.

Prayer

As we establish ourselves on this Holy Ground, we realize we have something that was before our bodies and before this world — "Even before Abraham was, I am. I am the beginning and the end. I am forever. I belong to something which is indestructible. I am that which controls all.

I am looking for a life from above down, recognizing that which is within is also above. That which is above is within. We are created in the image of God. Let us be reminded that we are the children of a loving God, that we have the privilege of living in God's kingdom. Let us ever have that desire to make a better life, that each day may be a better day and that we may be better persons before God and our fellow man.

We realize now that all is well when we accept that truth. We go forth. We have risen. We shine in the Light. And this is the Light that never fails. It is the LIGHT of GOD. And let it be so.

The Greatest Words in the Dictionary

To bless and be thankful
To forgive and forget
To direct your powers
To be still
To recognize
To be aware of
To glow
To grow
To radiate
To be joyful
To be serene, tranquil,loving and
To seek repose.

Chapter 21

God Is Bigger Than The Last Number

Everybody is looking for a
good doctor.
I am looking for a
good patient.

We have to learn to care enough about ourselves to reach out for the spiritual values. If people don't learn to care for themselves, they'll soon need a doctor to care for them. And, you know, doctors are helpless without good patients. If I had to choose just one gift to give to a patient, do you know what it would be? An untroubled spirit. A patient with an untroubled spirit would be a patient who cares enough for others to take good care of himself. Think about that for a moment. That is the kind of patient I'm looking for — one who really cares.

We talk a lot about taking care of our physical bodies because that is the down-to-earth basis for good health. We have to have good health to have comfort and contentment. And we all want these things. When we are suffering from aches, pain and disease, it seems impossible to be comfortable.

Contentment is also something we want for the mind and the spirit. Milk advertisements sometimes talk about "contented cows." We don't want milk from mean cows, do we? We don't want milk from nervous cows, do we? Mental and spiritual attitudes affect every gland in the body, every digestive juice in the body. These are unseen qualities, unknown factors. Yet they are very real. Everything that goes forth from the person with the contented mind and spirit is higher and better in quality.

In my profession we work with what are called "trigger symptoms." We want to know what first triggered a particular disease or ailment. We want to know what triggered the effects that we observe as symptoms in a patient's body.

For example, a lady brought her five-year-old daughter who was having tonsil trouble in to see me. I examined her, asked the mother a few questions and saw that one of the major problems was in the child's dict. So I said, "We'll go on a catarrhal free diet to eliminate the catarrh, phlegm and mucus developing in this little girl's body." We started on the diet, but a week later the girl's father came in, obviously disturbed. He said, "My wife just took our daughter to the family doctor, and he says the tonsils have to come out. But you told her they don't have to come out."

"Yes, that's right." I said, smiling at him. "I can see you are a little upset over this. I can certainly understand why, since you want to do the right thing for your daughter. Please sit down."

When he'd made himself more comfortable he sighed and admitted, "I'm really disturbed right now because I have to decide whether to take your advice or the family doctor's advice. I have to think this over."

Now, this man was thinking of a loved one, and when thoughts get mixed up with loved ones, people can become quite upset. If you have loved ones, you know what I mean. A parent always wants to do what's best for the children, but that isn't always easy.

"As you think about this," I said, "I suggest that you consider what might be causing the tonsil trouble. Ask yourself whether removing the tonsils would get at the real cause of the problem."

That seemed to catch him by surprise. "I hadn't thought of it that way," he said. "What do you think is causing the problem?"

"I'd rather have you ask that question to the doctor who wants to remove the tonsils," I said. "Why don't you give him a call?"

He used the phone in my office and when he'd finished the conversation he looked at me, elated. "Our doctor says it's stomach trouble that's causing the tonsilitis. He said my daughter's digestion is probably poor."

"That is very interesting," I replied. "Now I'd like you to call him back and ask him what's causing the digestion problem."

The look of elation disappeared from his face. I knew the answer but I wanted him to discover it for himself in a way that would leave absolutely no room for doubt in his mind. He phoned his doctor again and after talking with him a few minutes, hung up. He didn't appear entirely happy but I could see he was much more relaxed.

"My doctor said that my daughter's diet was causing the digestion problem," he said. "When I asked him why he didn't just change her diet instead of suggesting that the tonsils be removed, he couldn't give me a straight answer. I can see now that my daughter is in the right place."

Can you see how the emotions can complicate a situation like this? Great distress can arise just from thinking about such a problem, whether it involves health, family finances or our jobs.

People who become dissatisfied with their jobs often grow extremely irritable and mean-tempered. Then they bring this attitude into their homes at the end of the day and take it out on their families. After a while the wife begins saying, "I just can't stand being around John any more. He upsets me terribly. I've got to get away from him." We have seen this happen all too often. The unseen things of this world have a great deal of power over our lives.

At the Ranch a lady once said to me, "How can anyone have troubles here? The weather is beautiful, the garden is beautiful — everything is simply lovely!" One moment we know that God's in His heaven, and all's right with the world, and the next moment we remember the mortgage or the bad-tempered husband or the stingy boss, and down we go again.

Can you understand how thoughts can be involved in physical problems? Let's get our thinking straightened out. We know that God's in His heaven, and all's right with the world, so let's take a good look at ourselves. If we feel something wrong in our lives, that means it's time for a change. You must start thinking right for the sake of your nervous system, your health. If you don't cultivate good thoughts, you'll end up at your doctor's office, and he'll have to treat your nervous system.

We Need To Be Kind To Our Nerves

The network of nerves throughout your body is just like the electrical system that provides power for a city. Electric current flows through these "wires." When we are thinking good thoughts, the amount of electrical current is just right to animate life in the various parts of the body. Have you ever seen a flood or powerful windstorm tear down electrical poles and wires? A big flash accompanies the blowing out of power transformers, and sparks fly as wires are shorted out. Emotional storms and floods do much the same thing to our nervous systems. Then we have a nervous breakdown, a nervous blowout. I make a living on burned-out nervous systems, nervous systems that have had too much high-voltage on them too often.

That is why people run to resorts. We have

a health resort to lift people out of their problems and to get them to think better thoughts, to visualize brighter days ahead.

If we feel right now that we are in hell, we must seek better ways. This may seem easier said than done, but know that it is possible. Know that you *can* do it. You must learn to think good thoughts even when you are surrounded by confusion and disturbance. If you can't learn to remain calm when you owe money, when people don't treat you right or when the weather is miserable, you are asking for trouble with your nervous system.

Have you heard the expression, "He got up on the wrong side of the bed this morning"? Which side is that? Now, I don't know which is the "right" side and which is the "wrong" side. But I do know that if you get out of bed with the right thought, you will always get out on the right side.

You may reach a point where you say, "I can't take it any more. I can't take this world!" And, if I were there with you, do you know what I would say? I would say, "Congratulations! You have just learned the most important lesson that life can teach us!" The Good Book says you have to lose your life to save it. You have to let go. You have to "let go and let God." Why wait for a painfully devastating crisis to bring you to this point? Why not let go right now? God doesn't ever run destructive surges of electric current through our nervous systems. We are His children — and He loves us.

A loving father always wants what is best for his children. The difference between human fathers and the heavenly Father is that the heavenly Father always *knows* what is best for us. He doesn't have to guess at or agonize over complicated decisions. He *knows*! When we are living according to the will of the Father, he takes care that nothing comes our way that we can't handle. Nothing. But you know, every once in a while we move away from God's will. We get away from God consciousness. Then we stumble. We run into a stone wall. These are the lessons that show us we have taken a wrong turn on the path.

You must learn to take it easy on your nervous system. It wasn't created to take high-voltage. This is often a hard and uneasy world to live in. We have to rise above it. Christ said, "I am in this world but I am not of it." From the spiritual standpoint there are two worlds. We have to get out of this lower world to get into the higher one. We have to lose our life to save it.

A little girl once sent me a valentine on which she had written, "Dr. Jensen, you're out of this world!" That was her way of expressing a delightful compliment, but you know the old saying, "Out of the mouths of babes, wisdom is spoken."

"Yet show I unto you a more excellent way," wrote the Apostle Paul. And Solomon put it this way: "Happy is the man that findeth wisdom and the man that getteth understanding." Paul, Solomon and all the great spiritual teachers throughout history are pointing out the way for us. They can only point it out. Nobody can make us take it. We remain asleep until we gain enough wisdom to awaken. Then we see it. There are two worlds — the physical and the spiritual. The choice between them is up to you.

Why Do We Need Love?

Deep inside we all know we need love. This is an intuitional thing, an inborn awareness given to everyone. But if I asked you, "Do you know why you need love," what would you say? Most likely you would say something about companionship or romance. But I'm not talking about companionship or romance. I am talking about something much deeper.

Let's look at this another way. To simply love your friends and family members isn't enough. To simply love even your enemies isn't enough. *You must learn to love everyone you meet on the path of life.* Why? First and most simply, because it is right. Secondly, because you live on what you are giving forth. To love is necessary for your own good, for your own peace of mind, for your own health.

When we love we are harmonizing our relationship with both the spiritual world and the physical world. When we love we don't have to worry about what anyone has said or what anyone has done. What you say or do to me will always be all right — because I love you. Can you see that? And love is something you don't run out of by giving too much away. There is an endless supply, you know.

God is bigger than anything we can think of, did you know that? God became much bigger to me after I studied the universe and the galaxies and pondered the millions upon millions of stars and planets in the heavens. As a child I thought the earth was the only planet. Of course, I saw the sun make its rounds every day and the twinkling stars at night but I gave them little thought. It took my five-year-old son David to awaken me to the immensity of all this and the immensity of the God that created it.

While we were out walking one night I mentioned something to David about how many stars were out and how beautiful they were, and David asked, "How many are up there, daddy?"

"I don't know," I had to say.

"Well, you ought to know. You're my dad," he said. I had to chuckle at that and I thought, yes, perhaps I ought to know. But I don't. Then David looked up and said, "I'll bet the last number is up there."

The *last number*! Can you think in terms that great? And I'll bet David is right about that!

"God is love," we are told. If God is greater than "the last number," greater than all the stars and planets in all the galaxies, then we don't ever have to worry about running out of love.

Do You Need A Mental Adjustment?

I can give you an adjustment of the spine, but what you may need is an adjustment in your thinking. I could give you a colonic irrigation, but what you may need is to clean out your thinking. Whatever we do from the physical standpoint has its counterpart in the mental and spiritual realms. Personally, I don't believe we must become so spiritual that we neglect the physical aspect. But, I don't believe that the spiritual is more important, more fundamental than the physical. To me the physical is the effect, the end result of what we are doing at a mental and spiritual level. The physical condition is important because through it we can tell whether we are going the right way mentally and spiritually. Our physical state acts as a barometer, so to speak, that tells us how the weather is in the invisible realms of mind and spirit.

One of my teachers once told me you can never do anything for anyone except *awaken* him. Then he must do the rest himself. How do we awaken? You can start by telling yourself a few things: "I want to be able to see more. I want to expand and become a better person. I want to be able to accomplish more. I want to be able to see truth." Now you have asked for an awakening. The Good Book tells us, "Ask and ye shall receive." We have to ask for the right things. It is good to ask God for wisdom, guidance, light, vision and strength. Then you can handle anything.

When you find yourself having difficulty with a problem and you ask God to take it away, another problem will come in its place. Why? You have a lesson to learn with each problem that comes before you. It is unlikely that you will ever be entirely free of problems, until you begin to see and accept them as opportunities for growth.

Put A Little Light On The Problem

We should pray for light when we are having a hard time with a problem. Christ said, "I am the light of the world." He came to bring Truth to the world and He will not lead you astray. But He isn't going to do much for you unless you do your share. That's why you need to awaken to the Light. If you have a problem, you need to awaken to the lesson in it. Then it will leave and never return.

Don't run from problems. Don't try to avoid them. Put some light on the subject. Then you will sleep like a baby. Then you will find rest. We need a rested nervous system and we will never have one until we get away from worldly thinking.

Positive thinking is wonderful for the nervous system. Enter into the other world — the spiritual world. Let what you find there flow into and throughout your nervous system and you will be marvelously refreshed. You will encounter fewer troubles and handle them better. You will get well quickly when you have a physical problem. That is one reason why I like Christ's teachings. They are wonderful for the mind and the nervous system.

Seek The Still Waters

People who have frequent emotional storms in the sea of their lives really don't have the right spiritual atmosphere. You need to seek the still waters.

I'm sure God is quiet. The still, small voice that guides us doesn't come like thunder. You hear it in stillness. You will never hear it until you become very still. And there is a marvelous side benefit in this stillness. The body heals quickly when you learn to become really and truly still.

If you will practice quieting the mind, the bowel will become better. Your system will begin to recuperate. In a matter of a week or so you will change. Whenever any physical ailment you have is getting better, let this good news be known. Tell yourself and those around you, "I'm getting better!" This speeds up the healing even more.

A lady I know was telling me about the negative attitude of her house maid. She said, "All she talks about is how her misery is bothering her — misery this and misery that! Finally, I couldn't stand it any longer. I sat down with her and tried to teach her your approach to positive thinking. I asked her to try saying, 'I feel wonderful' as often as possible. I really wanted my home to feel better and I wanted her to feel better. Then she took a week off, and I guess with my complaining about her attitude she must have thought she might lose her job if she didn't show some interest in what I'd tried to teach her. When she came back to work I asked, 'How are you?' And she looked at me with a kind of funny expression and said, 'Hell, I'm well!' "

You Have To Feel Better Before You Can Feel Better

This is intended to be a world of joy. There is joy in serving others. There is joy in doing good for other people. There is joy in accomplishing things that benefit others. But you can't be sullen and experience joy. You can't be hateful and experience joy. Two conflicting emotions can't occupy the same mind at the same time. Can you see that?

It is impossible to feel good when you hate someone. I suspect there are people who "love" to hate people, who "love" to see people get hurt. But this is a sick kind of love. It would be better described as a twisted kind of pleasure rather than love. It is certainly not God's love they are expressing. Probably such people have a deeper hunger for love themselves but don't know how to open up and receive it. They need to let go and let God awaken them to the real joy of life.

When you feel better, I feel better. Did you know that? When my patients are getting better and share the good news with me, that is the nicest pay I could receive. It does something wonderful for me. When I have patients who are feeling worse, I go home and sometimes have difficulty sleeping, because their problems are my problems. When they are feeling better, I rejoice inside.

Even when I see you broken down, not thinking correctly, I still know there is a rose inside you. I still know there is a wonderful person inside you. And I know that you will become well as these qualities come forth to express what you really are.

All the power of the heavens has been vested within you. God is within you. Everything peaceful and harmonious and good is within you. If you let your body know this, you would be well. I am talking about a very physical manifestation. You people who have nervous problems, stop it — $10 please. You people who have heart problems, stop it — $10 please. You people who have sinus problems, stop it — $10 please. Can you understand this?

If you can get this idea working, it will change your life. You will walk down the street a new person. People who knew you before will blink in surprise and say to themselves, "I never realized anyone could change so much!" You have shed your old troubles. You have shed your negative attitudes. And you can say, "I FEEL WONDERFUL!"

Right now this is possible. But it must come from the spiritual realm to the mental realm before you can experience it at the physical level. And you must awaken first for this to happen. I can't sell it to you and say, "$10 please." I can't make it happen for you. The remedy is within, and only you can go there.

I have heard people say of me, "He carries a heavy load," but they are wrong. I am carrying beautiful opportunities — and sometimes I am carried along by them! I could never run the Ranch, I could never lecture, I could never write books, I could never treat as many as fifty patients a day, I could never do this day in and day out — unless I was moving right through life taking problems as they come, cutting them off and leaving them behind. I learned from one of my teachers a very important secret: "When you pray and give problems to your heavenly Father to take care of, leave them there!" Most people who take problems to the heavenly Father grab them right back within ten minutes after praying! They don't seem to find the faith it takes to leave them there. But now we are going to do it the right way.

Prayer

Father, as we give ourselves to Thee, we recognize that we walk in purity and goodness; we walk knowing that all is well. We recognize that with this wonderful sunshine and loveliness and these good people, it is a privilege to be living. We are thankful, and in this thankfulness, we are good to ourselves.

Father, we are thankful to Thee for showing us all this good. We are thankful for guidance that comes from on high. May we ever be acceptable in Thy sight in all that we do. Help us be good to one another.

Strengthen our belief in Thee and bring us close to Thee. I know that Thou wilt never forsake us.

From the Doctor's Pen . . .

TOGETHER

The road we travel in the days ahead
May be smooth for this moment, and hard the next
But as we walk, run or stand, go forward or backward—
The road today will be easier together.

The house we conceive and the bricks we carry
The struggle to get all the pieces to match
A million problems—as we struggle to finish the job—
But I love this, because we do it together.

We look and plan, and are pushed from pillar to post
Some moments are light, but a darkness comes
Then darkness fades, and the road opens up
When your hand's in mine, and we travel together.

God be with us in each moment of sight
Let us not plan, travel or build without seeking His guidance
Then whatever happens, till the end of the road
Let's keep on keeping on—God, you and I, together.

The path of the masters was trackless;
They left no before or a past.
All at once I awakened within me
And thanked God I knew I existed,
And had a presence among those that had mastered.
I saw my gesture reach out and become.

My training became helpless as I wandered;
My knowledge grew into existence to help me.
Confusion laid a path most people walk over,
But I took a seat and waited for wisdom to carry me.

My faith was as solid as the earth that held me;
I was as solid as the space that pressed me into shape;
I was as meek as the seed that knew its destiny;
I was as humble as the leaf bowing before the breeze.

I attended the music of the spheres in silent tribute
For my being was collected in the ears of feeling;
My knees no longer existed—
I was kneeling in the awareness of Law.

I hurried my spirit to the front seat occupation
But the stillness of all that surrounded me
Stopped all of restless travels, to the eye
That saw all from any point of vision.

Chapter 22

Peace: What Hast Thou To Do With Me?

We live on what we project from our inner self.

Do we have peace in the world today? As I looked at a newspaper recently, I noticed that inflation troubles continue, the president has serious problems and conflicts between nations are still going on. Peace with our neighbors? No, we don't have it. We don't have peace in our country. We don't have peace among people. Where does all this chaos begin? How can we ever hope to put an end to it?

We will have peace in the world when we first have peace in our own hearts. Peace starts with you. Peace starts with me.

In my experience I believe that very few people would seek health if sickness and disease were not so painful, inconvenient and indisposing. Most people are capable of just letting that war go on inside their bodies if only it wouldn't interfere with their pleasures and their jobs. When we are flat on our backs in bed or suffering from arthritis pains, we are limited in our pursuit of physical pleasures. There's something wrong with life. People want to be cured so they can get right back on that same old merry-go-round of poor eating habits and poor living habits.

Do you suppose it is possible that when we become sick, God might be trying to tell us something?

What Do You See In Life?

At this moment very few of us are aware of spirit working in and through us. We take it for granted as an unseen power but we pay very little attention to it. Yet, what is unseen is the most important power in the world. From the unseen, all form comes forth. Everything has to be in thought before it is actually brought into physical existence. It should be obvious to us that what is brought forth from selfish thought will be very different from what is brought forth from selfless thought. And it should be just as obvious that spiritual power and spiritual principles can only come into existence through selfless thinking.

When you look into the mirror you may think that what you see is all there is. But it is not. If we could learn to let the spiritual power flow down into the physical body, our physical problems would begin to heal. We can do this by just being quiet. Did you know that quietness can cure more people than anything else?

Many of the important qualities of life lie beyond the reach of the physical senses. Still, they definitely exist. Honesty exists, but what color is it? Peace exists, but how tall is it? These things don't have physical qualities. How do we get honesty? You acquire it. You appropriate honesty. It is yours for the asking, yours for the receiving. So is peace.

Some qualities must be earned; others are free. Life comes as a gift. Quietness comes as a gift. Peace comes as a gift. These things are free. But many people don't value a thing unless it has a price tag on it. Many people don't value a thing unless they have to fight for it. They might want peace if you told them they would have to pay for it or fight for it, but those are exactly the attitudes that destroy peace.

It's Time to Declare Peace

Covetousness and strife have nothing to do with peace. Peace is free and easy flowing. When you reach the center of stillness inside yourself, peace and quiet are there. When you have that peace, that quietness, covetousness and strife disappear. Peace and quiet are wonderful for the physical body. People in this country take tranquilizers in an attempt to find peace, but pills don't bring them peace. They need peace from their jobs, bosses, children, husbands or wives, friends and the hectic world around them. They are allowing themselves to be destroyed by the turbulence around them. Yet, all this time peace and quiet are available for the asking. We need to attract more quietness, peace and harmony into our lives. That's the best tranquilizer you'll ever find. How do we do it? We go within. When we find that inner peace and let it flow out we will find that the outer physical life changes. We attract more peace when we express it by letting it flow out.

Your doctor should give you hope. There is peace in hope. There is quietness in hope. We feel better in hope. That's why we study nature, isn't it? In the constant renewal of living things, in the constant return of spring, there is hope. Can you hear the grass grow? Can you hear a poppy open in the morning sun? How peacefully the poppy opens! The wonderfully fragrant apple blossoms take four days to open, but when they come out there is no big noise.

In human culture it is always the squeaking wheel that gets the grease. It is always the crying babe that gets the milk. We are running after all these noises. These noises make us jump and get moving. Yet if we greased the axle when we should, if we fed the babe before it cried, we wouldn't have these noises, would we? Can you see where these noises are coming from?

Can we stand in peace? Can we walk in peace through the valley of the shadow of death? Of course we can.

How To Attain Peace

When we are in the process of acquiring a good physical body, we must remember that every single thought, every single emotion, affects that process. These mental activities accumulate day by day, instant by instant, to build a better body.

If you want good health, you can make a change in "a twinkling of an eye." You can take a new path. You can have peace and quiet and harmony. We start at the spiritual level. Now, I can't change your physical body in the twinkling of an eye because in the physical world we are creatures of time. It takes time for the effects of the mental and spiritual work to affect the body. But there is no time in spirit.

Spirit, life and eternity are here to stay. It is we who go. Truth is always here — it never changes. We grow impatient with the physical body because we are creatures of change. When I treat my patients, my goal for them is a peaceful mind.

As we begin to see what is best for us, we begin to seek peace and harmony. Peace is the remedy that cures. Drugs, with their cumulative effects upon the body and their harmful side-effects, will not change your mind at all.

Today we hear talk about the conquest of space. We send astronauts to the moon in rockets, but they land just as frustrated as when they left the earth. The space we need to explore most is the space between our ears! This is the space we need to know more about — not outer space but inner space. We need to take a rocket journey there.

I would say that fifty percent of all the troubles that come to me are space problems — the space between the ears. We haven't conquered that frontier yet. We are going *out* for the cure when we should be going *in* for it. To find the cure that is needed, we have to probe into deep space: deep inner space. Where will we find peace? Within.

Can you conceive of the kingdom of heaven in turmoil? Can you conceive of the kingdom of heaven without peace? No, you cannot. Know that the kingdom of heaven is in you now. An untroubled mind is the one gift I would like to give you more than any other. An untroubled mind is a peaceful mind.

The Prince Of Peace

The *Bible* speaks of Christ as the Prince of Peace. Is there anything we need more than peace? The Prince of Peace came to tell us that the kingdom of heaven is within. He came to tell us that is where we must go to find peace.

Yet, we live on a warring, hating planet. Mars, called the angry red planet, was named after the Roman god of war. Maybe the planet earth was wrongly named. Everybody is fighting for a living. Everybody is fighting for the dollar. You even have to fight to keep your man or woman. Everybody seems to be fighting for everything.

We see fighting everywhere. Look at the divorce rate in this country. Look at television, the movies, the newspapers. No peace. No harmony. Once a year Christmas comes, Christmas goes. The Prince of Peace comes into this world and dies again the following day.

If it weren't for the fact that people live so wretchedly for 364 days of the year, I wouldn't be making a living. Why don't you start cheating me out of a living? I dare you to. But, the only way you can keep me from making a living is to live a peaceful life.

You have to find peace in your garden. You have to find peace in vegetables and fruit. If you eat green apricots or green apples you won't find peace. If you eat the wrong foods you won't find peace. There is no peace in drinking, smoking or wrong living. So, the first order of business is to turn around. Change inside and begin going the right direction. Get rid of the turmoil you are harboring inside. If you want a better outlook, get a better inlook. Start going inside, then come outward.

Do you think you can find peace in coffee and donuts? I'll tell you that you can't live on these kinds of foods and have peace in this world. You will never have peace until you start living right and eating right. We will never have peace in the world until we have peace in our own homes first. Peace begins in the spiritual plane then moves through the mental plane before it comes into physical existence.

Many wars, I believe, start right in the coffee pot. A chain-smoker has brown fingertips from the nicotine. If his fingers are brown, what do his lung and brain tissue look like? Can you think clean and smoke? No, you can't. You can't live a clean life on coffee and donuts. Only the person who lives a clean life can find peace and good health.

If we are going to have peace in this life we'll have to cut out white flour and white sugar, too. People become miserable as a result of eating foods with these ingredients. A miserable person does not walk in peace and harmony. You have to face truth to produce peace. You have to face truth in your inner nature. You have to face truth with your food and your attitudes. We are talking partly from the physical standpoint but we need spiritual ideals to lift us from these poor habits.

Good Attitudes Bring Peace

The average person has very little conscience or consciousness, although we occasionally come upon some inspiring examples. I wonder why Abraham Lincoln walked seven miles to return three cents to a customer he overcharged. I wonder why Ghandi took the path of nonviolence in a world where violence is so prevalent. Are the people in our mental institutions going to walk out in peace when they live on pork chops, fried potatoes and canned foods? No. These foods are keeping those people in there.

There is no hope without peace and there is no peace without hope. It has to start with good attitudes. There is no hope in a way of life that breeds conflict and stress. I can't offer you anything if you are going to live in an unnatural way. It is simply impossible. I know of people once given three weeks to live who are still walking around today. They made a change in their lives. They saw a new way, a new path — and they took up the challenge. They felt that in right thinking, right attitudes, God was with them.

If there is going to be any healing, it is going to be in harmony with the way of God. This may sound unorthodox, but it is the only way I know how to put it. Today we too often look to the wisdom of man for the solutions to our problems. It isn't enough. It has never been enough.

Do you know that the word *peace* used to be a salutation when people met? When they came together and when they parted they said, "Peace be unto you." Isn't that a fine gesture of good will? "Peace be to this house." What a greeting! But these days we say, "How are you?" Then people proceed to unload their problems and troubles on us. That is a far departure from peace.

I would like to bring some helpful thoughts to you today. I want you to have peace. I want you to have harmony. If we were to meet face-to-face, I would say, "Peace be unto you." If you ask me, "How are you?" I'm going to respond by saying, "I feel wonderful!" You don't have time to think about your troubles when you are thinking and talking like that. You are too busy looking for something wonderful.

Peace Must Begin With You

Most people say we will have peace when we have disarmament. That's wrong. Disarmament comes as a result of peace. We hear people say, "I'll treat you right if you treat me right." But you have to treat people right even if they don't treat you right. Someone has to start right. Let peace begin with you. Share it with friends. Share it with me. Why don't we start an epidemic of peace in this country?

The problem is, we don't know how to walk in the godly light. In a telephone booth one day I found a notebook with a note in it that said, "Be sure to call Dan tonight and cuss him out." We don't know what it is to follow the godly channel. We are not bringing peace to ourselves.

Peace has to begin with you. You can't have good will toward a person and hate him at the same time. "Peace on earth, good will toward men." You find your prayers are answered when you express good will toward others. Prayers are answered through people. People return what you give to them.

Everybody is waiting around for somebody to make the first move toward peace. Every time you begin a peaceful activity, your life is changed and your family and neighbors are changed. It spreads. This is what I mean by an epidemic of peace.

Sometimes food for the mind is what we need, the kind of food that brings peace. "Oh, you're a sight for sore eyes!" "Your voice is music to my ears!" These are words of comfort. Comfort brings peace. "I like to be with you." It's a peaceful union, a peaceful connection, a peaceful communion. We bring the best out in each other. We bring peace out in each other. Isn't that what we want?

Where Is Peace?

To have peace, you have to pick good friends. You have to pick the right people and stay away from spitty, spiteful, mean people who try to hurt you. Let them hurt each other. Let them find their own level. Get away from them, find people who make you feel good and you'll find health. Marriages can make well people sick and marriages can make sick people well. When we need each other and love each other, the effect is healing. When we need each other we look for the harmony each can bring the other. But if we rub each other the wrong way, we produce sickness.

Love and harmony bring up a blood count faster than anything else. Money can't do it. A banker may be handling a million dollars a day. Is his life any better, any happier, any more peaceful for it?

It is said, "Peace on earth," and "Thy will be done on earth as it is in heaven." Too many of you think you have to die to reach the kingdom of heaven. If you really want to live right, you're going to find the kingdom of heaven in this life. You're going to find peace on earth *right now.*

Wouldn't it be wonderful for your mind to be transformed to the mind of the Prince of Peace? Wouldn't it be beautiful to have a transformed mind and to walk in peace?

One of the scenes pictured in the Good Book is, "The land was wide, quiet and peaceable." Isn't that a lovely description? There's a lot of territory to walk through in this life, and as you walk through, no matter how wide the land is, walk quietly.

The *Bible* says, "My people shall dwell in a peaceable habitation," and that verse has a special meaning to me. When I was in Vancouver, Canada, someone asked how large my Ranch was and how many people I could seat in the dining room. I explained that our dining room was small and could only seat about sixteen people and I looked forward to the day I could enlarge it to a seating capacity for eighty to a hundred people.

One man stood up and said, "I am a contractor and I would come to California to build you a larger dining room if I had help." Another man rose and said, "I'd be glad to go down with you and help build the dining room." Still another said, "I'd like to help, too." Can you guess how our dining room here at the Ranch was built?

Twelve men came from British Columbia and built that dining room. It was built out of love. These people were wide in consciousness. They worked quietly. It was done very peaceably, very lovingly. These men led a quiet and peaceable life. They speak peaceably with God. They live peaceably with their fellow men. The Good Book says, "Blessed are the peacemakers, for they shall be called the children of God."

Whenever you bring peace to another person, you can't bring hurt. If you are not bringing peace, there is hurt. Remember that.

I would like to leave you with this thought: "What hast thou to do with peace?" Think about this. What have *you* to do with peace? The secret of your health is found in peace. Heaven is found in peace. The Prince of Peace has come to you.

Let our hearts and minds be filled with peace. I know and you know that if peace is going to come into existence today, it must start within each of us. Let us realize that we have a God of Peace. Let us live close to that God of Peace today, for we know that God will never let us down. We need this peace. We walk in peace and harmony.

It is by yourself without ambassador that God speaks to you. You are as one who has a private door that leads him to the king's chamber.
— Ralph Waldo Emerson

From the Doctor's Pen . . .

LOVE

Love seasons all of our movements;
Love flavors each word of the tongue;
Love is the honey in kindness;
Love is the time we live well.

Love sends each word on to heaven;
Love balances the day to make good;
Love is the wrapper we put on the gift,
And makes it a gift of God.

Love makes life's pictures worth seeing;
Love soothes the hurt of the hand
Love is the substance in mixture,
Needed in talk, in walk and in deed.

Love gives power to friendship;
Love lifts the fall of the sparrow;
Love is the care we build life with;
Love gives touch the hand cannot feel.

Love is the heart of a Master;
Love is the garment he wears;
Love is the substance he heals with
And resurrects life to the highest up there.

Love is the attraction in color;
Love gives the gardener his care;
Love is the growth that lifts us upward
So gardener and garden toil together up there.

Chapter 23

Let's Go In Peace—NOT In Pieces!

The more truth you have, the more alone you go.

When I get up to greet each new day I like to say, "G...o...o...d morning" to every person I meet. Why are mornings so wonderful? Once someone gave me a reason that I think is marvelous — *the sun!* The sun is the most uplifting power we have on this earth. Can you think of anything more uplifting, more energizing, than that first glimmer of golden morning sunlight that sets the dewdrops sparkling on the grass and flowers?

With all due respect for April showers and rain in general, I could do without it. But not the sun! When we can't have the sun, we really feel that something has been taken away from us. There are people who pray for rain, and sometimes I wish they wouldn't. But we never stop praying for the sunshine. Sunshine is one of the greatest needs we have. It is a giver of life.

Sunshine represents happiness to us. It lightens our day. It makes us feel better. We recognize that we need to feel good, and the sun makes us feel good just as our friends make us feel good.

In fact, we pick out certain people as friends because they make us feel good, don't we? You have to be around good people. You have to avoid negative people who constantly rub you the wrong way, because they can destroy you. They can hurt you. They run you *down*, so to speak. When you find yourself with people who leave you "down in the mouth" or "down in the dumps," you must realize that you shouldn't have been with them in the first place. For your own good it is necessary for you to choose your companions with care. I don't think anything ever "just happens." I think everything "happens just."

After all — we must be good to ourselves. Your feelings are very important. So are mine. When we stop and think about this, we will take care of one another's feelings. So, when I say, "I feel good," don't spoil that. Don't tell me something that will drag me down or destroy my good feelings. Feelings are among the most powerful things in the world. You can tell when a person is feeling good by the way he or she looks, can't you? Down in New Zealand when they meet someone, they say, "You look like a box of birds this morning!" Isn't that a wonderful expression? The person's feelings are showing. And if you don't look and feel very well, this is what they say: "You look like seven miles of bad road."

Our feelings show in our faces, in our expressions. This is what I want you to see — we start with the mind to get to the body. Most people think the opposite way. Most people want the carrot juice first. They believe if the body feels all right, then they will feel good mentally. We have to start feeling right mentally first.

You see, when most of you want something, you think that after you get it you'll feel good. But the law of the mind is this: You have everything you need *right now* to feel good. If you don't feel good, it is your fault.

So we want to be developing these feelings of good, we want to be getting into this world of feelings, changing our life so that this physical body — made of the dust of the earth — isn't shattered. People come to me as nervous wrecks. They say, "Look at me, shaking and all tired out." They haven't started right mentally.

Mental feelings can't be bought. I can put it this way: You acquire them by appropriation. This is a difficult point to get across. The feelings are already there inside you, potentially available. You just appropriate them.

Money, so it is said, is a comfort to the nerves. Most people go through life seeking a mountain of money and a mountain of tangible things that give them a feeling of security. But truly, the person who already has contentment is the richest person in the world. Contentment starts with peace and harmony. These are things you can't buy. You earn them. You acquire peace and harmony. You are aware of peace and harmony. There isn't a doctor or drug store in the world that can give you these things.

There is only one person who can help you. Two thousand years ago, a man was making his way through a thick crowd of people when a woman reached out and touched the hem of his garment. He stopped and said, "Who touched my clothes?" The woman, trembling, came forward and confessed that she had touched his garment, certain that by doing so she would be healed of a problem many doctors had been unable to cure. The man was Christ, and He said, "Daughter, thy faith hath made thee whole." And, she was cured. Now, He didn't say, "*I* have made thee whole." Christ came to tell us we have to do it ourselves. You have to do it yourself. You have to reach. You have to touch. You have to have faith that it will happen. You know, we could sit in the lap of the Christ and never get healed. Or, if we did, we would soon get sick again if we still believed and behaved in the same old ways. This is a hard fact to get across, but you must realize that you yourself are the only person who can make the basic changes necessary to bring wholeness and health into your life.

What Do You Believe In?

I want to share with you some of the truths I really believe in. When I say, "Really believe in," I must add that I believe in good food, exercise and other physical aspects of healthy living. Don't think for a minute that I don't believe in carrot juice! But I'm not talking about carrot juice this time. I'm going to give that business a rest.

I have something else to say, and that is about the relation of our physical body to our spiritual attitude. How rich can a person be? I think the richest person knows what it is to walk forward in absolute peace.

It is said, "If you give a person a piece of your mind, you lose your peace of mind." We are talking about agitation. We are talking about violence. We are talking about war. Some people are at war with themselves. They are living in violence within themselves. Now, we want to go in peace, not in pieces.

Wouldn't it be wonderful to live with peace within yourself?

Have you ever been to a funeral? Friends and relatives pass by the coffin and say, "Doesn't he look peaceful?" Wouldn't it be nice if we could possess that calmness, that peace, while we are still alive? Wouldn't it be nice to have that peace in your marriage, your work and your relationships with friends? I am very serious about this idea. Peace is not just something that we receive only after the physical life is over. We are meant to have peace in this life.

When patients come to me with their "war" problems, I am reminded of the story about the man who went to the psychiatrist and said, "Doctor, I have fleas all over me!" As he began vigorously brushing himself off, the psychiatrist objected, "Don't brush them off on me!" Don't brush your troubles off on me — or anyone else. You have to be very strong today to go through life and not take on other people's problems.

The wisest man is the one who leaves other people alone. Leave the other person alone. I don't want to raise you. That was your mother's job. I am not going to take care of you. But there is one thing I am going to do, I am going to learn to agree with you so there is no agitation between us. The Good Book says, "Agree with thine adversary." When you do that, there is no adversary, is there? It always takes two to argue. If one stops, there's no more argument. "If you can't fight them, join them," the saying goes. There are no winners in fights, arguments or wars. There are only losers.

People Need Spiritual Glasses

If people can't see what you are trying to tell them, you must have enough compassion to understand that at their level, they just can't see. This is a point you have to realize. That is why we have to bless even the people who steal from us. They don't know any better. That is why you even have to bless the one who "sits" on you because he doesn't know any better. But there isn't anything he can do to disturb or break up the peace and harmony that you carry inside yourself. He can't touch what is inside you unless you let him. Now, I don't really care whether you want peace of mind or not. But I want you to know that your body needs it — for the sake of your health.

Most doctors don't care if you have peace, or they would end up in the unemployment line. Doctors make a living from the chaos in your life.

I say this because I would like you to get closer to the idea of peace. That heavenly Voice speaks to us only through that inner silence during times of peace and calm. It does not speak through chaos. The Voice doesn't come from the devil or hell; it doesn't come from the enemy. I have to say it comes from God. It has to come from a spiritual standpoint.

That is why we have to be aware of the spiritual presence, and I think it is a matter of looking again. Get out of that hellish mess you are in. Get out of your agitation and war. As I have mentioned many times before, the Good Book tells you, "Lift up your eyes and look on the fields, for they are white already to harvest." It's all right here. The fields are white. The harvest is here, and it is ready now!

Recently a man said to me, "I saw a doctor a year ago, and he said that in a year's time I would have a terrible glandular condition, and you know, it has been weighing on my mind ever since." It has been weighing on his mind ever since! Look at what we accept! We accept a doctor's interpretation, and it can so weigh on our minds that it can actually come to pass. Whatever we fear, we bring into existence.

One of the doctors at the Ranch used to tell patients, "I'm afraid you're going to be happy!" Wouldn't it be interesting to go around telling patients, "I'm afraid you're going to be well"? But, you know, it is never going to happen until you take it upon yourself to do it. The cure is not in the doctor but in you. We can treat you, but you have to cure yourself.

Reach For What You Want

Everybody is looking for a good doctor, and every doctor is looking for a good patient. I have to find a good patient, because otherwise where are my efforts going to lead? Do you think I want to waste my time? Is health going to pass right by you because you can't take it? Is it going to miss you today because you don't want it? Is health going to skip you because you're not ready? What a terrible thought!

We have to reach, now. We have to touch truth and we have to accept it. When you come in to see me, the first thing I am interested in checking is the body's vital organs. I am most interested in your heart. Your complaint might be of pain in the toe, but I want to see if the heart problem is causing the toe problem. So, I am interested in the heart. I am interested in the kidneys, which could be causing uric acid problems. This could cause rheumatism. And you may say, "My knees are bad" or "I have a shoulder problem." So, I have to check the kidneys. I have to watch those vital organs.

If a person comes to me with a terrible headache, I might look at his head, but what could I possibly put on it to help that headache? A mud pack? Am I going to work with the head or am I going to look for the cause of the headache? Perhaps the cause is in a vital organ. So, I am going to look for the vital spot, the vital problem at the root of this thing. Now, my next step is this: If you come to me a nervous wreck complaining of stomach problems, I know what I have to deal with. The most vital cause here is your thoughts.

I am going to say that thoughts are real. I can't tell you what shape they are, but when I previously mentioned the man whose problem had been "weighing" on his mind for a year, I believe it must have had some weight. Weight is a property of "reality," isn't it? He bemoans the fact — or is he afraid to think of it? These are mind inventions. These are vital facts. These are solid facts that we have to face.

I go to the mind in such a case to change the body. But when you are in my office, I first check the vital organs — the heart, the kidneys, the liver. I want to know exactly what is going on there.

You are worrying about symptoms today. I can tell you that most high blood pressures are from the head, from the thinking. Half of your vital organ problems result from the kind of thinking you do. These thoughts, in themselves, may not even be bad. You know, a person can be too sincere for his own good, too serious for his own good. He can overdo. *He can be too harsh on himself in doing good.* I have seen many people apply so much pressure on themselves to do what is right that they wear themselves out. They are hard on their body, hard on their feelings. Even efforts to do good must be in moderation. My dad used to have a sign on his door that said, "If you can't do it perfectly, don't do it!" He wanted us kids to do right so much that he would beat the devil out of us to make us do it.

Discipline Your Mind

I think discipline has its place, but instead of the discipline that comes from a strap or the back of a hairbrush, I want to discuss the discipline of the mind in relation to taking in what is right or wrong. You can give yourself a terrible licking when you don't go the right way mentally. You get back what you give, you see. You attract what you give out. I want to emphasize that one of the greatest spiritual and mental principles is that we live on what we give out — what we pour forth. We determine the feelings within our body by what we give out. I know this. It is one of the greatest revelations I have ever come upon.

It is a simple fact that I can only give you what I have. I am what I am. To me this is a wonderful axiom. Let us have a little "truth serum" for the mind's sake, because eventually it is going to get to the body. There isn't anything you think that isn't finally going to affect the body.

Do you know how lie detectors work? They measure the breathing rate, the electrical conductivity of the skin and the blood pressure. You sit in a chair, and the police attach these gadgets to you that are hooked up to the lie detector machine. Then they ask, "Did you do this? Did you shoot this man?" If you lie, your blood pressure goes up and your breathing rate and skin conductivity change, sometimes off the scale of the machine. Your body knows what you have inside your mind. When you tell a lie, physiological changes take place in the body. You can't fool your body, and your body can't fool that machine.

All thoughts affect the body. That is why it is definitely to your advantage to straighten out what is within you. My teacher taught me that what you are deepest, you really are. Do you know how deep that is? All the way to the center of your life. All the way to where life begins to come out. I have seen people weep tears of joy. I have seen people weep tears of sorrow. These mental extremes cause corresponding physical reactions in the body.

I wonder where your blood pressure comes from? Where does your twitching come from? Where does that ulcer come from? What are you taking into your life? What are you giving forth? That's something to stop and think about.

Recently I heard about a man who died on the witness stand while testifying against his wife in the divorce court. We have to be careful how we testify. In the larger court of life we must testify and witness to all the good we possibly can.

Exalt The Within

Now I am going to tell you something very important — we must start from within and exalt the within. In the exaltation of the within we lift the body to greater harmony and better health. This I know. This I really and truly know.

In the process of doing this we relax and bring relief to the physical body. Some people need glasses, and I think you should wear glasses if the alternative is a strain on your nervous system. The glasses can be used to relieve a strain. But look what so many doctors are doing to relieve strain and stress. If you are nervous and upset they will prescribe tranquilizers for you. They are treating your symptoms but they aren't raising your consciousness. They are treating you but they aren't teaching you to live a better life.

As you go through life, you should be a better person for every single day's living. You should be a better man or woman today than you were yesterday. I am going to be a better man an hour from now. I must be. Otherwise, what's the point of living? If you are just taking in everything you can, you must take whatever consequences come to you.

Life deals out consequences. When I have gone the right direction with you, I want those consequences to come. When I have gone the wrong direction, I don't want those consequences. The whole point is, we must do what is right. We walk that path and we walk it gently and compassionately, reflecting the guidance of that Voice from heaven.

Whatever comes to me, I am going to accept — good or bad. There are many people who can walk the right path for a while. Then you hear, "I don't like what he did," and they get sick over it. You should be a happy person. You have earned that right. You have given everything you have, so kick the dust from your heels and go right on. When you have given your very best to a person, that is all you can do.

Let's take the weight off the body and the mind right now. We can start with peace — peace and harmony.

What is peace? My dictionary says it is "a state of quietness or tranquility." Most doctors want their patients to be tranquil. Otherwise, why would they give them tranquilizers? So, why don't you start developing your own state of tranquility? You don't have to move from the state of New York to some other place. Just stay right where you are and move into a new state of mind. We'll call that the 51st state! And you will have to establish it by appropriating it. You will have to make it yourself from within.

Congress will never legislate this state into existence. You'll have to create this environment yourself. No lawmaker can legislate good feelings. No king or queen can grant you happiness. You may think that if you were a king you could be happy. But I know kings who have their problems, too. The answer isn't wealth or power, because these things can so easily bring misery.

Long ago, King Charles of England was out riding with a group of his courtiers when he saw an old man walking down the road. Though dressed like a beggar, the old man carried himself with unusual dignity, so King Charles rode up beside him, dismounted from his white charger and asked, "Who are you?"

"I am a king," the old man replied.

"A king? What are you king of?" asked the surprised King of England.

"I'm king of myself," came the dignified answer.

You are king of yourself today or queen of yourself. But you can't be a king or a queen unless you express it and let it come forth. Let it come forth!

Cultivate Your Own "Ten Acres"

In a sense, your inner world is your own plot of ground, your own "ten acres" to cultivate as you choose. If you start treating that "ten acres" as your own personal kingdom and cultivate it properly, it will bear good fruit for you. You will have freedom from disturbance, freedom from agitation. You will have peace and harmony and agreement all around you. Now, it isn't an easy task to be in agreement with life, considering the way the world is these days. The question to be determined is what, exactly, your area of responsibility is.

Your responsibility is to start with your own "ten acres" and to begin improving the world by improving yourself. Let peace be in this world, but let it start with you and me. I don't want to do it all. I can't do it all. Sometimes it seems as though we are all alone in this task, and then we ask ourselves, "What's the use?" It seems that it is just too much for us. But we can't let ourselves think this way. There is much good in this world if we open our eyes to it and keep up with our own responsibilities. You just take care of your own "ten acres." You can make that "ten acres" into the most beautiful place in the world, and then everything else will take care of itself. Your job is to bring that beautiful "ten acres" into existence.

When we talk about existence, isn't it interesting that the prefix "ex" means to go out? Existence is the outside reality. Why don't we invent the word "inistence"? Inistence would be the inner reality. That's a new word, one that Webster hasn't come to yet. But if we start with a good inistence and come forward from that, we'll have a good existence, because the outside depends upon the inside. I know people who have had poor health, and they live for many years because they have such a wonderful inner self. They have a good inistence; they are going in the right direction.

It would be useful for those who concentrate on the spiritual life, the inner life, to know that it is also necessary to take good care of the physical body. It would be wonderful if they knew how to eat right as well as to pray right and think right. Wouldn't it be marvelous to put these things all together, to really be a "whole" person in every sense of the word? Today there are people praying one minute and drinking a can of soda pop the next minute. I feel this is a crime.

On the other hand, just to go through all the physical motions of health — eating good wholesome salads and other nutritious foods — isn't enough. What kind of existence can you have without love in your heart? So you see we are talking about an all-inclusive philosophy of life. If heaven is just a spiritual concept, then why do we pray, "Thy will be done on earth as it is in heaven"? No, heaven is not just a spiritual concept. The heavenly state is when you are in good health physically, mentally and spiritually. This is heaven.

The world cannot have heaven as long as there is revolution. And you are not in heaven when there is a revolution going on in your stomach. Just try to meditate when you are in pain! Physical life is important, but we can't emphasize the physical life to the exclusion of the mental and spiritual life. Don't give it 100 percent. Give it just its rightful one-third and another third each to the spiritual and the mental.

You know, the Christ never called himself "the Christ." He said, "Whom say ye that I am?" He leaves you to decide what you see in Him. He said, "He that hath seen me hath seen the Father" — that is, if you are "seeing" right. That is why you can't afford to see anything but good in people. "I forgive you. I love you." If you can't accept my forgiveness, if you can't accept my love, then where are you? At what level are you thinking?

Take A Drive Down Love Street

I choose to go the way of love, and if you don't want to meet me at that level, I guess we don't belong together. But you're missing something. You're missing something, and so am I when we are not at the right level. Presumably, we have learned to be human. Let us learn to be godly.

To be human is to let go once in a while. They say that "to err is human." But is this the idea? No — we're going to find the higher way.

Peace is a state of calm and repose. Just calm yourself. Don't "blow your top." Don't "flip your lid." Kids today know what they are talking about, and they have the language for it.

We have to develop a peaceable relationship with one another. We have to have freedom from violence, freedom from crime, riots and war. There must be a cessation of these things. I'll tell you what peace is. Peace is spiritual contentment. Of all the truths I have shared with you about health, I want you to remember one point in particular. You will *never* get well until you realize that the body needs plenty of rest, good feelings and contentment.

So, I return to my original statement that feeling is one of the most important things in the world. We have to learn to agree, yet lead. We have to realize that feeling begins in the mind, in our attitude, in our altitude. Your attitude is your altitude. We have to know what it is to let go of the human way and to go the godly way. Now, nobody should go around saying, "I am God." People who say that sort of thing still have much to learn. You don't need a label on your lapel to explain who you are or what you believe. People will know that by what you do.

When you stop and think, God is beyond all human concepts of size, beyond all human concepts of time and space. We say He is omnipresent, everywhere all the time. Don't think of God as a power just to be used at your own convenience. Some people have a "spare tire God," whom they leave in the trunk until they have a blowout or flat. Let God be a constantly working Principle within you. As I say, this comes from practicing good thinking and self-exaltation.

You will hear many people saying, "I am broke. I've been left out. Look at him and what he's got. He's so lucky." Let's get away from feeling sorry for ourselves and from looking for sympathy. Let us find our own good. You have to cultivate your own "ten acres" because nobody else is going to do it for you. Do it right and you will be standing on holy ground. That's the only way to see it.

The World Is A Stage — And Heaven Is Watching

You have excellent qualities. I know that. I've found them in everyone. A short time ago in England, an actor explained his brilliant success by saying, "When I act, I act as though I am playing to the king." We are all actors and actresses — and we must realize that we are acting before the King of kings, the Father in heaven.

Many years ago I learned from mother that we must love friends, enemies and everyone else — not for their sake — but for our own sake. It's not that your enemy *needs* your love; sometimes they seem to need a good "shaking up" instead. But you need to have that love pouring forth from you for your own good. Leave the "shaking up" to the Law. " 'Vengeance is mine,' saith the Lord." The Lord is the Law. When you do the God-approved deed, it comes back to you. Let people reap their own consequences until they learn better. Aren't you glad you're finished with lying, cheating and stealing? People don't know how wonderful life can be until they have left these things behind.

The person who is tearing himself down is a misfit within himself. He becomes a physical wreck. I treat the physical body. You bring your physical body to me, and I say, "You can have a new body — but you will have to go back into your real self and exalt the God within you." I know that with God all things are possible.

Many of us don't take time to build ourselves up. We think of ourselves as "second class" human beings. Many people believe that they aren't really any good, that they haven't much of a future. They have no hope, nothing to live for. Let's get rid of this. Let's let our living soul shine forth. Our body needs and deserves a good tenant — not a beggar, but a king or a queen. Don't let that beautiful soul of yours lie dormant and unexpressed. Let it come forth.

As we go forward we recognize that God has made the path of our life possible by "breaking trail," by clearing the way, in front of us. He has the answers even before we ask the questions. We must work toward higher ideals constantly. We have to hold and keep our peace. We find God in everything, in every act, word and deed.

Let us walk the high way, the peaceful way. I am sure that all good will come to us. Let us realize that we need peace. As we think about this and as we come before God, we realize that we can only touch God as we become godly. We can have what is lofty only as we become lofty. Our acts, words and deeds come forth in direct proportion to the loftiness of our thoughts and the spirit we carry within.

We recognize that we need this and we ask that we may have it. But, in this same moment, let us recognize that to have this means we must share it with others, we must give it forth, to allow the complete circulation of life to take place.

So, as we have received, let us give that which we know is good. As children of God, let us live in His heavenly abode. Let us give of that heaven as we have received from it. Let us know what it is to relax in Him who knows our way and our path. Let us recognize this as the beginning of all healing, of all peace and harmony in our society today. Let us bless those around us and be thankful for that which we have. Let us enjoy that which we have, as little or as much as that may be.

Prayer

Let us recognize that we are rich when we have Thee, our heavenly Father. We go today in peace and harmony. We have been blessed.

One serves God best,
who serves his fellow man.

—Thomas Paine

Chapter 24

Laws Govern Our Lives

"No one sees his shadow who faces the sun."

We all know there are certain laws we have to live by. There are federal, state and local laws. There are criminal laws and tax laws and traffic laws. In nature we have the law of gravity, and we know that if we try to defy it we can break a leg or worse. In natural laws like the law of gravity we begin to encounter built-in punishments for violations. But in an even more subtle realm, there are laws of life itself. Now, there are no courts, no policemen, to enforce these laws. Just the same, if we disobey them, there are powerful consequences.

I would like to talk about some of these laws by which we live. You know if you go the wrong way on a one-way street in your car, you will be caught and punished if you don't have an accident first. There will be consequences. Who is going to decide what will happen to you if you go the wrong way in life?

Have you ever heard people say, "He brought it on himself"? Why did he bring it on himself? Is there a *law of attraction* by which you bring certain experiences to yourself? Yes, there is. If you recognize this law, you can use it to bring the better things into your life. And, there are many other laws.

"You Can Have Anything You Want In Life, But . . ."

If you don't like your life the way it is, you will have to change your direction. From the direction you choose, you will attract life experiences accordingly. That's the way the law works. I've mentioned before what my mother used to say: "You can have anything you want in life, but you have to take everything that goes with it."

If you live on coffee and donuts, I can tell you what consequences go with them. If you eat nice salads, I can tell you what consequences go with them, too. Eating the good foods brings good consequences. That is why you need to know the laws of life. You have to know what they are and how to follow them. When you get tired of being tired, when you get sick of being sick, you will realize that it is time for you to get back on the right side of the laws of life. You have been on the wrong side if you are often tired, sick or beset with troubles and problems.

You can thank these negative experiences for bringing you to the realization that you need to bring about a change in your life. Some of you will never make a change until you can't stand living the way you are. Do you know the story about the little frog who became trapped in a deep rut along a dirt road? This little frog spent almost half an hour trying to jump out of that rut, but it was too deep. His friends tried to help him get out, but everything they tried was in vain. However, an hour later his friends were surprised to see him hopping along the side of the road chuckling to himself and happy as could be. They rushed up to him and said, "My goodness, how did you ever get out of that deep rut?" And the little frog said, "Well, a truck came along — and I *had* to get out!" This is what happens to us.

We have to get out of the rut. But as long as we are holding on to our old habits, the law of attraction is going to keep bringing the same old consequences. You are going to keep your anxiety, fear and distress. So it's time for you to attract something else, something better. You can't change the law but you can get on the right side of it. Who is the lawyer to seek for help? The lawyer is you, putting the rules into action! Can you understand that?

You cannot disregard the laws. If you do, you lose every time! There are certain laws by which we must live. We may not like some of these laws, but we can't change them. We can only change the way we use them. Perhaps we like to live the way we do because it's become a habit or we don't know any better or maybe we're too lazy to make changes. Going into a new field is always difficult. Sometimes we automatically oppose anything new. We don't like to go into the unknown. But if we want to improve our lives we must live right. And that means living within the law.

That Good May Follow You . . .

We have a good many laws that are given to us from the ancient prophets. The Ten Commandments are laws. We obey them and when we do we find that something good happens. That is why Moses gave us the Ten Commandments — that we might follow a good way, so that good might follow us the rest of our lives. Isn't this what you want? I'm sure you do! All of us want good to follow us.

Many people think they can go the wrong way and still have good follow them. They have to learn the hard way. A God of good consequences doesn't work that way. A God of good consequences works in laws. He is always protected who lives within the Law.

I give those people who come to the Ranch a law which I'd like to tell you about. It is a law you see working all the time. It's called *Hering's Law of Cure*. Dr. Hering's Law of Cure tells us that all cure comes from within out, from the head down and in reverse order as symptoms first appeared.

When I use Hering's Law of Cure, I start with you where you are today. I have to change the acid-alkaline balance in your body. When I change this balance to one of less acid, all the tissues and cells of the body change to a different expression of health. Then I change these acids still more and add more chlorophyll and more of the resistance elements such as fluorine and calcium. Then I add more of the magnetic elements such as silicon. With all of these changes, the chronic condition begins to leave. Toxins are eliminated from the body, and tissue begins to rejuvenate. We have more health, more resistance.

To accomplish this, the body goes through healing crises in which old symptoms return for a few days as toxins are thrown off.

To take care of one part of the body, we must take care of the whole body and all its parts. This is a law. The Greek philosopher Plato made this proclamation over two thousand years ago. Any one part of your body cannot be well unless you care for the whole body.

To be well we must take care of ourselves through a life more abundant — not just through foods, not just through mechanical measures, not just through chiropractic, not just through osteopathy.

Many people have the idea that curing takes place only when the pain disappears or when stress disappears. This is not so! Many times when we start right living we have begun to get rid of the disease, but the pain does not leave on the first day. It hangs on. When the disease finally goes you are still healing for some time. When you get well you are going to have something to be thankful for during the remainder of your life. But if you get rid of a pain immediately and go back to the same old habits you had before, the same old condition—or a worse one—will return. That is what is wrong with drug therapy by and large. There is no reason to cure you just so you can return to the same old trouble. Why not get rid of it for all time?

The Mind Can Cure Or Kill

In the Good Book we find the law of belief used many, many times. Christ put it this way: "As thou hast believed, so be it done unto thee." We use this law constantly whether we realize it or not, and it works even under very surprising and unusual circumstances, as in the following stories, true episodes from medical history.

A man who had become very ill went to his doctor for an examination. Afterward, the doctor wrote up a report for this man in which he said that the fellow only had two weeks to live and that he should go up to the mountains — away from people — to enjoy these last days of his life.

Another man in good health came to the same doctor for an exam, and again the doctor wrote up a report. This one stated that the man was in excellent health and that he should live a good life, laugh and enjoy himself, get the best from life.

Somehow these two medical reports became mixed up and went to the wrong men. The sick man received the report of excellent health. The healthy man was told he only had two weeks to live. And, each followed the instructions he received. The healthy man went to the mountains to spend the last days of his life. The sick man followed instructions to live life to the fullest — and he regained good health.

In another true story in the medical records, approximately 200 people were dining in a French restaurant when the chef ran in from the kitchen, pale and distraught, and announced, "I am terribly sorry — there has been an accident. Arsenic has somehow been put into the food!" Immediately the diners became acutely ill with stomach cramps, and all were taken to hospitals. In the meantime the chef returned to the kitchen to investigate the circumstances of the accident and found that he had been mistaken! No arsenic had been used in preparing the food!

He telephoned all the hospitals and gave them the news. All of the 200 people who had been admitted in great pain and suffering made rapid and complete recoveries when they heard the news, walking out of the hospitals overjoyed that they hadn't, in fact, been poisoned. The law of belief is extremely powerful, and we must be careful about what we believe.

Once seven men were condemned to death by firing squad. Somehow blanks had been placed in the rifles instead of real bullets. The seven men were lined up against a wall, blindfolded, and the count was begun: "One, two, three . . . fire!" The rifle shots echoed, and six of the seven condemned men remained standing. But one of them had crumpled to the ground, killed by his own belief.

"Get Thee Behind Me, Satan"

The law of attraction is a most wonderful law. You must realize that whatever you bring to yourself you have earned and you are in need of that. The nice thing about this law is that as you progress and make the law work for you by changing your pattern of living, you bring on a good life and a good body with it. The body follows the mind, and you can make it do anything you want to. Whatever you are seeking in life is also seeking you. This is the law, and it is a wonderful law we can depend on.

We also have a law of denial. Some people prefer to go through life denying, doubting, scoffing at anything that isn't "scientifically proven" or anything they haven't seen with their own eyes. Now, the law of denial is valid when we apply it to untruth; but when we apply it to truth we begin living a lie. Because our beliefs can blind us to faults in our own thinking, we can live according to what is false for quite some time. Eventually, however, we are caught up in the consequences of our false beliefs. Consequences always try to point us back toward the truth, and that is how we learn from our mistakes.

Some people prefer to deny the existence of the devil. I believe it is not well to do this, but I think we can put the devil where he belongs by saying, "Get thee behind me," and by putting something good in the devil's place.

Nothing exists unless we give it life. You can give a lot of credence and support to what should not exist in your life. But to live in lies is to be lost; we can only find our way by following truth. That is why we must deny certain ways. We do this by not putting our minds on them. We cannot give them a thought. Thoughts grow when we focus our minds on them.

Wrong use of the law of denial simply blocks out much joy from life — and, it can make us more vulnerable to the things we want to deny. We must be very careful with this law.

Nothing Is Lost In God's Kingdom

There are no losses in life. There is nothing lost in God's kingdom. God's kingdom is life, and there is no way we can subtract one iota of life from that kingdom. So, you see, you can really build up what is beautiful in your life.

Yet, some people live in their losses all the time — "I lost my boy friend." "I lost my money." People live in and grieve over their losses. We say, "There goes a poor lost soul."

There is an old story about a well-known spiritual teacher in India who was on his deathbed. His students all gathered around him weeping and moaning. "Don't leave us, Master," they wept. "We don't want to lose you!" The teacher opened his eyes and looked at them. "Don't be silly," he said with a smile. "Where could I possibly go?"

Get away from this "lost" business. You don't lose anything in God's kingdom! Believe that when we set ourselves on the right channel, when we live by the law, we cannot lose anything. Nothing can oppose your good if you go in the right direction. With God all things are possible. This is a law. Believe it!

Emerson wrote one of the finest essays I have ever read. If you would like to be mentally rejuvenated, read "The Law of Compensation" by Ralph Waldo Emerson. Where there is silence, there is compensation. When we are thankful, there is compensation. Everything we do brings something back to us. Throwing your bread upon the waters has its compensation. Giving out good thoughts brings back something good.

To Forgive And To Forget

The *law of forgiveness* — to forgive and to forget — is one of the greatest laws. When we refuse to forgive, we hold within ourselves the burning poison of anger and resentment. Who is hurt by this? We are. Loosen up and let it go. Don't let anything hang on. Carry on with a new thought. When we do this, we are seeking the higher thought. This is how we work toward the law of love. We must forgive others as we would have them forgive us. Then we bring in the *law of love.*

When love enters, distress leaves us, and we don't have to be treated for a physical ailment later. This is the way the law of love works physically.

There are all kinds of laws. The *law of retribution* tells us that it is not the person who is killed that suffers. It is the one who does the killing. Because of regret and remorse he suffers a living hell. " 'Vengeance is mine,' saith the Lord."

Be Thankful For Your Problems

There is a *law of thankfulness* that will release us from stress and strain faster than anything else. Be thankful for your problem, even if you don't understand it. Be thankful for what has happened to you, for it will show you another way and start you in another direction. It will bring you into relationships where something better may happen. I sincerely believe that being thankful is part of the cure for any ailment.

The *law of release* is certainly one of the more important laws. We have to release people to God. We have to release our problems — we have to let them go. There is no need to have problems and troubles if you would just release them. If you want to have freedom in your life, you will have to free other people, release them. The moment you release other people, you free yourself.

The Law Of Love

We find that we must stand on Holy Ground if we are to get away from disease. The *Bible* is made up of laws given us to live by. Moses gave us some great laws, but there are even greater laws. The law that Christ brought us goes beyond the "eye for an eye and a tooth for a tooth" law. We hear people say, in effect, "You treat me right and I'll treat you right." No! we must go beyond this law! You must treat the other person right even though he or she doesn't treat you right. We must go beyond the law of the "even trade,"

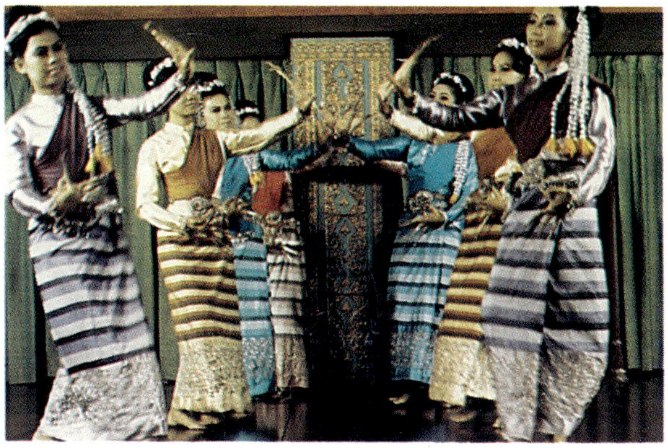

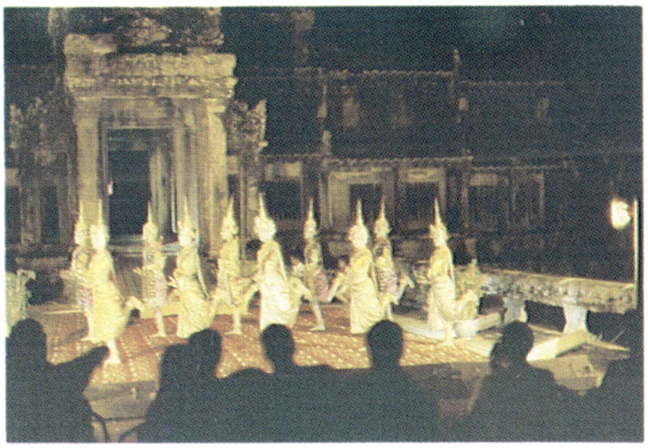

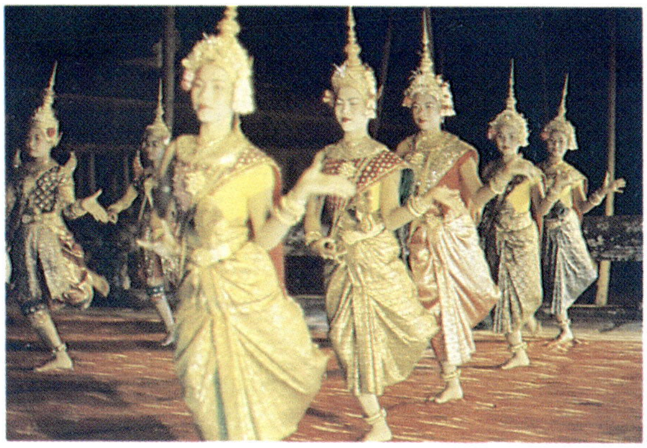

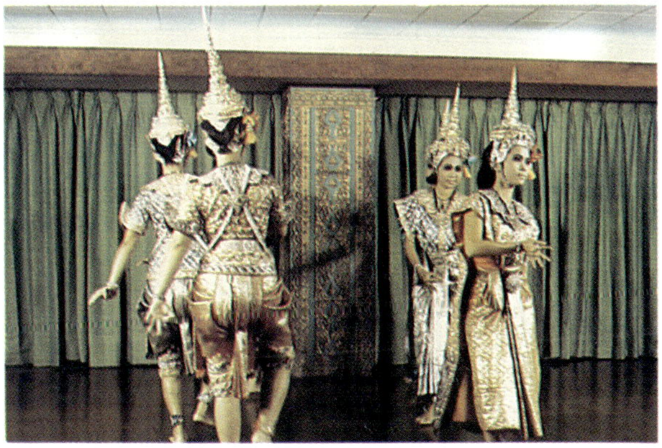

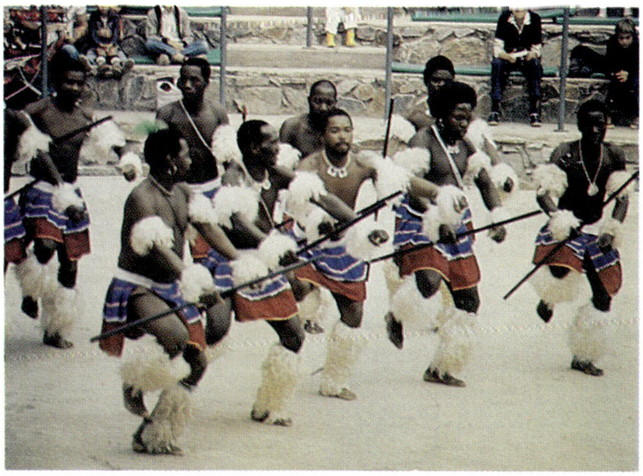

Dancing in Thailand. These costumes may take 2 hours to put on. They are sewn to fit the body perfectly. The dancing at night in the temples was beautiful. While this was going on, less than 50 miles away, bombs were exploding that actually shook us off our chairs at times. Life goes on and beauty will always live. Dancing can be considered a remedy. It can cure a headache. Dancing is a matter of our vibration, lifting us into another rhythm of life. We are vibrant beings and we can change the vibration of our bodies by dancing.

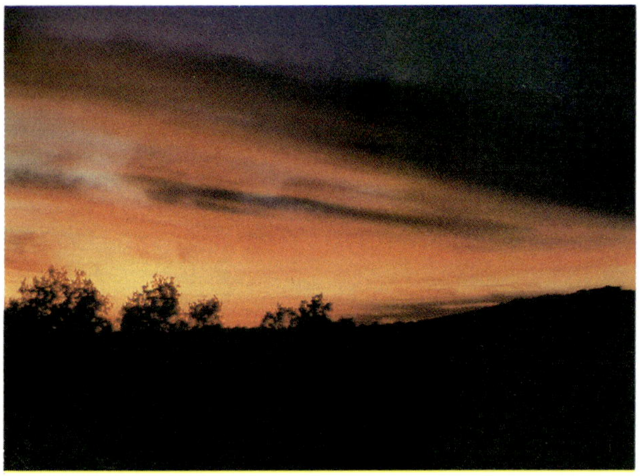
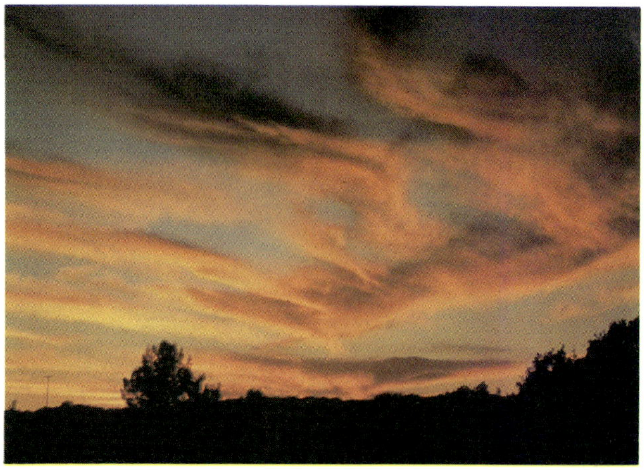
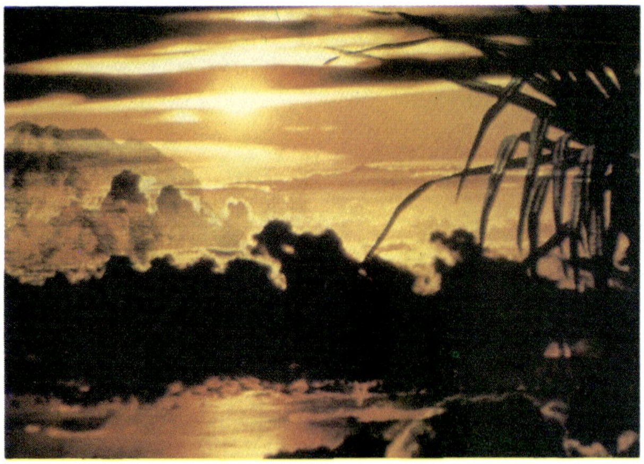
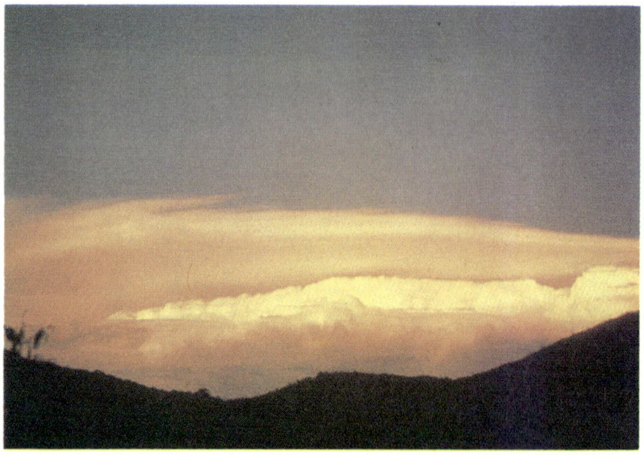
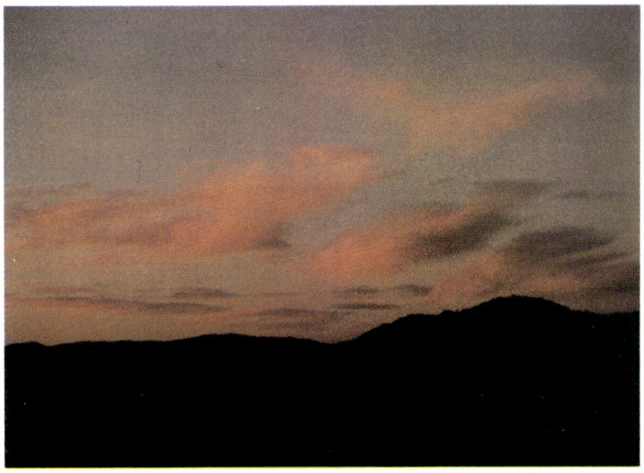
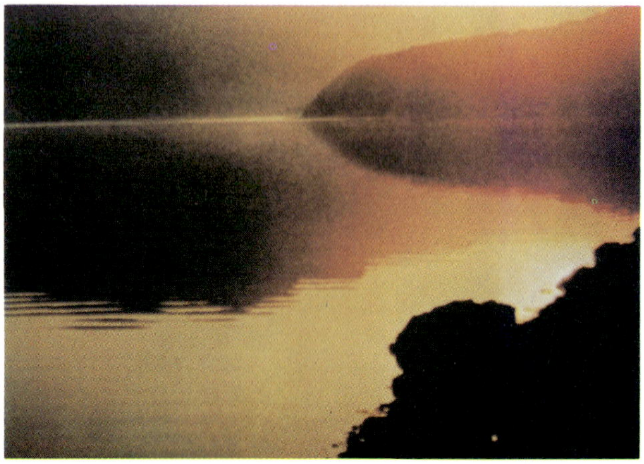

Sunsets bring out some of the most beautiful colors known to man. Color is a food for the mind and soul, and has healing qualities for those deficient in the "beauty" vitamins and minerals.

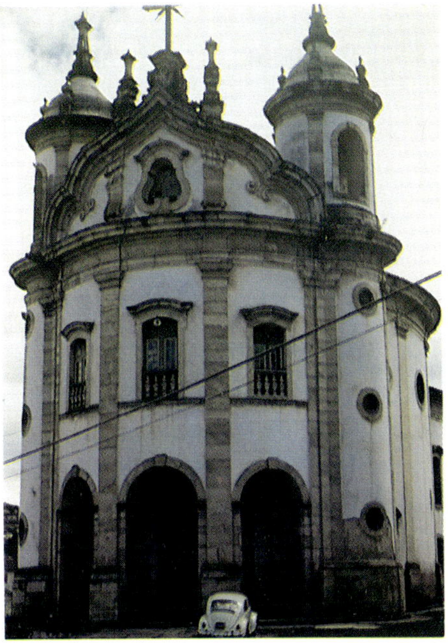

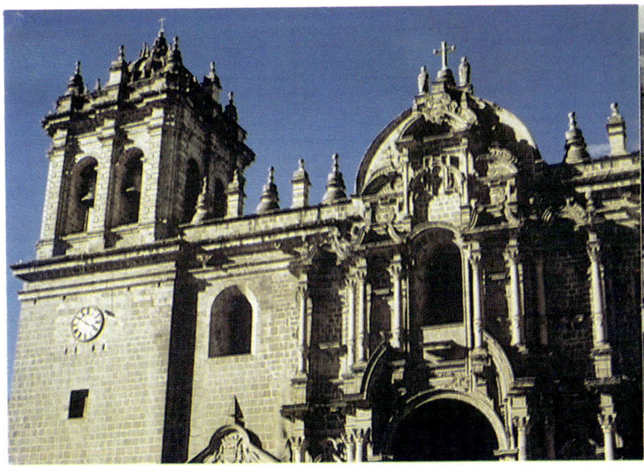

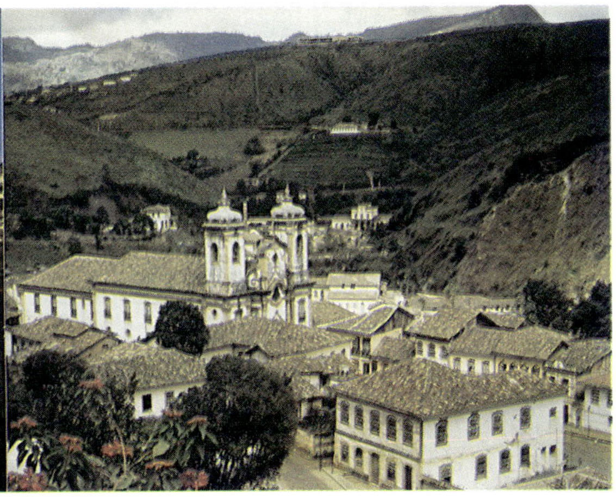

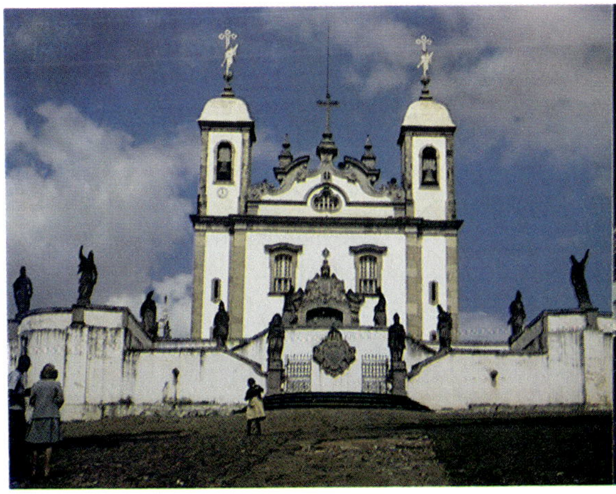

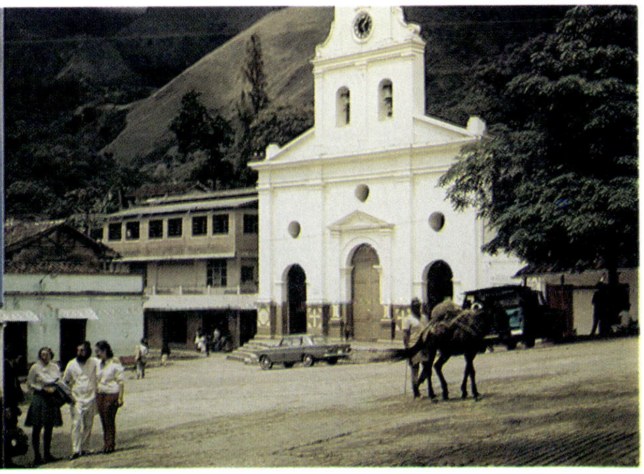

Top: This church, so I was told, was built round, so the devil couldn't corner anyone who went there. Bottom: There are many old churches in Latin America, lovely churches where people come to worship and pray.

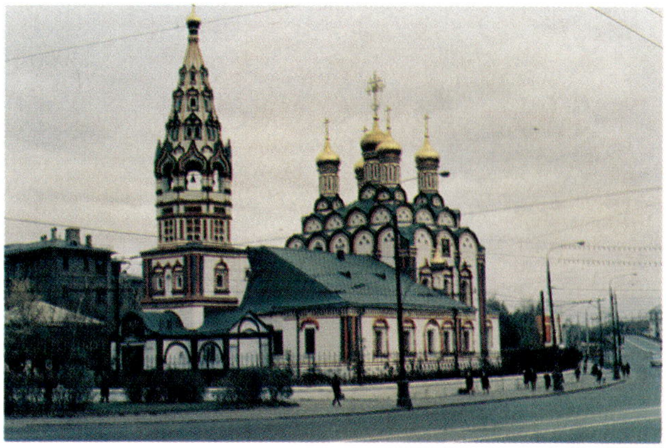

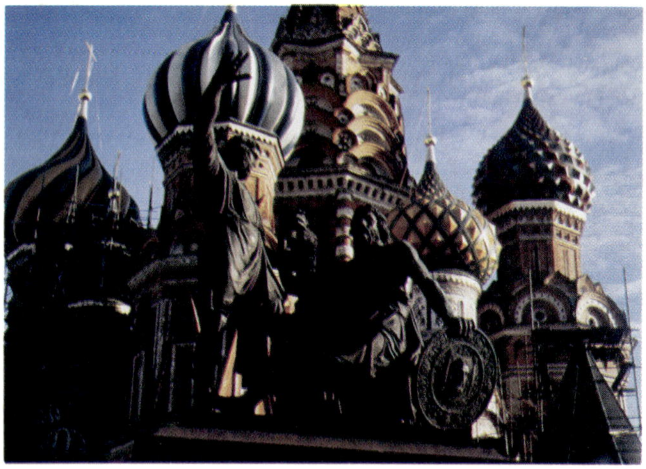

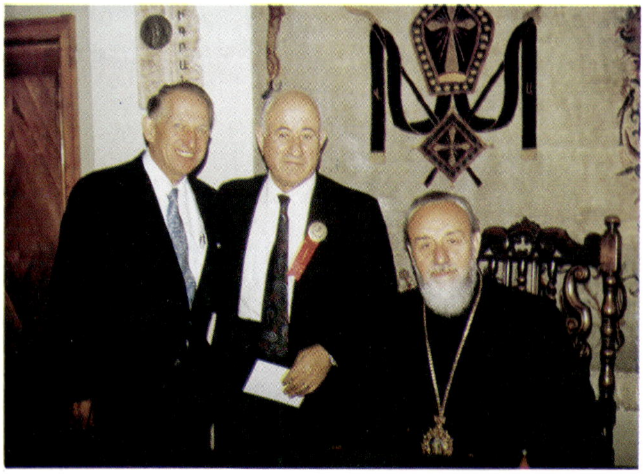

Top: This church is said to be where Tolstoi, the famous Russian author, was married. Center: Russian Orthodox churches in many places had this distinctive architectural style. Bottom: Here I am, with a friend, meeting with a bishop of the Rumanian church.

the law of "If you give me something, I'll give you something."

The greatest law, as Christ said, is "Thou shalt love the Lord thy God with all thy heart, with all thy soul, with all thy mind and with all thy strength." This means we must love the Law itself, because God is Truth, and His Truth is the ultimate law.

The second greatest law is "thou shalt love thy neighbor as thyself." It takes a lot to love a neighbor who spits in your face. It takes a lot of fortitude. It took a lot of love for Christ to wash the feet of the one He knew would betray Him — the one who caused Him to bear the cross the very next day. Christ did this — he demonstrated such love! I think this is one of the greatest examples of love in history.

Love Is The Key To Healing

Love is the key to healing. Love is like a soothing hand. Love relaxes and harmonizes. Where love is, you will find no tension. We find often that those who are ailing have stopped loving themselves. They have lost their feeling of self worth. Yet God, the greatest being in all existence, still loves them as He loves all human beings. We hear, "God is love." If we are loved by the One who knows everything, even the deepest secrets of our hearts, then we are always worth loving. We must not stop loving ourselves.

We must not wait to apply the *law of love*. Why should we live a long miserable life when love is right inside us? We must turn it on — right away! Love should be the highest attribute in our minds. The top priorities on our list should be: Speak love. Give love. Generate love.

Can Unrequited Love Affect Your Health?

Do you realize that many overweight people are suffering from a lack of love? Their substitute for love is food. They eat continually, trying to satisfy a lack that can never be fulfilled by food. When there is no love in our lives, we often go in some other direction in an attempt to compensate, to satisfy ourselves.

Love is one of the powers we should study more than anything else. Love must come from within and go out. Most people try to seek love on the outside. They say, "I just want someone to love me." Love has to be generated inside a person, and as we generate love, it comes forth, and we live on it. Then we attract the love of others. Our body molds to the love that we generate from within. Love is the sweet warm earth from which the flower of joy grows and blossoms!

Many effects are attributed to the law of love. Love makes us over. Love makes us new. Love gives us a renewal of cell structure. This is a tangible force that we must recognize!

This is the healing thought that I want to give you: If you cannot understand the laws of life, if you cannot agree with what is going on in your life, you must still love it — for your own good. I know this to be true. We not only must love our neighbors and our enemies and our friends, but we must love all people for our own good. By doing this, we heal ourselves from within, and love comes forward.

The Healing Pattern Of Love

God is within — closer than breathing, nearer than hands and feet. When we know that, we are our own healers. We are our own cell protectors. We are our own ease producers. Dis-ease, dis-harmony — these are the producers of mental and physical sicknesses. You must have your mind on love to generate health and wholeness. You must put yourself in a healing pattern.

I think that we should recognize that we are a focal point, that we are close enough to God to talk with Him and ask Him for guidance. As we ask for His guidance, let us realize that the most divine place to go is the deepest place within us.

As a person changes his or her mind Godward, turns all life plans Godward, that person is going healing-ward. The cell structure throughout the entire body is being adjusted by the change in the pattern of thinking.

As we think about Him — coming close to Him — we recognize that God's love will adjust our lives and make us whole. As we recognize that the wholeness of life has to be considered in the healing, we take in all of life to make us whole.

Peace and harmony abide within us. If you will accept love's blessing, you are blessed!

Chapter 25

The Father Principle

> *"It is your Father's good pleasure*
> *to give you the kingdom . . ."*
> *Luke 12:32*

It's wonderful to be a father. I have six children. Five of them are married, and I have fourteen grandchildren. So I am certainly speaking from experience when I say that children can certainly bring a lot of both pleasures and problems to you. But, I absolutely know that they come to teach parents lessons. We need them to give us lessons. You never really learn to love until you have children around. You'll never really develop patience until your children force you to just wait and wait and wait.

When we stop and think about this word "Father," we think back to our forefathers. If we keep going back, we pass through Adam to God, our First Father. We know God as the First Principle, the Father Principle.

Many times we do not follow the First Principle of Life, the Father Principle of Life, in order to be well physically. The Father Principle is a Spirit Principle, an embodiment of the Law. Some of us say, "It's the Lord that we follow." Some of us exaggerate this aspect to the extent that we "Lord it over" our children to show our authority. But you can accept authority from a father with love rather than resentment. It is only when we express our human nature instead of our spiritual nature that we have resentment. Many times we have to drop this human thing and recognize that "Father knows best."

Let us stop and think for a moment. Most of us not only don't look before we leap, we don't think while we're looking. We leap into problems and then we have to deal with them. We leap into a disease and then we seek a cure for it. Very few have reached the place where they think that preventing a disease is more important than curing it. Many people would like to know, after they have the disease, what they can do about it. I can tell you, to wait until after you have cancer is a sad time to begin doing something about it. When you've had arthritis twenty or thirty years, that's a sad time to do something about it. We haven't done enough thinking in life, and I realize the reason for this is that in school our teachers didn't teach us how to use words properly.

We think in words. When I say, "Ham and eggs," immediately your mind thinks and remembers the sight, smell and taste of ham and eggs. When someone calls you an uncomplimentary name, your mind responds right away. When somebody gives you a compliment, you also respond right away, but much differently. It's wonderful to be able to say, "I love you," isn't it? Yet, if I walked up to a stranger on the street and said, "I love you," I might well get locked up! Words are very powerful, and we have to be careful how we use them.

Whether the stranger on the street knows it or not, I really do love him. I love people, although I know it isn't wise to say some of the things I think. I think in the form of love for my own body's good. I think in the form of good. I think in the Father Principle, the Principle of Life, because it is the Father within who helps me to be well. Words affect us deeply, and that is why I am telling you that you have to think from the First Principle, the Father Principle. We live by the Word!

Words are formed in the thinking mind even before they get to your tongue or lips. "Kindness was on his tongue." "Love was on his lips." Where do words start? Inside us. Peace is made inside us. It makes no difference what the exterior is, it is what you are within yourself that matters.

In talking about this mental and spiritual principle from a health standpoint, I want you to think and stretch—stretch your mind. Do you realize that we gesture with our minds?

Thought Comes First — Action Follows

I never move my arm until the thought moves in my brain. I have never gone anyplace until my mind went there first. What wonderful trust we would have if we could realize that the Father goes ahead of us to make sure of the way. He is within you and going ahead of you, so there is nothing to worry about. Isn't this a blessing? It's this inside worry that we have to take care of. We have to trust the Father.

As you read this, your mind takes it in and responds. We find that all we have to do is suggest a word to someone — just say "candy," for example — and you may remember back to the age of five when somebody took some candy away from you. Or, you may think about the fudge you ate at a carnival once, the best you ever tasted. You may remember your children licking the bowl after you made candy. When I say "candy," look where you go. Look where you go with just this one word!

Thoughts attract other thoughts, don't they? You have to train yourself to make these thoughts go in the proper direction. If you don't, you'll ruin your nervous system. You will ruin your body. You can produce prostate troubles through fear and anger. Wrong thinking can ruin your kidneys. You have to be sure you are not producing hemorrhages, colitis or ulcers with the kind of thoughts you have. Are you following me?

I watch people making nervous wrecks out of themselves because they are "uptight." They are pushing too hard; they are trying to make life happen. They are not letting life happen in themselves. To have life and to have the life more abundant, you have to think from the Father Principle of Life. Whether in your work or your relationships, just letting that life flow through you is good for you.

The other day I said a little prayer: "God, now this is your job." Then I thought for just a minute. Am I neglecting my duty? Then I said to God, "This is my job as I see it. Do you want to help me with this, or am I going to help you?" Can you understand this way of thinking?

We need to know just what God's job is, and what our job is. Thinking isn't easy to learn. We stir up people, we get suggestions, we mull things over. Very few people go far enough in their thinking. But every now and then, some precious insight dawns on us.

Do you know how your mind works? We often think in terms of word associations — either opposites or similarities. If I mention "light" some people will think of darkness or even dungeons while others will think of rainbows or sunrises. Some people will take a word and make the worst of it. Others will try to make the best of it. When I say "black," what should you think of it? What's the opposite of black? White, isn't it? When you think of white, what do you think about? Rightness, angels, heavenly good? Let's learn to think in the right direction. Let's learn to change any word, any thought, any problem, to something better. Always work toward what is higher and better.

The fearful person is often sure that something terrible is going to happen to him. And it does. What you fear comes upon you, and it never fails. This is an example of a wrong thinking habit. The fearful person says, "I was afraid to answer the phone. I was afraid something awful had happened." Go answer the telephone with a cheery "Hello." You are going to have to resolve any problem that comes before you, whether you encounter it immediately by telephone or later by letter or telegram. If God is there with you, you can handle anything. If you are there with your Father, you will answer it and answer it right.

During the war along one of the battlefronts, civilians were going across the front lines every night with wheelbarrows full of straw. The inspectors would go through the straw every time, but they could discover nothing. "If we slack off," the inspectors told one another, "they'll be smuggling radios or other valuable material in that straw, and we'll miss it." But they never found a thing. After the war was over, an inspector spotted one of the civilians who used to cross the lines with the wheelbarrows of straw. He went up to him and asked, "What were you trying to smuggle to the other side in that straw?" The man grinned and replied, "We weren't smuggling anything in that straw. We were smuggling wheelbarrows!" Can you see what people tend to do? They miss the obvious. They just don't see it.

You Must Give Before You Receive

Sometimes I wonder if in our lives we miss the wisdom that is sitting right next to us. Whenever one man says to another, "I'll treat you like a gentleman if you treat me like one," he is missing something.

"Lift up your eyes and look on the fields, for they are white already to harvest." The Christ said that, but the ordinary person says, "If you treat me right, I'll treat you right." The ordinary person is not raising the situation to a higher level. I will tell you that you have to treat the other person right even if he doesn't treat you right. The ordinary person sits right next to the very truth that would help him, but he just doesn't see it. He misses the main principle. He looks in the straw but forgets the wheelbarrow.

It's always the young men who get excited about fighting a war. Do you know what an old man says about war? He says, "War is hell." He knows what he is talking about. He is the wise one. He has seen war-shattered nerves, the death and meaningless destruction. We have to go to the Father to get our information. We have to get our wisdom and understanding from the Father.

You know, Christmas may come just once a year, but the heavenly Father is here all year around. He is ever present, and I am thankful for that. I need His Presence more than once a year, more than once a day — I need Him all the time! I don't know how we could live without the Father Principle of Life.

What kind of being is this Father Principle? First of all, He is a loving Father. His love goes far beyond that of any human father. Would you want your children to live in problems and troubles? Would you want your children to be diseased? Of course not! The heavenly Father is just and loving. No diseases come from the Father Principle. We bring them on ourselves. We have to get back to this First Principle.

Sunshine And Light Are Healers

God said, "Let there be light," and there was light. If you want to get well, so it is said, get a goat and live on the south side of a hill. That's the sunny side. The south side of the hill is where the citrus fruits grow best. The south side of the hill is where we get the best reflections of God's good sunlight for our bodies and our minds.

Hippocrates, sometimes called "the father of medicine," gave us the oath that medical doctors follow today, an oath that requires physicians to follow the highest ethical standards. What about those who are not trained in the healing arts? One of the first principles for everyone is to take care of your body. In Hippocrates' time, sunshine and light were recognized as having powerful healing effects. They still do.

If you have studied the finer forces in life, you know that sunshine, ordinary light, is a mixture of all the light vibrations that make up the colors of the rainbow, and even beyond. All color comes from light. All living things depend on light for their existence, either directly or indirectly. We say that we come out of the darkness into the light. If there were no light, we would have only darkness. There is no life in darkness.

Light assists in controlling calcium in the body, the element that gives us tone, energy, power to work with. Would you want to be a jellyfish? You can't live without tone and energy in the muscle structure, and this comes from light. Sunbathing was recognized as good for the health by Hippocrates, and we can thank the father of medicine for this principle.

What about the fathers of our country? What first principles did they give to us? Does the Declaration of Independence guarantee us happiness? No, it doesn't. We are guaranteed only the right of the pursuit of happiness. Yet, even though we run and chase after it, many of us don't catch it. We get worn out chasing after something that can only be found inside us. The fathers of our country, the makers of our Constitution, gave us the first principle of freedom under law. But most of us don't know how to use this freedom to find happiness.

Jesus Christ came to give us a first principle. "I and my Father are One," He said. You find this first principle in many religions throughout the world. Here is another first principle: "Do unto others as you would have them do unto you." Does it make any difference how this first principle comes? It comes to the Chinese, to the Africans, to the Germans. It comes to the Hindu and the Christian. We are all brothers and sisters because we have the same Father. You and I have to look to the same Father. But today we separate ourselves because of so many different ideas, so many different religions, so many different channels in the healing art.

Everybody is fighting everybody else. So many fences, so many beliefs separate us. Yet we are all one. We are one because of the Father Principle. But we can only separate ourselves from a human standpoint. God didn't make that separation. We did. That's why we talk about atonement — At-One-ment. Attunement. Atonement is to come into At-Oneness, to come into attunement. That is what we must have.

One of my former professors, a wonderful man who passed away a short time ago, was a gland specialist. In our bodies we have a system of glands called the endocrine system: the pituitary, thyroid, parathyroids, pancreas, adrenals, ovaries and testes. The master gland, the one that controls the functioning of all the others, is the pituitary gland. One day this professor taught me something very interesting. He said, "This master gland, the pituitary, is just like God in the body. It is the Father Principle in the body, lord over all the other glands in the system. If the thyroid is overactive, the pituitary becomes underactive to bring balance." Many people who neglect health principles, who neglect caring for the physical temple, are the ones who don't have balance in life.

It isn't enough to care only for the mental life. Psychiatrists find that over sixty percent of the suicides in any particular profession are those who concentrate on the mental life. More people are in mental institutions because of religion than anything else. The Father Principle, like the master gland of the endocrine system, will bring balance into our lives if we accept His guidance. We can't do it by going man's way. To balance body, mind and spirit we have to be in tune with the Father. It isn't enough just to give lip service to the spiritual principles. It isn't enough just to go to church on Sundays.

You can really become happy only when you have a healthy body. You can be close to God with a healthy body. Have you ever tried to meditate with a toothache? Can you have sweet thoughts with a sour stomach? No, you can't. We must see that the physical, mental and spiritual go together.

You will find that you can end a lot of problems right now. The solution is simple. Go back to nature. Go back to the garden. Go back to God, the First Principle of Life.

A Garden Is The Cloak Of God

God is working through nature. God is working through the garden. God is working through you. But God can only do for you what He can do through you. You have to recognize this because if you were left by yourself, without God, I don't know where you'd go, what you'd choose or how you'd progress. How could you live without faith, without love, without guidance? What do you think a godless life would be like? You know, I can't even imagine a godless vegetable, because the Divine Principles are there. The Divine Architect works in those vegetables; the Divine Chemist works in the chemistry of these foods. Man can't duplicate parsley, carrots or tomatoes. We should thank God for our vegetables, for the natural things we have. We should get connected with those vegetables. They were here before we were. Christ said, "Before Abraham was, *I am.*" That is a long time, friends. Without the Father Principle, nothing is kept in order. This house we live in has to be kept in order.

When we come back to the First Principle, the Father Principle, we find no disease there, no sickness. We start the disease. We start the troubles. We do this by turning away from the Father Principle. Some people can't even talk about the Father Principle. They can't reason together.

There Is Power In Agreement

You know, there are a lot of people who argue. They argue because they think this point isn't right and that point isn't right. But the Good Book says, "Agree with thine adversary quickly." You need to do that for your nerves. I treat wrecked nerves because people can't bring themselves to agree with their adversaries. Let them go. Let God take care of them. You have enough to do to lift yourself. What a wreck many of you have made of your lives! It is time that you did something good for yourself. The Father Principle is the greatest principle we have, and it works within us, it molds us, it gives us a better body. Do yourself a favor: Go back to the Father Principle.

Have you ever seen a picture of "father time"? He is represented as an old man with long white whiskers, holding a scythe in his hand. Some people picture God that way. But our heavenly Father is above and beyond time. There is only eternity with the Father. Time is a human invention. We think back to last year and we remember this and that happened. If God ever thought about "last year," it would be such a tiny little speck as compared to eternity that it would seem He could hardly find it.

Do you want to become timeless, part of the agelessness of eternity? Then tune in to the Father Principle. That's where eternity is. Actually, I get scared once in a while when people ask, "How old are you?" I tell them and then I think, "My goodness, I'm just as young as when I was twenty!" The principles I have are just as young as when I was twenty. When I say that, I mean I am in better health now than I was at twenty. At that age I lost my health, and the doctors only gave me a matter of weeks to live. Then I found some of the principles that saved my life.

I learned about the story of the Prodigal Son. There was a Father Principle at work in that story. The Prodigal Son took his inheritance, spent it foolishly and ended up in the gutter. But it was in that same gutter that he realized his true inheritance and decided to return to his Father. Do you understand that?

Let me shock you a little bit. You can have anything in life you want, but if you just cling to the material possessions and to this physical life, you will end up in the gutter. At the physical level we can only have things that thieves can steal, rust can decay, fire can burn. Even the gutter will decay in time, so you won't even have it to cling to. In other words, this is where it ends. We can choose to take the road down or the road up. When we think about it, we realize that we don't want to go any way but up.

When we don't think about it, we get involved in the daily grind. We say, "I'm going to get this job done if it kills me." And it kills us. Choose a living that won't kill you. Learn to work with the Father Principle that sees to it that your life remains balanced. The Father is the beginning and end of all life.

Our earthly fathers taught us self-reliance and how to take care of ourselves, as well as they knew. Then, perhaps, we go to college and while we are in our twenties we think we know it all. Twenty years later, we begin to realize that we really don't know very much. So, we have to return to the Father's house because He has principles so much greater than those taught in any college or university.

You know, near the end of the second world war, scientific researchers developed DDT and claimed that it would revolutionize agriculture. It worked very well at killing insects that damaged farmers' crops, but it turned out that it killed many other things as well. It killed birds and animals. It collected in our underground water supply. It ran into our rivers and into the oceans, poisoning the fish. The government wasn't in a big hurry, but DDT was finally banned, or it might have begun killing human beings. This is what happens with manmade "miracles." This is why we have to follow the Father Principle instead. We can take the first step right now into the higher life. We can make a change "in the twinkling of an eye."

Helping Others Costs Nothing

Are we working with first principles? One of the first principles is that we must take care of our brother. Some people think that it is enough trouble just taking care of themselves. But if you give your brother kindness, it doesn't cost you anything. Caring for others is a principle that comes from the Father.

Many of these principles that are expounded in church on Sunday are left right there in church when people go back home. They think these principles are too hard to apply. It would be too difficult to do these things. But we don't have to do them. The Christ said, "It is the Father in me, He doeth the works." We just let the Father work through us. Do you see this? Do you think I'm expressing truth? No. It is the Father in me that expresses the truth.

You've heard of financial settlements and legal settlements, haven't you? Well, we have to make a mental settlement in our lives. I think we make a mental settlement when we agree with our adversaries quickly. When I do right by you, I make a mental settlement because I want the right thing to be done for me. But if I make what I do for you dependent on what you do for me, that's just a business transaction. Do you see the difference? That latter kind of mental settlement isn't going to bring you good health; the former one will.

Earlier I mentioned that children come to teach us. These lessons are good for us. This human development is one of the stages of eternal unfoldment, eternal progress, eternal growth. As human beings, I think that we are in a very young stage as compared with what is yet to come in the unfoldment of the Father Principle.

One expression of the Father Principle is, "I feed my sheep." But that doesn't mean God is going to write out a check for you or pay off your mortgage. It works this way: If you have a business, *you* are the business end of the business. The business doesn't support you, you support the business. The Father Principle is the spiritual power working within you that puts all life in good order. You may not have bread, but you'll be cared for. Do you understand that? You'll be cared for.

God was here first. That's why we speak of Him as First Principle. God is wisdom. He knows all about everything we are going through. This is why we have to turn to God for that which we need, right now. We can have faith because we have a Father we can turn to and trust. But first we have to find this First Principle — or we wouldn't have any basis for our faith. The Father Principle comes first.

Let Go And Let God

When we hear, "The Father that dwelleth in me, He doeth the works," the principle it embodies is this: "*Let go and let God.*" Let the Father in you do the work, Christ advises us, and He goes on to say, "Greater works than these shall ye do." Can you see how this thing works? You have to get your "self" out of the way and let the Father do it. So, when you see me, I'm letting the Father do the work. Where do you think miracles come from? They come from God, not from man. If you want the miracle, if you want the healing, if you want the change, turn to the Father Principle. We need the Father Principle; our bodies, made of the dust of the earth, don't know which way to go.

We recognize that we can do nothing without the Father Principle. The Father knows all thoughts, and this is why we have Truth. To find this Truth we have to seek its origin, and it was born in our Father. That is where we have to go.

The Prodigal Son story has a wonderful lesson to it. When he went back home, the Father saw him from afar and came to meet him, rejoicing. What a lovely scene that is! When the student is ready, the master appears. Before you ask, He has the answer. As God's children, all we have to do is to be like children — give up the old human faults such as pride, vanity, selfishness. We have to give up all the human frailties that hinder our development. Let the Father Principle come through.

When you stop and think about this, it will take care of your inheritance. We have our problems with our human "dad." I found that the moment I realized I didn't have to follow the way of my human "dad," I was released from a great burden. Since I finally realized that my dad had the same Father I did, he became my brother. This is when you evolve, when you go to the highest path. This is the Principle that will help you become well.

The Good Book says, "The things which are impossible with men are possible with God." The reward is there. You can claim it "in the twinkling of an eye." It belongs to you.

If therefore ye are intent upon wisdom,
A lamp will not be wanting,
And a shepherd will not fail,
And the fountain will not dry up.
— *Anonymous*

From the Doctor's Study . . .

MIND AND SPIRIT

In discussing mind and spirit, many people do not realize that the mind has to draw from experience to learn how to live. But, where does it draw on to learn right and wrong? Spiritually speaking, to develop correct concepts of right and wrong, we have to draw from a mind that works right. We find that many minds are dominated by fear. Others are dominated by achievement. But if the mind finds no meaning in life, if it is not exposed to the higher values in life, we are not happy. In the deep self, you will find we can never be happy without touching the higher values with our lives.

Some appear happy with wealth. But no one is happier than the person who knows that what he or she is doing is helping others. Is there anyone who is not touched deeply when he sees the life of a child he has helped greatly improved?

Mind healing is just as important as physical healing. We can touch wood, metal, stones and gems, because they have physical substance. They all have value. Yet happiness and unhappiness have values, too. We can't touch them in a physical sense, but we are "touched" by them as they flow through the mind.

It is the spirit which has to evolve to bring about a good mind or to bring about a good body. If we can recognize that the mind is ready to unfold and to do what the spirit directs it, we are ready to progress. The spirit is always ready to do its job.

People say, "I'll see you later, God willing." Well, God is always willing. Within the God-consciousness there is no sickness, either mental or physical. We have to recognize that the spiritual path or consciousness is found latent and equal in each person. The only thing necessary is to awaken this quality.

It is when we say, "Now I see," that the awakening process is upon us. We might wonder, "Why didn't I see this before? Where have I been?" Worlds I never knew existed have come to me. This is what is meant by the saying, "I have ways ye know not of." "I go to prepare a place for you."

We would all like to know about the places prepared for us, but it can only come by revelation and it can only come by seeking the higher values in life. I am positive this is accessible to each and every one of us. It is available when the need comes and when our consciousness is awakened. Very few people have found the need for the spiritual things in life who have all they want mentally and physically.

The spirit is on a level above the mind, and it does things for the mind and for the body that the mind and body cannot do for themselves.

Once I heard there was one thing that a rich man would never experience what the poor man feels—who has just made his final car payment. It is this "feeling world" that we can't adequately express in words or measure or accumulate. This spiritual thing passes through us as a consciousness that everyone has. Until we become actually aware that this exists, we cannot reach the highest pinnacle of service to mankind—feelings for ourself, keeping ourself in the best of health and knowing what it is to walk a more godly life.

There is more to this book than a certain number of pages. For those who can read between the lines, for those who can perceive the feeling behind the thought, for those who can sense the spirit of this endeavor, this book will have no end.

This book describes much more than the path I have walked. It points to a universal truth, the truth that there is a higher path, a right path for every individual. If you can get to this by meditating upon what I have presented here, you will find this is a book you will never finish.

Chapter 26

Stand On Holy Ground

Listen — or thy tongue will keep thee deaf.
— American Indian saying

Back in the days when kids could go to the Saturday afternoon matinee at the local movie theater for a dime, the entertainment fare was almost always a cartoon or two and a couple of cowboy movies and a serial episode. The serial always ended with the hero or heroine hanging from a cliff or tied to the railroad tracks before the words "continued next week" came on the screen. You could always tell who the good guys were, because they wore white hats. The bad guys wore black hats. There was always at least one chase scene in every cowboy movie. A band of Indians or outlaws would be chasing the good guys, and the hero would yell to his sidekicks, "Head for high ground up yonder — we'll have to take our stand up there."

When problems and troubles are surrounding us, we have to take our stand on high ground, don't we? We have to rise above them. We have to plant our two feet firmly on Holy Ground to find peace and safety.

Once I visited a patient whose little five-year-old girl was saying a prayer that night before going to bed. At the end of her prayer she said, "And God, please make me a good little girl, for goodness sake!" I couldn't help but be deeply touched. It was partly the way she said it and partly the words she used. I thought, "Let us *all* be good, for goodness sake!"

The way the world is going these days, it takes a lot of nerve to dare to be good — for goodness sake. But we must be good — for the sake of our nerves. It takes a lot of goodness to heal nerves that are battered and depleted by problems and troubles. Our nervous systems cry out for peace and harmony and goodness.

Have you ever seen a wrecking crew tearing down an old building? Sometimes they have one of those tall cranes with a heavy steel ball hanging from a long cable, and they swing that steel ball until it is smashing down the sides of the building they are wrecking. Many people today are employed on wrecking crews. Only instead of wrecking old buildings, they are systematically wrecking their own nerves and the nerves of those around them. They have the wrecking attitude. Another thing that can wreck your nervous system is bad food.

There is food, of course, that can soothe the nervous system. There are foods that can improve the nerves. But I believe the food we feed our minds is more important — the food for thought we have developed through our philosophy, through our reading and studying, through our contact with people. Just as there is food that stills the stomach, there is food that stills the mind. Don't you feel good when you know that everything is all right? Don't you feel good when everything around you is in harmony?

One of the most important laws we must realize as we look at life and at our environment is that we must adapt ourselves to those aspects of our environment that we cannot change. When there is something we cannot change in the outside world, we must make our peace with it. We must make the changes within ourselves.

Many hates may come and go within us. At times we hate our jobs, our taxes, our bosses, certain relatives, people of different races, colors, politics or religions. These hates are inside us. To change these things, we must change ourselves.

Now, hate is a heavy, burdensome thing. To get rid of it takes a good deal of strength or the right kind of leverage. Have you ever tried to push a car that is stuck in sand or mud? You can't do it. Your feet keep sliding and slipping from under you. You don't have control. You need some firm ground to stand upon. To gain control of the mental attitudes, there is only one ground I know of that will give us the proper footing. We must stand on Holy Ground.

Are You Prepared To Face Life?

Let us make an effort to get settled in our faith, to find and to get settled on Holy Ground. Then, no matter what happens in this world, we are set for it, we are equipped for it. We may think of life as a pilgrimage through Holy Land, and there are certain ways that we can prepare for this pilgrimage.

You wouldn't start out to climb a mountain without rope, climbing gear and a knapsack of good high-energy foods. In the same way, we must equip ourselves with knowledge, wisdom and growth so we can get over the ridges and rough spots of life. We are all pilgrims. We all have mountains to climb, rivers to cross, deserts through which we must pass. We have difficult and unpleasant people to deal with. I believe these obstacles are placed in life for just one reason, and that is to give us all an opportunity to grow. Instead of learning from problems, many people look for someone or something to blame for them. This doesn't work. When you try to place blame outside yourself, the blame will eventually come back to you. "The chickens will all come back to roost," the farmers say. We must realize that these problems and obstacles are put here for our own strengthening, not to drag us down.

Many adults become upset at children and young people. But children and young people are here for our own good. We learn from them. Because of them we are forced to grow. We have children at a time when we know relatively little of life. Children come to teach us, and we certainly need teaching!

Accept What Comes Before You

We must prepare ourselves for that which is yet to come. Let us get started on this preparation as quickly as possible. Let us equip ourselves.

It is said that the last enemy to overcome is death. One time a man came to my office with heart trouble, and after our consultation he left the office. Three hours later when it was time for me to leave, I found him still sitting out in front. I asked, "What's the matter, John?" He said, "I'm afraid of dying. I'm afraid my heart might stop. I want to be around you."

I gently assured him that when his heart stopped I would be unable to help him. It took me a couple of hours to get the fear of death from this man's mind. He is still living — and that was twenty years ago.

It is very difficult to take care of a person who holds onto thoughts of dying. They can kill themselves just by dwelling on their fear of death.

I know a lady who spent three years going from doctor to doctor, she was so afraid of dying. Then she came to me. What could I tell her? It seemed impossible to get this idea out of her head. After she had voiced her fear at some length, I looked right at her and said, "Yes, you are going to die."

She paled. "You certainly are not helping me," she responded angrily.

I replied, "Well, you *are* going to die. And *I* am going to die. I will probably die before you do." I continued to talk to her and assured her we all had to learn to accept death, and that after we had accepted the fact that someday we are going to die, we should just forget it, put it aside. Running from doctor to doctor is not only hard on your pocketbook, it is hard on your nerves.

The Body Is A Wonderful Instrument

While we are walking through life on this Holy Ground, we are handling and operating a Holy Instrument — our body. Did you ever stop to think who gave the human body that ultimate shove, that first shove, that initial, all-important shove that sent it into life and light? Did you ever stop to think that you are an instrument with millions of strings, nerve pathways that are used for everything from tying your shoes to playing the piano? It's easy to add them up. Consider that you have over a million nerves leading from each eye to the brain, 26,000 nerves leading from the ears to the brain, and these are only a small part of the entire nervous system. When I was in college, they were talking about a discovery in Sweden which implied that one nerve carried 2,700 more nerve fibers. We are all "musicians," playing an instrument of a million strings! We really have been put together wonderfully!

We are not usually aware of the wonders of our bodies — nor do we need to be under most circumstances. The only time you become aware of your heart is when something goes wrong with it. The only time you become aware of your foot is when a shoe pinches it. Generally, we only become aware of our bodies when something is wrong with them. You are not supposed to know of the body's physical existence. You are supposed to be absent from the body; absent from your toes, your knees, your stomach, your lungs. Why are you supposed to be absent from the body? To be present with the Law!

A man who was dying of cancer called his minister, saying, "I must go back to first principles. I want to return to the first principles in life and start right." Now is the time we should start right. Then we will not have our minds concentrated on ailments. No ailments will follow us if we follow the Law. We can run and not be weary. We will not have these physical problems if we get back to first principles, get back to Law.

Good Rest Means Longer Life

Most people today are trying to see how far they can go with this body. I'm a bad one at that. I want to see how long I can go before I have to climb in bed. I want to see how much I can read, how much I can study, how much I can get out of this body.

But that isn't wise. Go to bed at a reasonable time. Take care of your body while you still feel good. You shouldn't continue to push the body until you are tired. When you become tired you start using your reserve energy, and when you are using that reserve, you start using the marrow of the bone. You start taking it out of the bone marrow and the nervous system, and then you become vulnerable to ailments.

It is possible to rest the nervous system by repairing your attitude, regenerating and rebuilding it.

So, let's take your attitude into the garage today. Let's lift it up on the hoist. Let's grease and oil it. Let's give the radiator some water. Let's recharge the battery. It isn't the environment that you drive your car or attitude through that harms it, it is what is being processed inside it that wears our the physical parts.

By repairing the nervous system, you can stop the destruction before it kills you. Nothing can harm me, for I do not consent to be harmed. I recognize that this is a wonderfully made body, a very finely tuned instrument, an instrument that can't take much shock or excessive harm. I refuse to become interested in anything of an inferior nature. I will not permit anyone to come into my life and upset my nervous system because I stand on Holy Ground.

We Need A Good Outlook

This body and this mind need a good outlook, a good attitude. If you come to me sick, my attitude is that I would like to show you how to regain good health and how to keep it. You made your sickness. You can rid yourself of it. In fact, only you can do it. Even Christ didn't claim to be able to heal people. He would say, "Your faith has made you whole." He puts it back on you. So do something about it; get yourself tuned up in "good faith." Keep this fine instrument in good order. You can do this with faith. This hasn't anything to do with carrot juice, my friend. It has to do with something much bigger — your mental attitude. When you get your attitude cleared up, your nervous system will clear up.

When people ask me which church I belong to, I tell them I am trying to live so that any church would like to have me as a member. I believe that is as it should be. We must all live by what is right, no matter who lives around us. It is not "who" is right but "what" is right. We have so many lines of demarcation, so many directions to choose from. If you must belong to something, start by belonging to the right attitude; and what is right must be right for all of us.

We must balance our lives. We have to let extremism and fussiness go in order to let the finer experiences come to us. I know that some of you are getting into trouble with extremism. Don't go that way! Take the central path, the middle path. If you can't get your combinations perfect, try to get them as natural as possible. Think the best thoughts possible. Get as much knowledge as possible, especially regarding food.

Too Many Mental Pains

When you gain control over yourself through a good mental attitude, you don't feel tied up and tense. Tension can restrict the flow of blood, affecting your entire circulatory system. Fear and anger cut down the supply of blood to the heart. How can you get a blush in your cheek without a good mental attitude? Many times congestion of the blood in any part of the body, such as the liver, is caused by our mental attitude. Attitude is one of the important health prerequisites. Get it fixed up!

I stopped a patient at the Ranch once and told him, "The only time you are allowed to feel miserable here is when you are in my office. When you are not with me, feel happy." We shouldn't get into our troubles with anyone but our doctor.

In the Good Book, Paul tells us, "I am exceeding joyful in all tribulation." Paul had overcome tribulation. He had risen to pure joy. Wouldn't it be wonderful to greet our trials with pure joy? Joy is wonderful, and it is nothing more or less than an attitude. We could, like Paul, use joy to greet problems or troubles. I doubt that Paul ever laughed at his trials, but I don't doubt for a minute that he greeted them with joy.

I can't laugh at my troubles either, but I have found that if I look at them without tension or resentment and go after them with a firm attitude, I can handle them quite well. You may want to try facing your troubles in this same manner — without resentment.

What we will do is to put light in the dark places. While I was in Germany studying iridology, they spoke of black as compared to the devil of hell, while light was compared with the angels of heaven. When I see white lines come into the iris of the eye, I know you are going the right way. The more white lines you acquire in the eye, the more acute, active and better function you will have. That's what we are after, isn't it? We must put light in all the dark places: We must learn; we must study; and we must adopt better attitudes in our lives to replace the harmful negative attitudes.

If God is going to help us "even to the marrow of our bones," we must have some spiritual nourishment. This is very important. We must recognize that in the beginning we had a shove from eternity to get us started. We had help to get us going, but there is much we must do to keep this instrument of a million strings in good shape, internally and externally. You don't put your nice paintings out in the sun to get burned, do you? You don't let the roof go unrepaired until the rain comes in, do you? You can't leave these things to nature. We say that nature cures — and it does; but nature can be very hard on those who will not lend a helping hand in the process. I could send you down to the beach for some beneficial sunshine, but if you came back like crisp bacon, that wouldn't be good for you. Nature can harm as well as heal.

Don't Let Your Mind Destroy You

A lady came in to me the other day and said, "I just came from the bakery where I bought a dozen donuts, but when I opened the bag there were only eleven! I could just kill that clerk!" Now, there's an attitude for you! Thinking of killing a person over one donut! We know she didn't mean she was literally capable of going back and killing someone, but it is important to notice just what expressions we use. She chose to talk about killing that person. Why didn't she go back and tell the clerk about his mistake? He would believe her in most cases. We've all made mistakes. And if the clerk didn't believe her, she should have just forgotten the incident. One donut isn't worth it. We must protect our attitudes by watching our responses.

Put more trust in God. We can leave our problems with God, and they will pass from us. "This, too, shall pass away!" There are certain ideas we have to trust and believe in. You have a God who takes care of you even when you don't have bread. With God we know that our life goes on — there is no stopping, and it goes on beautifully. It runs without effort.

When we get into trouble it is because we are trying to force things to happen. We must not try to *make* life happen; we must *let* it happen. These are days of anxiety. Doctors are treating more people for anxiety neuroses than anything else. They call it an "effort syndrome." It just isn't necessary.

So don't put too much effort into trying to make life happen, and if you overdo it for an hour or so, rest for the next hour to make up for it. Go through life smoothly for the good of your nervous system, everything will be all right. "A merry heart doeth good like a medicine." What we need is cheerfulness! A heart of mirth is the best antidote for stress, a tonic for the nerves.

We had a man here at the Ranch whom everyone refused to sit with at mealtimes. If he sat down, people would get up and leave the table. When I asked several people what was wrong, they said, "Every time he comes through the room, the air gets so blue you could lean against it." Puzzled, I said, "What do you mean?" And they said, "Go over and sit with him and see for yourself." So I did.

He had to be simply the most negative person I have met in my entire life. I asked him if we could go for a little walk together, and he suspiciously replied, "What's the idea of going for a walk?" I told him I wanted to talk to him — that I wanted to tell him why people didn't like to sit with him at the table. He said, "I don't care whether they sit with me or not." I told him he couldn't expect to take up a whole table himself when we were so crowded. He said, "I'm paying for it, am I not?" I told him, "Yes, you are paying for it, but I think it would be good for you to feel happy." He asked, "Well, what's so important about happiness?"

I finally persuaded him to go for a walk. I reeled off a few humorous stories and jokes, but there wasn't a laugh in the man. Finally I said, "You know, it says in the Good Book, 'a merry heart doeth good like a medicine.' " He replied, "Don't quote the *Bible* to me — I'm an elder in my church. I'll tell you one: 'I've gone to prepare a place for you.' So, why be happy here?" He was determined he was not going to be happy here — he was going to wait and be happy in the hereafter!

We are all meant to be happy here. Anyone who has a loving Father who cares for him can be happy. We can be happy because we have the gift of life itself. We have the privilege of expressing our talents. We have the privilege of knowing one another. We can be happy knowing that we are being prepared by our experiences for something greater than we now have.

Let us look forward to the marvelous things yet to come, but let us not ignore the joy revealed to us each day. Let's change our attitudes, friends. One out of every seven people in the United States is taking tranquilizers, seeking peace "through better chemistry" — the bottled kind. How unfortunate that people are stumbling dazed through life on this "slap-happy" idea. They don't realize we have the privilege of working with the body. We can accomplish marvels with this body. We have goals to meet, ideals to up hold. We have so many gifts to express with this body that we can all be assured of the peace, happiness and joy to be found in unadulterated life without any artificial coloring, sweeteners or preservatives.

I'd like to quote you a reason for my belief that life can be beautiful. I'm not certain who wrote this, but it is lovely.

I will not worry, fret or be unhappy over you.
I will not be anxious concerning you.
I will not be afraid of you.
I will not give up on you.
I will not blame you, criticize you or condemn you.
I will remember first, last and always that you are God's child,
And have His Spirit in you.
I will trust this Spirit to take care of you,
To be a light in your path,

To provide for your needs.
I will think of you always as being surrounded by God's loving presence,
As being enfolded in His protecting care,
As being kept safe and secure in Him.
I will be patient with you.
I will have confidence in you.
I will stand by in faith and stand by you in my prayers,
Knowing you are growing,
Knowing you are finding the help you need.
I have only good feelings in my heart about you,
For I am willing to let you live your life as you see fit.
Your way may not be my way,
But I will trust the Spirit of God in you
To show you the way of your highest good.

What a beautiful thought that is! We must leave other people alone, knowing they can have the presence of God expressing within. Let us try to bring the godliness out in other people. We say, "I bring out the worst in him." But let us turn to bring the best out of others. Let us go about uplifting other people. Let us give them the best that we have within ourselves.

We must come back into ourselves to take inventory of who we are. What are our capacities? What are our privileges in life? We must come to realize that we have a beautiful body — wonderfully and fearfully made — a body that is capable of expressing itself in many different directions. Let us realize that we have the privilege of writing a certain amount of history as we go through life, as we walk on Holy Ground. Let us make the kind of history that finds its approval in God.

Prayer

May our expression of life on this Holy Ground be guided in a direction that will reveal the will of God within and through all those we meet along the way. Let us realize that God is love, that God's church is the church of life created within us as we let His love and His truth flow through us. May your pursuit of life and wisdom have the blessing of God.

From the Doctor's Pen . . .

Time is the space my consciousness dwells in;
It's the moment we have, knowing life is here;
Our senses come forth to express themselves—
We go on, but immortal time will stay.

Time can be squeezed by our anxious self;
Fear in our heart says this moment is cruel;
The hate we have as we travel the space of life
Makes us conscious of time, and we don't want to feel it.

The quickness of thought or the slowness of speech
Gives us conception of traveling the space;
But we're using ourselves to exist and just be—
Time stays here—and we travel on.

Discontent squeezes each cell in our body;
The time we go through can be misspent
For we live in a pull, a push or a pain—
How do you live this time as you travel on?

Rejoice this moment, for it is all you have,
What is gone has been lived and belongs to the past.
Don't reach or strain yourself to a future—
You're traveling too fast—time is this moment.

Happiness can fill the wall of this moment
Till time can become so obscure that it is not.
And we awaken to find our living is life—
It is we who travel and it is we who are time.

Chapter 27

The Two Powers of Man

What we are deepest, we really are.

We all know of many pairs of opposites in life: positive and negative, light and darkness, health and sickness, profit and loss, high and low, male and female. Western philosophers call this system of opposites dualism. Eastern thinkers regard these pairs of opposites as connected polarities, half of each pair belonging to the *yin* or female principle, and the other half to the *yang* or male principle. But together, they form a whole, a oneness.

Now, some people believe that every silver lining has a dark cloud above it. They look for disaster to follow a joyful or happy event, and if this is the way you view the law of polarities or dualism, that is what will happen to you. As you believe, so it will be done to you. But I am going to tell you this is wrong thinking. I am going to tell you this belief comes from the lower path, the earth-bound path.

Of course, if you stuff yourself with rich food as some do, you will suffer later. If you fill your poor stomach with coffee and donuts, you will reap the consequences. And the "plop-plop, fizz-fizz" drug store remedy will not solve the basic problem. To do that you will have to correct your mental attitude. You will have to reach out to the spiritual values. Then you will realize that the "silver lining" has a cloud above it to bring life-giving rain to the beautiful flowers and green trees you and I enjoy so much. Then you will begin to walk the higher path.

We all know there are right attitudes and wrong attitudes. Every moment we have the choice of being cheerful or being down in the dumps, totally depressed, reaching up to touch bottom.

We know that the person who cannot be cheerful and mirthful is not walking the right and positive path. Depression is about as natural as a man trying to catch up with his correspondence writing on an upside-down desk.

I promote the spiritual attitude because I have seen what happens to people who live without it. Now, the spiritual attitude is an ideal, just as perfect health is an ideal, and we must have these ideals as goals in order to go forward. These ideals and goals are especially necessary because the environment in which we live is both positive and negative. We must constantly choose the right attitude, the right ideal, the right goal. Most of us know people who are sick all the time. Doctors sometimes refer to them as hypochondriacs. They claim sickness as their own. They say, "I am sick," and they say it often. We must be very careful about what we claim. When we know about these things, we claim health. We claim the best for ourselves.

We would not have much action in life without the polarity principles, the dualistic opposites, the positive and negative. Some of you have to be scared before you act; others have to feel positive and confident before they make a move in life. I'm speaking of positive and negative because everything in life is positive or negative to some degree. Men are positive and women are negative by this way of thinking. When I say that women are negative, I don't mean they are "negative-minded." I am not talking about good and bad or right and wrong. What I mean is that women are more passive and yielding in their nature, more like the attracting pole of a magnet. Men are more outgoing, more go-getting, more dynamic, like the repelling pole of a magnet. Each person, man or woman, is actually a mixture of the positive and negative principles in varying degrees; but men, in general, tend more toward the positive principle, and women, in general, tend more toward the negative principle. That's what makes the world go around, as they say.

Crowd Our Negatives with Positives

All of life follows the polarity principles. What do you believe in? Is your mind positive or negative? When I work with my health principles, I think upon one principle: Good health is the greatest preventative for disease. So, what about you? Are you chasing a cure for disease, or are you going to build good health? You must build good health until there is no room for disease!

Another principle I want to stress applies to the spiritual level. If you can keep your mind on God, there will be no room for the devil. What lessons are you going to carry forward? Are you going to follow the positive or the negative route?

I recall as a child walking through a little forest on the way to and from church at night. Coming and going through that dark forest we would loudly sing, "God Will Take Care of You." I don't know what we thought might be lurking in that forest, but as I look back, I can remember one double-minded young creature wavering and glancing over his shoulder at every turn, faith in one hand, doubt in the other. We are like that — we waver in this kingdom of good health by mixing the negative with the positive. We drink soda pop along with an otherwise nutritious meal.

When we follow the right path, when we make the right choices, the right experiences will come to us. Our bodies will change and positive results will come forth. We start this process mentally by crowding out the negative thoughts and bringing in the positive thoughts.

During my work time with patients, I reflect on what is wrong with the person — what is affecting the shoulders, the knees or various other parts of the body. When I learn that the foods he has been eating are working in the negative direction, I start by putting something positive in their place. It's a replacement therapy that I work with. We start by replacing the thinking, slipping bright, new positive thoughts in place of the worn-out negative thoughts. We put God in place of the devil. We accentuate the positive, not the negative. We go the right instead of the wrong direction. God takes care of us all when we choose the right path, for we have a God of good consequences. But we cannot do wrong and expect a God of good consequences to bail us out. This is an impossibility. I believe that is why many people are not healing as well as they should. They are praying for good health with God in one hand and soda pop in the other.

Right Foods Bring Right Results

A lady came to me complaining of trouble with her eyes. After I had examined her, she asked, "What are you going to do about my condition?"

I told her, "We are going to change your diet."

Immediately this lady became indignant and recited to me a well known *Bible* verse: "It isn't what goes into the body that defiles it — it's what comes out." Then she continued, "I didn't come here to have my diet changed. I came because I heard you were a spiritual person and I thought you would have the spiritual key to making the necessary changes in my body." When I told her I believed a change in diet was the only alternative for improvement, she said, "Son, I'd like to tell you something. I can live on *anything*! I can live on coffee and donuts and make perfect tissue for my body!"

I replied, "Do you seriously mean to tell me that you can live on coffee and donuts?"

"Yes, I can," she insisted. "With prayer and the right spiritual attitude I can make perfect tissue!" I assured her that I didn't believe that to be true, and she said, "Well, son, I would like to prove it to you."

"You're going to have to," I said.

We agreed that if, within ten days, she could bring about a healthy body by living only on coffee and donuts, I would change my thinking. On the morning of the tenth day I awaited this lady's visit with considerable curiosity, as you can imagine. While I was waiting, the telepone rang. "You win," said a rather meek voice on the other end of the line. She went on to explain that her knees had swollen up as big as her head, making it impossible for her to come to my office.

"I didn't win," I told her. "God won, just as He always does. The natural way, the right way — they always win. You see, all natural laws are designed by the Divine Architect, and they carry the spiritual principles within them. It takes a Divine Architect to make carrots and parsley and to put the green chlorophyll in the parsley. When you really think about it the natural foods fit right in with the spiritual laws."

"I see what you mean," she said. "I'm convinced there isn't a godly atom of good left in coffee and donuts!"

You know, she's right. The godly thought, the godly good, is only in the natural foods. That is why you have to come back to God and nature in order to have a good body. I could give you example after example of how the positive and the negative work in a health program. Conditions always change for the better in the body when natural foods are used. Symptoms of illness leave a person who changes to the whole, pure natural foods.

It is said, "A merry heart doeth good like a medicine." We should have a good merry heart. You must plant the seed of happiness in yourself to bear the fruit of smiles and laughter that can be shared with others. This is a must for our nervous systems. The negative of this is what we have previously called "the wrecking crew." The construction crew is on the merry side of life — the side you should get on.

It is sometimes very difficult for me to get on that merry side. When I know that something has to be done and done fast, I get serious. I can get carried away with seriousness. I enjoy humor and I love being happy — but to keep my sense of humor and remain happy has been difficult for me at times when I have many responsibilities to take care of.

Good Health And Spiritual Wealth Go Hand In Hand

Often we don't stop to realize that life is nothing more or less than an experience. What do you experience from moment to moment? The person who can grasp the spiritual concept is being good to his nervous system. That is one reason it is necessary for you to have a spiritual experience, a spiritual contact, a spiritual study. This does not need to be an emotional experience, nor does it necessarily have to happen in a church. It does have to be an experience where you know, where you feel, that you and God are one, that you are following the godly path, walking the positive road. When you feel you are right and godly, you will be released from problems and troubles. None of the negative "hang-ons" or "hang-overs" can destroy or break you down. A person who lives in truth will be free, indeed!

I remember a remark one of my spiritual teachers made to me one time when I was half an hour late and started telling him about all my freeway troubles. He said, "That's your problem — you keep it."

When you want to make a success out of life, an important principle applies. You cannot condemn anyone or debase another person, thinking that you are improving your own image, for that will not bring success. Instead, you must build others up. You must just be yourself. Don't pretend to be someone you aren't, just be yourself. What is yours will know your face and will be attracted to you. Likewise, don't try to get something that doesn't belong to you. Just take that which is yours. Too many people are trying to get what belongs to others in addition to their own share. Don't try to grab the other person's bread. Bake your own. This is the way to make a success out of life, for everyone must bear the consequences for the way he lives in this world of cause and effect. It is true that you can have what you wish, but you have to take everything that goes with it.

Don't accept anything less than the best you have within yourself. If you have a spiritual ideal in your life, if you are giving out spiritual love, you will attract, you will contract, you will set up a regular epidemic of just what you give out — and this is as it should be. If you want to spread an epidemic of joy, you must start it yourself. Spiritual power is within you, and it should be wrapped up in a happy feeling so it will be easy for you to start a joyful epidemic.

Don't Accept Anything But Good

When we believe the devil will get us if we don't watch out, when we believe in hellfire and brimstone, we are forgetting about the loving heavenly Father, the forgiving Father. And we are forgetting about the wonderful gifts we receive when we are close to our heavenly Father. He says, "All that I have is thine." Since it gives the Father such great pleasure to give us His kingdom, why settle for anything less?

There is a great happiness awaiting you if you can accept this spiritual belief. While you are seeking it you must assume it. While you are striving for it you must appropriate it. Otherwise you will become discouraged and fail. You must place yourself right in the midst of it and stake your claim. You must say, "This is mine. I am one with the Father." When you do this and accept this spiritual feeling, you can forget any unpleasantness around you, any disease and poverty. Do this quickly; assert yourself in the positive!

Life is not only an experience, but it is also a demonstration. You are here to demonstrate this life and you can demonstrate life in a pleasant way as soon as you get on the positive road. We are not trapped in a perpetual series of up and down cycles. There is no such law of life. We don't have to accept the incorrect belief that every happy event is followed by some major or minor disaster. When you stop giving in to the negative powers and accept the positive powers, you will be able to demonstrate life to its fullest.

Many people are living with both the power of evil and the power of good at the same time. Many have mixed the power of doubt with the power of faith. Many of us say, "God will take care of me," all the time wondering if He really will. We say we are getting well, but inside we secretly feel we are still sick. We pray for a job and get one but we are afraid it won't last for more than a week. We must change these attitudes and accept *only* the power of good.

We are all more or less like the Prodigal Son. Leaving a place where we actually had everything, we stride out into the world seeking some magical place that we imagine must be much more wonderful than the one we left. Instead, we find that the new life is hell. Finally, we go home. The trouble is, most of us return home after we have spent our life, our money and our vitality. When we've lost everything, we say, "Now what am I going to do?" And that is the time we turn.

But we should not and need not wait until we are drowning in a sea of troubles and problems. We should turn to our God as soon as possible and stay with Him. We should keep our bodies fortified and healthy at all times so that we can meet problems and troubles when they come and take them in stride. Many people only turn to spiritual help when they are bombarded with troubles — they say our churches are always crowded during a time of war. But if we dwell on the positive attitudes all the time, we will keep our inner selves in constant repair so we can face anything with calmness.

Only you can decide where you are going to put your power — in the negative or in the positive. If you choose to put your power into the positive channel, if you choose to do that which is right, you can develop anything you wish. It is the law of the mind that anything you put your attention to grows and develops.

All Power Is Given to You

If we truly accept and believe we are one with the Father, we are the most powerful beings in the world. When you are following the natural way of life, when you adhere to the laws dictated by nature, you are the most powerful person in the world.

You can get rid of aches and pains very quickly with an aspirin, but that method only gives temporary relief of symptoms. When the pain returns, you have to head for the aspirin bottle again. If you want to get rid of the aches and pains for all time, you must get on the right path. Some of you, I know, hope to have this happen in a hurry. You must remember that whatever you accumulate for good, doing the right deeds, is forever.

"He that abideth in me, and I in him, the same bringeth forth much fruit." If we are to be cheerful, we must work on God's side. If we are to know mirth and happiness, we must work on God's side. If we are to be uplifted, we must work with truth. If we are to have healthy bodies, we must work with nature. If we are to have fewer problems with people, we must join the godly team. When you live truth, and when God is with you, you will not worry about what other people say to do. If we make ourselves right, all else will be right.

For the first time in our life, when we do that which is right, we can leave the rest to God. "Let go and let God." That which God does through you, He will do for you. For once in our lives, our problems are in the right hands — God's. He knows no disease. He knows only perfection, success, that which is good. The person who accepts that life will have good health, prosperity and success. To do that which is approved by God each day allows us to leave the rest to Him. Then we will know that whatever is yet to come will be that for which we can be thankful, for it is the will of God.

Joy — you understand so little of the Joy of Life! You perform so many of your daily avocations as burdensome tasks instead of labors of love. Be like little children filled with secret wonder and joy and the Spirit of High Adventure.

— Author Unknown

From the Doctor's Pen . . .

LIFE'S RICHES

The riches of life are locked in a vault;
You carry them deeply within.
The riches you spend with the finger's touch
Are sought by the senses again and again.

The riches you acquire and add to your heart
Can be used to take you far and near.
It's truly a passport and will see you through,
For what you have inmost should be spent now and here.

Riches could be buried, never used,
And piled high to overflowing;
The value of the riches you have within
Is how you spend it on your fellowmen.

You are the bank to deposit your riches;
Make a deposit whenever you can.
Do this by giving of the riches buried
From past deposits made deep in your heart.

How many times have you heard it said,
"I'll give you my very last dollar?"
But when you give of yourself from within
You can give it over and over again and again.

Chapter 28

Easter Sunday

Miracles happen, not in opposition
to nature, but in opposition to
what we know of nature.
— St. Augustine

It is especially appropriate to consider Easter in terms of life and health, because Easter and Christ's resurrection are a celebration of the life principle. Healthful living in spirit, mind and body means we can overcome suffering of all kinds and rise again to build a better physical body, a better mind, and, of course, better relations with other human beings. This renewal can give you your most valuable asset in life, a realization that there is no such thing as a final end, no such thing as death. Christ's greatest gift to humanity was his wonderful demonstration that we transcend even death, passing from this life into a new life.

I think the greatest thing in this world is to be able to transcend and rise from whatever conditions we are living in right now.

Because we are all interested in the truth, we should be interested in transcending, in resurrection, in coming out of the old and moving into the new.

Today I will talk of transcending, of resurrecting this thing that we call the body, this body that is constantly breaking down and that we are constantly working to save and to keep from deterioration.

Here is something for us to think about: The moment that we transcend whatever is bothering us, the body will begin to rejuvenate and regenerate of its own accord. The comic strip character Pogo in the newspapers once announced to his friends, "We have met the enemy — and he is *us*!" So often that is true. Well, why don't we just turn around mentally so that we can be our own best friend? Wouldn't it be marvelous to have your best friend right at your elbow whenever you needed a friend? You can be your own best friend.

People come into my office saying, "Doctor, my memory is going downhill." "I can't concentrate anymore." "I'm in financial difficulties." "I don't think I'll make it." "What is wrong with me, doctor? I have lost so much." I have seen many losses, many problems and troubles, and I want to tell you we live our sufferings in our minds more than we know. We don't live in the body as much as we do in our mind. Our mind is going nonstop morning, noon and night, even during sleep. When you are absent from the body, this busy mind is still working. You go to bed tired and worn from your daily activities, and if you don't release yourself from these, you wake up in the morning under the covers just as disturbed as you were the day before. People are suffering today, and it is time to remind ourselves of the great lesson the Christ tried to teach us. We can rise above suffering. We can transcend it.

One of the most important things I have to tell you is this: The body follows the mind. I put my hand on the piano. Who put it there? I kick this book. Who kicked this book? We don't realize what moves this hand or these feet. We have to remind ourselves over and over again that *everything* the body does begins in the *mind.* This is the lesson we have to learn: We must rise from suffering in the mind before we can rise from suffering in the body. We must have an untroubled mind.

Would You Like An Untroubled Mind?

We always have to start from where we are to get to where we want to go. Our destination is an untroubled mind, but for most people the starting point is a troubled mind. "But how do I get there?" you may ask. I would just love to be able to reach inside my desk drawer and hand you a map. I would just love to be able to say, "This map will show you the way to an untroubled mind." Now, the best I can do is to show you the general direction you must take. The rest is up to you.

Fifty per cent of your physical sufferings would leave if you had an untroubled mind. At least half of the high blood pressure problems start in the head, and the same is true for colitis and kidney trouble. All stress and strain, which interfere with good circulation, come from the head. Your heart just can't beat right with negative thoughts going through the head. If I could give you an untroubled mind, it would be one of the most wonderful gifts you could possibly receive.

We live lives of anxiety. We suffer overwhelming feelings of fear, tension and frustration. We have them all day long. We are afraid of what is yet to come. Too many of us haven't fixed up our lives — we are either afraid that we will live a long time in suffering or that death will come too soon. We're afraid of death. We're afraid of life. We're afraid to take on the challenges life offers us. If you'll just stop and think of one single thing that you *can* take on with confidence each morning, you'll find out that your whole body will be released. You'll start the day with an untroubled mind and peace. And once you start right, it will stay with you as you shift to other tasks. Take them one at a time.

I can tell you many true stories about people who are crucifying themselves on a cross of harsh thoughts. They are ruining their nervous systems. When the nervous system is ruined, you ruin your stomach activity, your kidney activity, your power of concentration and your memory. You ruin your whole life and you drag down those around you.

This is why you have to rise to something new that will bring peace as it flows through your mind. This is not an easy idea to understand, but I believe there was a time when mankind was actually spiritual. I believe that when we were created in God's image, we were spiritual. And I believe we can get back to that higher way.

We have all heard about the "fall of man," the fall of Adam and Eve from the Garden of Eden. I believe this was a falling from the spiritual level to the physical, a falling to the human level. The first children of Adam and Eve were Cain and Abel. Cain slew Abel, the first murder since the dawn of Creation. Somewhere along the line our ideals were lowered. Why did Cain slay Abel? Was it envy? Envy that turned into a murderous wrath? Where does envy come from? Where does anger come from? How is it that the human race came to wear the thorny crown of violence? We have fallen heir to human faults and failings which we must rise above before we can regain good physical and mental health.

You Must Make The Decision

This will be somewhat abstract, and you must take time to figure it out along with me. You will have to decide this day, this very day, who you are and where you are going. This can only be done in your mind.

Somehow or other, when we start this life we don't seem to know all the better things. I can't tell you why this is, but my children were always fighting when they were little. I would say to them, "Where did you learn all this fighting? I didn't teach you to fight." As we get older, as we develop wisdom, as we grow closer to spiritual thinking, we try to leave our childish ways behind. Now, this is the *real* life. This is the *normal* life. The real life and the normal life are the spiritual life. Can you see this? Many have not realized this yet.

We may have studied but we may not have learned. Most of us don't know that our minds take on a certain shape. They are just like muffins! We pour batter into the muffin tin, and the muffins are shaped exactly like the mold. They cannot be different. The shape of the mind determines the shape of things to come in our lives.

There are two things that give the mind its shape over all the rest: doubt and faith. Doubt attracts fear. Faith never does this. People have fears in their minds today, and then tomorrow they will add others to these, and next week they add still more fears. They go from one fear to another. Doubt shapes the mind, fear pours into it, and the result is suffering, pain, disease. Perhaps you should change the shape of your muffin tin. Perhaps you should try a little faith. I think you should and I think you can. However, you still have to decide what you are going to pour into it.

I don't feel sorry for the person who dies; I feel sorry for the person who has never lived. Living is the thing we have to grasp. Living means so much to us. And we live by faith. When we doubt that good will come to us, we go through life manipulating this scene and that scene. We manipulate this person and that person. Then doubt creeps in again, and we try to change the scene. We try to get it out of our mind or we try to picture something else. What are we doing? We are running away from life. We go next door to avoid a person we don't like who is coming to our house. Or, we pull down the shades and refuse to answer the doorbell. We get so we can't stand other people, and the first thing we know, we just can't stand ourselves. We have never lived. We are imprisoned behind a wall of doubt, tortured by fears of our own creation. This is our darkest hour — and some of us must get to this point before we begin to see the light, before our eyes begin to open to the great lesson in all of this. We have nowhere to go but up. And the only ladder around us is faith.

Faith Is Like A Ladder — It Leads Up

"Faith," says the Good Book, "is the substance of things hoped for, the evidence of things not seen." We begin by planting the seed of faith in our own heart. We stop relying on others to give us the good life on a silver platter. We stop blaming, nagging, complaining. How many times have I told you to leave other people alone? Build a life of your own. You can rise from your problems and become a new man or woman. Some of you never study. Some have never been out of the town or city they live in today. The worm in the horseradish thinks it is the sweetest place in the world. Get out into the sunshine. Discover the world. Find out about all the wonderful people and places in it! There is a lovely place to go, and we can go there if we desire it. If you are not where you should be, you must begin to evolve. I would like to tell you about some of these wonderful new possiblilities.

We become so busy that we heal one part of the body only. Tomorrow we find some other part of the body that requires healing. If we straighten out our mind, the whole body can follow a wonderful new routine. The body follows the mind — but what does the mind follow? The mind follows the spirit if we let it, and we can let spirit pour into the mind. If the mind accepts it, it expresses spirit and brings it forth. All the physical things are an expression of your mind and your spirit. Your mind is an expression of the spirit. If you are troubled mentally, what are you in spirit?

To be transformed in mind we have to have a spiritual change, that is, an outgoing, a divine flow of something through this mind and body. I wonder if you realize that the mind and the body are instruments of the spirit. They are instruments to be used. Have you used your mind? Have you opened up to the working of the spirit? We start by planting a mustard seed of faith. Then we watch it grow.

The Apostle Paul wrote, "Whatsoever things are true, whatsoever things are honest, whatsoever things are just, whatsoever things are pure, whatsoever things are lovely, whatsoever things are of good report — if there be any virtue and if there be any praise, think of these things." Put your mind on these things and you will find that nothing can disturb you.

Usually, we let the mind run rampant. We

let its thoughts scramble around like a bunch of wild children. Whatever happens here, we run to take care of it; whatever happens there, we run back to take care of it too. But do we really? We can put this mind under control. We can direct it toward good. "He blew up," they say. Where are you going when you blow up? "It was such a peaceful experience to be with that person." "What you say is music to my ears." "You are a sight for sore eyes!" These are mental things. You have to have something besides just muffin batter in your head, and you have to have something besides fear and hate.

I think Christ (this might sound strange to you) hated a lot of the things people did, but He never struck a person. He loved the people. His love for people was greater than His hate for what they did. I don't like some of the situations people get into, or even get me into, but I can't hate them for it. I can hate the situation. I can hate the result that man has produced. But I don't hate the man. I love the man.

Our Spiritual Center

We have a center. Call it a spiritual center if you will. When I offer you a choice between a poison pickle and a ripe apricot, which will you choose? There is something in the center of you saying, "I deserve the very best there is." I am sure there is something, too, that says, "If you are frustrated, if you are fearful, fear not. I have not given thee fear. I have given thee loveliness. I have given thee a sound mind. I have given thee purity." You have a center from which to realize that something good is here. If you didn't have that spiritual center, if each one of you didn't have a Christ consciousness, you wouldn't recognize that Christ was sincere, that He was working for mankind's upliftment. You must have something good in there because you were built in the image of God. That is why you have this godly center in you.

I stuttered and stammered for nearly seventeen years. I know what it feels like to burn up when you see people. I never realized people couldn't hurt me. They hurt me — but, who let it happen? I did! I allowed people to put me in a shell. I locked myself up in my shell and wouldn't come out. I would try, just a little, and my voice would stutter. I couldn't make those words come because I was afraid. I took about thirty public speaking classes, each one lasting for the extent of one evening because I would become so frustrated trying to speak that I would quit. I didn't want the same person to see me twice.

The best thing that ever happened to me during those speech classes was when a teacher awakened me. He said, "Tonight you are going to have a topic. You are going to speak on 'How to Remove the Garbage Dump from Oakland, California and Make a Clean City Out of It.'" Of all the topics to talk about! But, I took it very seriously. I was going to renew that city.

That night I walked up in front of the class and did it. I was right in the middle of my speech about cleaning up Oakland when a student interrupted and said, "I don't like the color of your tie." Then someone else said, "Why don't you tie your shoelaces with a different kind of knot?" Then a third person said, "You know, I think you are a nut." For a while I kept on talking. But then in the midst of that increasing heckling, I stopped.

That wise teacher of mine said, "Don't stop — go! Don't stop now. Go on, get out of that!" And, I'll tell you, I went right on and I said, "I want you to listen to me. I spent a lot of time preparing for this speech." I broke right out of my shell and I have had no stuttering or stammering since. I was completely free! Now I can say, "I feel wonderful!" I have a new life. I am not afraid to go anyplace and speak now. I always say a little prayer ahead of time. The greatest thing is being free — having that wonderful feeling of being free! I know what it is to break out of bondage. I know what it is to get out of a stranglehold. People lock themselves in that prison. They are caught inside those shells. They are caught inside an Easter Egg. Why not break out of that shell and be free?

Want To Break Out Of Your Shell?

This is the time for me to tell you how to break out of your shell. Or are you going to remain an egg for the rest of your life? Did you ever hear of a "bad egg"? A bad egg is someone who has never come forth into the good life. But you can have the seed of rebirth. You can become something in the new generation. You can have the resurrection; you can have the new life. If you refuse to break out of your shell, you will have to remain there for the rest of your life. Oh, you can color your shell up like a fancy Easter Egg. You can wear lovely clothes and beautiful hats, but what are you on the inside? To be a beautiful soul, you must know that life and goodness come from within and these are what your nervous system is crying out for.

Some of us only live half a life. We don't even know what we control with this nervous system. You can take that nervous system and let *joy* have an Easter Parade through it! It will change almost immediately. The nervous system is asking for peace and joy and harmony. It is asking for resurrection. It is asking for Easter. It is asking for springtime. It is asking for something new to come forth. This is what Easter should mean from a health standpoint.

I can't make anything happen for you. I can't get you out of your eggshell. You can only break it from the inside. I broke out of mine, but then I crawled into another one. I'm breaking out of that one, too. I'm going to break out of that one because I have learned that eggs never stop. Chickens never stop laying, either. Which was first — the chicken or the egg? You go from chicken to egg, egg to chicken. That is what life is all about. It goes on and on. It never stops. Life is never ending. Life is eternal.

What is flowing through your mind? Did you ever hear expressions like, "I am a child of God;" "I am here to bring peace and harmony to other people;" "I'm here to be kind"? Is this spirit working in you? Or, are you void? Are you empty? The only good God can do for you is in what He can do through you.

Do you want to end your dis-ease? End your disease by dissolving that little problem you have, whether it is in finances, in your job or in your marriage. You can end many problems by the right mental and spiritual attitude. You can go the successful way spiritually as well as the positive way mentally.

You see, too often we are trying to start from the bottom up. Why don't we start from the top? You have been going at this thing backward. I speak of this because I see so many people who are trying to make this transition in the mind. They are making this transition through plotting and scheming and overcoming and trying to *think* their way out. You have been taught that thoughts are things, and now you are trying to manipulate your thinking. But manipulation is hard on a person. You try this today, only to have to try something else tomorrow. You're getting tired out from trying. You're all "tried out." You're tired from trying.

The mind gives us health one day and sickness another day. It wavers. We have faith in one hand, doubt in the other. This is the mind, but the spirit is constant. We wouldn't have all these ups and downs if we straightened out our minds. We must transcend mind, we have to go above mind.

I once had to treat a patient for high blood pressure, kidney trouble, stomach trouble and an ulcer. This man had been very rich but had lost all of his money except for $10,000. He had to lay off his cook. He no longer had a chauffeur and had to drive his own car. He was really a poor man from many standpoints. His insurance coverage had to be dropped; it cost too much. He said, "Look at me. I amount to nothing. I only have $10,000." This man wasn't easy to treat, because he was practically a mental case. "Fix my stomach. Fix my kidneys. I can't sleep any more." Mental depression had come upon him. He knew he was weary and worn out from thinking.

Another man came in some time later and said, "I'm the happiest man in the world, doctor!" He slapped me on the back and continued, "Is there something I can do for you?" Well, this was quite a switch, coming into my office asking if he could do something for me! He added, "I'm so happy — I bought a couple of old houses, fixed them up and sold them, and I have $10,000 in the bank! I'm the happiest man in the world!"

The first man was the most dejected man in the world because he had only $10,000, but the second man was the happiest man in the world with his $10,000!

It's Your Mind That Does It

This is mind over matter. This is mind over platter. This is mind over the body. This is mind over disease. This is ease over dis-ease, love over hate, benevolence over fear and condemnation. This is charity over and above all the things the average person thinks about. But don't think too long, because if you get into tired, negative thinking, you're going to be in trouble. In your thinking you may decide that this muffin pan can only go so far and you can only put so much dough in it.

You have inherited the whole kingdom of love, peace, harmony, charity, benevolence, joy and happiness. "All that I have is thine" — the whole kingdom is yours! And look at what we bake — we bake a muffin and then we burn it in the oven! We don't realize that this narrow mind of ours needs to be enlarged. It's time we enlarged the borders of our sense. It's time for us to get a mind stretcher. It's time that we allow our minds to become big things in our lives.

We Must Learn To Rise To The Occasion

We must have a *rising* ability. We must be resurrected. It would be criminal to believe that life is all going to be snuffed out and taken away. This is not a matter to consider only toward the end of life. This is a daily consideration. We have to raise above situations day in and day out. We have to rise above that problem, rise above all negations that weigh upon us. Each negation is a little death that we have to rise from. We have to have rhythm, this "rising" ability. We have to have the rising sun , the realm of Spirit we can go to, a secret place of the Most High. We have to have the Upper Room, some place where God is. We have to go into the Great Within. This is the place where we have all been clamoring to be admitted. We hear, "If only he could understand me," or "If only I could understand him." We don't understand ourselves too well! If only we would go within, God is already there! You can't separate God from yourself. You try hard, you run mentally and you run physically, and by so doing you run away from the spirit center. We need to rise and to go back *into*!

That is why we have an Easter Sunday. The rising sun comes from the east, and we must look for that rising within ourselves. Easter would become more "Easterly" in our thinking — more "Easterly" in our sight. We've got to go Easterly. We've got to go toward the rising sun. There is no sunrise service outside unless it is first within you. There is no rising of the sun less it is within you. This is one of the greatest things I can tell you.

We cannot look to the mind any more for the good of our bodies. We cannot look to the mind any more for the good we want to spread to humanity. We can't look to the mind to get us out of these civilized problems we have today. We have to look to Spirit, to God.

When you come to me, and I adjust the second dorsal of the spine, it's very important. But I'm telling you that you need an even more important adjustment. I can change your diet from coffee and donuts but it's even more important that I change your worry, fear and hate to joy, peace and happiness. I have to change your thinking. This is something we have to raise more than anything else.

Mind is the effect! All is good with God. You have to start at the top, and the God point. Some people take this way of talking as "too religious," but I'm talking from the health standpoint. I say it this way because I know that the Truth and the Spirit give you something constant, something to believe in, something godly.

I know that whatever goes into the mind is going to have to flow out. If it doesn't flow out, you'll blow up. To be able to get things off your mind, you will have to have an open mind. We have to have an open mind and allow only good thoughts to come in before good can flow out.

So what you should ask for today, really, is more light, isn't it? You have to be the enlightened one. You must think about transcending the mind and going *into* more light. When you see more light, you're going to be easier on the rest of your body.

What Kind Of Light Do You Seek?

By showing color television to his laboratory rats, a scientist found that their pituitary glands dried up, and the rats became little hairless runts. The results of this experiment were taken to the federal government, after which 12,000 color television sets were withdrawn from the market, because they were determined to be detrimental to the human body.

Can anyone say that the spiritual light has ever had detrimental effects upon man? Quite the opposite. It is only the kind of light that man can create or invent that has harmful effects. This is what causes many people to seek their doctors — they have been overexposed to the wrong kind of light.

Today is a day to renew your faith that there is a greater day to come, that there is a better mind to live in, that there is a greater thought to harbor in the mind. There is something we have to seek from a Higher Source, a better source than we can create ourselves.

You know, many times I wonder how man can possibly believe in a new day. How can he believe in eternity? How can he believe in a deathless life? I look at all the trees. In the wintertime trees hibernate after losing all their leaves. Each spring I see the new leaf buds appear, and this is a wonderful sight to see. Sometimes I wonder — if I had never seen those leaves or blossoms come out before, would I believe? Because the leaves have appeared twice, I expect them to come out a third time, and they do. I know they will come out a fourth time, a fifth and so on. They will never cease. There will never be less than a spring, and spring always promises a summer. Let's resurrect our physical body into something new, something better. I'd like to emphasize that the time to start is *now*. I think one of the finest messages brought out in the *Bible* is, "Go to my brethren and say unto them, I ascend unto my Father and your Father, and to my God and your God."

Belinda Mary May Briggs wrote these words:

Easter? What is Easter's meaning for me?
Life. Life abundant, joyous and free.
Life in the brooding of seasonal mists;
Life in the crocus with cup sunkissed;
Life in the nectar searching of bees;
Life in the swelling of buds on the trees;
Life in the sparrow's inspiring song;
Life's quickening nature all the day long;
Life waking up from a cold winter's sleep;
Life in the land pressing close to the sheep;
Life resurrected in Jesus, our Lord;
Life's praises united ascending to God.
Oh, it is the Life in all that I see,
This is what Easter is meaning for me.

There is life in all she mentions in her poem. Of course, Easter is a Christian festival. It commemorates Christ's resurrection. This is supposed to be the spring equinox, or as close as they could get to it. At that time the sun rises upon the beginning of a new season.

I can't help but recall the scene of Mary at Christ's tomb when she saw that the rock blocking the entrance had been rolled away and His body was gone. Then Christ showed Himself to her. And she went to tell the people. "He is risen!" He had risen above death. If I could only convince you that you could rise above all sick ideas, above all these things that are given to you by mankind today! If you'd just seek to rise above all these things, you'd find a new life. A new life!

There is no end when it comes to God. That is why I would like simply to say: "*You are.*" You are a forever person; you are an eternal being. Don't ever get to the place where you think there's an end. Your world, your life, is your own ten acres: start plowing! Start spiritualizing. Let the Divine Spirit flow through you. When we allow it to flow through, we'll find that the physical will follow the spiritual. Good will follow good.

Seek this place called the kingdom — the king's domain of God. Then you will find all things added unto you. No disease will visit you because you will have arisen. You will have deserted the lower mind and "people" thinking and the hum-drum of everyday living. You will have a new life, and if you'll let this new life flow through you, you'll have joy. Remember that today you can be a new person. You can resurrect yourself as you become one with God.

Yes, something good is going to happen to you, because this is the beginning of a new day. You've taken a new life. Hereafter, you will walk and talk differently than you ever have before because you have something to live for! There is no end. There is no rejection. You will always be taken care of because you are one with God, the Eternal Being.

Stay with God. He will never forsake you!

"I have not given thee the spirit of fear but I have given thee power, a strong mind and love."

Chapter 29

Inheritance In Our Lives

Whatever strengthens and purifies the affections, enlarges the imagination, and adds Spirit to sense, is useful.

— Shelley

Whenever a new baby is born the relatives gather around and we hear, "He has his mother's eyes," or "He has his father's chin." Later, as the child grows, we may hear other things like, "He has his grandfather's quick temper," or "He certainly has the artistic talent that runs in the family." It is important to realize that inheritance is the starting point in our lives — physically, mentally and spiritually. But it is just as important to realize that it is not the end point. Our inheritance is not the primary determining thing in our lives.

Somehow, I have always felt that I have lived before, that I came into this life because I wanted to come, because I had a job to do. I have always been a seeker and have found that whenever I have been able to help another person live a better life, a happier life, I felt uplifted and happy myself. Now, there is something we can learn by applying this idea to our inheritance in life.

We will find this idea especially illuminating when we consider what many people call "tragic births" — those babies born deformed, deaf, blind, mentally retarded or with other congenital defects. The Good Book tells us, "All things work together for good to them that love God, to them who are called according to His purpose." It may be hard to see this thing, but we are all born with the same loving heavenly Father. Every child is born with a special purpose. We are all on this earth to learn, to develop, to grow. As I have mentioned before, I believe that one of the reasons children come is to teach the parents certain things. Some lessons are more difficult for us than others, but everything that comes before us on the path of life has something to teach us. Of course, that goes for the handicapped child and those around him as well as for his parents.

There is more to inheritance than meets the eye. There is the genetic inheritance that we have received from our parents, just as they did from their parents. We have the inheritance of the family environment, including the type of upbringing, the foods, the atmosphere of the home, whether harmonious and pleasant or chaotic and disturbing. We also have the cultural inheritance which brings in the schooling, the standard of living, the regional food preferences, the prevailing customs and religions. All of this is the child's inheritance.

Previously we have talked about the double meanings we find in many things of this life. Just as the child has a genetic inheritance, a family environment inheritance and a cultural inheritance, it works the other way, too. The parents have inherited the child, and the child will serve as a kind of mirror, so to speak, in which they will see some of their own characteristics in a new light. The family environment has inherited a new member, and it will change because of this. The culture, too, has inherited a new person, and each child born in this world will affect and change its culture in some way, small or great. Each child, we find, will both change and be changed by the lives of those people he or she meets on the path of life. But the deepest lessons will be those exchanged by the child and the parents. Some of the most difficult lessons of love, patience, forbearance, discipline and forgiveness are learned because of the strong bond between the parents and the child, and these lessons are necessary for us.

Marriage As A New Beginning

In most societies, including ours, men and women tend to marry young. This is the time when we are just a little bit brash, when we as yet lack wisdom, when our spiritual development has not yet advanced very far. Yet, this is also the time when the creative force of reproduction is the strongest, when we have high hopes for the future. What can the young husband, the young wife, give to the future? They can only give all that they have, all that they are. Their bodies are made up of the foods they have eaten up to that point in their lives, distributed into the physical constitution each has inherited from his or her parents. Their minds are made up of the accumulated thoughts, beliefs and attitudes that each has gathered so far, and we realize that these mental activities have affected the form and substance of the physical body.

We may ask, do this man and woman truly love one another? Are they well matched or mismatched? Is the attraction between them primarily physical, or is it balanced with the mental and spiritual? What are their living habits at this time? Do they harbor secret hopes or fears for the future? As we have said before, thoughts will affect every cell of the body — and this includes the reproductive cells.

All of this goes into the moment of conception. This is something to think about, isn't it?

I believe that nothing *just happens*; everything *happens just*. I believe that at the moment of conception there is a thought for the next generation in the mother and a thought for the next generation in the father. Somehow, the child born from this union is, in a divine sense, a thread that began with the dawn of the human race, a thread interwoven throughout the fabric of the family history, a thread running through the lives of the parents and on into the future.

We are born to learn and born to teach, whether we do it consciously or not. Often even a new baby will seem to sense when we are tiredest, when we have reached the lowest point, and at that time it will get the colic or a crying spell for some reason. Then we learn to draw on some reservoir of inner strength that we didn't know we had before, and we take care of that child. We learn lessons from our children that we would not be able to accept from anyone else, don't we? And they learn lessons from us that they would not accept from anyone else.

It is always best if lessons are learned in an atmosphere of love, but we must realize that the lessons will come even if love on the part of the parents — and sometimes the child — is lacking. That powerful parent-child bond is still there in even the harsh parent, the coarse parent. Many fathers seem to be this way, this unloving way. But they still get the lessons. They get the lessons because these lessons come from the higher realm, the realm of the Law, the realm of the heavenly Father.

I am convinced that we all look back and think that if we could live our lives over again, we would do better. We would change this or that. Many times I have thought that if I hadn't been so foolish in my living habits while I was young I would have a better body today. But, we must realize that every stumbling block can be turned into a stepping stone. Every obstacle can be turned into an opportunity. Our parents were doing the best they knew, just as we do with our children, and we must love them for that. If there is anything to forgive and forget, do that right now. Harvest the wheat and let go of the chaff, for your own good.

We must Honor Our Father And Mother — For Our Own Good

If you have harbored resentment against your parents, realize that there is ample reason why you were born to them and you must accept it whether you understand it or not. There is a deeper thing that lives within us and connects us with them from the past and with that which is yet to come. There is a life more abundant given to each of us, and we must be aware of this.

Now, often we regard our inherited strengths as blessings and our inherited weaknesses as curses. I have seen many conditions brought into life that caused me to wonder why these things happen. Why a retarded child? Why thyroid weaknesses? Why weak stomachs? I am sure there is a lesson to be learned in many of these cases, a lesson in overcoming, in taking hold of these weaknesses, in seeing what strengths we can make out of them.

We are on our way to wisdom when we overcome a physical problem such as an ulcer of the stomach. We are on our way to wisdom when we overcome the negative thoughts, the negative attitudes, we have picked up from our parents or from our society. This is one of our big challenges in life. Anyone who has brought his body from poor health to good health has much to be thankful for, much to be happy for. These are the moments in life that we're all trying to come to. So, whatever our weaknesses may be, I think they are there for a purpose. Let us use them to make a better life.

A lot is dependent upon our knowledge; more is dependent upon wisdom; and the greater amount is dependent upon the spiritual guidance that we seek in life. A weakness or physical handicap may be the means to steer us into the right job or occupation we should have in this life. In a similar way, a weakness may guide us to a particular place on this earth which is most beneficial to our health while at the same time bringing us together with people who need what we have to offer. It is well to know something about climate, altitude, humidity, ocean living, mountain living and ozone belts — things which help when we have certain weaknesses that are hard to overcome.

It is well to know that city life is not as beneficial as country life. It is well to know that green has a definite relaxing effect on the eye structure. The red that we find in cayenne pepper and tomatoes has a stimulating effect on the arterial system of the body. The yellow fruits and vegetables have a laxative effect upon the body.

I believe that our inherited weaknesses drive us to seek out the place and the way in which we can develop our highest potential. So we look at our weaknesses as stepping stones. We look at our weaknesses as incentives to polish our soul. We use them as motivations to learn more of nature and to get closer to God.

What you have is what you are. Birth is only one of the starting points in life. Right now is the beginning of the rest of your life.

The Well Mated And The Mismated

They say that marriages are made in heaven, and I believe they can be. But it seems that many marriages are made in some other place. The soaring divorce rate in this country shows us that there is a great lack of wisdom in the way that many people select their mates or conduct themselves in marriage. I believe that fifty percent of the marriages in this country are mismated; one person is fine and sensitive, the other is coarse and tough. In my experience with many thousands of patients, marriage works best when both persons are fine or both are coarse.

When I refer to a fine person I mean a sensitive person, finely put together as a precision Swiss watch. A coarse person is one who is rough and insensitive. There is a story about a farmer who was trying to train a new mule without the slightest success. The mule simply would not respond to anything the farmer tried to get it to do. When the neighbor came over, a man with a good deal of experience with mules, the farmer told him his problem. "Show me the mule," the man said. "I'll see what I can do." When they came up to the mule, the first thing the man did was to pick up a long piece of board and whack that mule across the rear end as hard as he could. "Goodness!" the farmer exclaimed."Is that how you train a mule?" His neighbor said, "No —

but first you have to get their attention. Now you can start training him." Of course, this is an exaggeration, but it is generally very difficult for a fine person to communicate with a coarse person.

Once a lady asked me to come to dinner and to meet her husband. She was in a quandary and needed help. She met me at the door wearing a nice dress with a lovely apron over it and said, "Come in. My husband is out back with the chickens, working."

I stepped inside and noticed that everything was clean and orderly, as I expected from what I knew of this woman. I could see her husband at work in back, stripped to the waist, barrel-chested, hairy and dripping with sweat. When dinner was ready, she called him to come in.

John tromped through the living room, trailing chicken dirt from his boots onto the beautiful clean pale green carpet. A coarse woman would have taught him not to do this by yelling at him and swatting him, but John's wife was too gentle and sensitive to do such a thing. He sat down at the table still sweaty, shirtless and unwashed until she asked him to go to the bathroom, wash up and put on a clean shirt she had laid out for him.

When he returned, his wife said, "John, I wanted you to meet Dr. Jensen so I invited him over to dinner."

"That's fine," John grunted and immediately began dishing food onto his plate without passing anything on. By the time his wife and I had started to eat, he was finished. He stood without excusing himself and retired to the living room where he promptly fell asleep on the couch. His wife was nearly in tears.

"Why did you marry this man?" I asked.

"We met at the Philadelphia Opera House," she said. "We both had season tickets and sat in adjoining seats. We both liked opera, so we became friends and soon afterward we were married."

They had one interest in common, and on the basis of that, they married. Obviously, this was not a healthy marriage for either of them, but since John was more "thick-skinned," he was far less disturbed than his wife was at the way things were going. There is no easy solution for this sort of marriage.

We Can Have What We Want — But We Have To Live With The Consequences

I have treated over 350,000 patients in the past fifty years. Half the people who came to me suffered from mismated marriages. That is anything but heaven. There is a lesson in this. We choose the person we marry and then we have to live with that choice. A certain amount of compromise is possible, but when it comes to a breakdown in health as a consequence of the marriage situation, a change must be made.

Fine people, due to the sensitivity of their thyroid glands, have a low tolerance for noise. Too much noise causes thyroid breakdown. Fine people need certain foods to remain healthy and must avoid foods such as fried eggs that aren't good for them. The foods that a fine person requires may not meet the needs of a coarse person. And when a coarse person tries to fit himself into the sensitively-tuned, orderly world of the fine person, he often feels as frustrated and unhappy as if he were in prison.

The children of this kind of mismated marriage have both their father's side and their mother's side. In one mood they are like their father, in another they are like their mother.

My mother was fine, and my father was coarse. He was a doctor, but she was the healer in the family. I have inherited characteristics from both.

Once a lady came to my father for a spinal adjustment, and when she laid down on the table, how he gave it to her! I thought her spine was going to sag down onto the floor, and when she recovered she said, "You don't adjust like Dr. Smith in Berkeley."

My father looked at her and said, "If you don't like it, you can get the hell out of here!"

She did, too.

I have found in my life that my mother's side dominates. When I'm refreshed and rested, I'm enthusiastic about things the way my mother was. I have her touch for healing. When I am at my best I can give you wisdom, which comes from my mother's nature. If I become tired, I turn into a bear, and that is my father's nature. Then I want to listen to music, as he did.

At the age of thirty my mother died of consumption and tuberculosis. I was born into the world with a weak lung structure, taking after my mother. To complicate matters, for three years of my late teens I practically lived on the worst of the "junk foods." Underweight for my age (or so I thought), I drank four milk shakes a day to put on enough weight to look like the "average" person. My health finally caved in, partly from the weak lung structure inherited from my mother, partly from my poor eating habits. The doctors gave me up to die in a matter of weeks.

This news sent me sprawling. They told me all I could do was rest — but I wasn't satisfied with that. I knew there must be a way. If there wasn't, I was in for a good long rest, so I moved subconsciously. I went into nutrition. I went through fasting programs, exercise programs. Using a breathing technique that I learned from Thomas Robert Gaines, I added four inches to my chest in six months. I could hardly believe that I could make such a change in my body. That was over fifty years ago, and now in my seventies I am in better health than I was then.

Seek What Is Right For Your Life

To a great extent we pick up many mental patterns and beliefs from our parents, and some of these are good while others are not. There are strengths and weaknesses at the mental level as well as at the physical level. In the previous portion of this book we have talked about overcoming the negative patterns, the negative beliefs. By now you know how to do this, so we will not go into it again here. We sometimes have to dismiss the weaknesses inherited from our mother and father and go directly to the heavenly Father where the greatest strength is and where the greatest wisdom is.

Sometimes we find a discomforting, disquieting feeling entering our lives and we just can't quite put our finger on what it is. This can be a time of great frustration. I am convinced that there are certain things we must do in this life to fulfill our purpose for being here, and if we do not do them, we become very unhappy. In a way, this is a sin of omission. This feeling comes from the failure to do what we are supposed to do. As in the case of the negative things that we must learn to overcome, we must also learn to overcome obstacles to what we are meant to do, the positive things.

When I was in Chicago taking a Homeopathy course with about fifty other doctors in the class, we were given the assignment of evaluating the symptoms of a person and then coming up with the right remedy.

One night we diagnosed the case of a woman married to one of the doctors in the class. She was tense, nervous, irritable, mean-tempered and quick to fly off the handle. Now there is usually a remedy for all problems, but when my turn came in class, I said that no remedy could cure this woman. I added that, from a homeopathic standpoint, a certain remedy might be helpful. But the cure was in another direction altogether.

This woman had been doing the work of a housewife, yet I could tell she was a born actress. The facial features, the eyes, the gestures, the voice — all these belonged to an actress. But this woman was not presently expressing her natural talent.

"Unless this lady becomes involved in dramatic work," I said, "either as an actress or drama teacher, her thyroid gland will have to be treated from now on." The thyroid gland is the emotional gland, and if it is not working properly we become mean and irritable. These physical things are dependent upon what is happening at the mental and spiritual levels.

This woman stood up, turned to her husband and said, "Did you hear what Dr. Jensen said? I've been telling you for years that this is what I wanted to do!"

"We have three kids," her husband protested. "You made the decision to get married and be a housewife."

"But I'm an unhappy housewife!" she asserted.

I added that she would have to have two careers, or she would never be happy. She loved to act. She was born to do it and she is doing it now.

These are things I know about. I've been a misfit myself. I have studied people carefully for many years and I know that no one will find his place in life until he knows who he is, where he is going, what his goals should be, what he is supposed to learn and what he is supposed to love. If we don't do some of the things we love to do, we will become miserable. That's the only way to put it.

The World's Diet Cultures

Part of our cultural inheritance, one that has

a very important effect on health, has to do with the foods that are emphasized in each part of the world and the ways of preparing these foods. When we decide to take the higher path in life, we realize that we must give our physical bodies the foods that are best for it.

The White Russian Doukhobors in Canada are among the best fed people in the world. When they take black bread and natural grains, they are caring for their bodies to the utmost. I visited them a few years ago and lived with them for awhile. They told me that when they first came to Canada they had no horses, so they hitched thirty women to plows to break the sod. These women did the work of horses. They are muscular, strong and have amazing stamina due to the way they eat. I think their diet inheritance is wonderful.

Other cultures have their problems. Switzerland has more cases of goiter than any country in the world due to a lack of iodine in the diet. Japan doesn't have goiter because the people eat fish and thus get the needed iodine. In India a certain type of stomach is called a "rice stomach." People develop a certain kind of body by the food they eat, and this is not always a healthy body. We have to be careful. We have to be selective. We know what habitual excessive beer drinking does to the stomach, don't we?

Whole countries, whole races, can mold to the foods they eat. During World War I a Danish scientist named Hinhede reduced meat consumption in that country by three-fourths, forcing the people to rely more on vegetables and whole-grain bread in their diet. As a result, Denmark was the only country to experience a decrease in its death rate during the war. Food chemists and nutritional experts are aware of experiments like this.

After the war the United States sent tons of white flour to Italy in an attempt to help its hungry people. But they developed gassy stomachs and poor bodies due to the low nutritional value of white flour. We must realize that people cannot be expected to be peaceful when their diet consists of disagreeable foods. I believe that war can actually be made almost inevitable when an entire nation or race is subsisting on the wrong foods. At the same time, we must realize that when a person's consciousness is raised, he or she will eat the better foods. To a considerable extent, poor food habits reflect a low level of consciousness. This, too, has a great deal to do with violent tendencies, warlike tendencies.

Germans love to drink beer. In this country we have our "coffee breaks." The Danes take their breaks to drink beer at ten in the morning and at three in the afternoon, but in this country we know them best for their "Danish pastry."

My mother was a good Danish cook, the best cook in the neighborhood. Everybody came to taste her pastry. But she killed herself with her good cooking, which complicated the problem of an already weak lung structure. It is sad that we have to go through such experiences but eventually we will all learn.

Good health is built gradually, just as disease is built gradually. If you keep on the right nutritional program, good results will eventually appear. I believe in vegetarianism very strongly. I believe that a vegetarian diet enhances a sense of peacefulness. One of my professors said that a mean, irritable, brutish person should never eat meat. It stimulates these characteristics. One of these days I believe we will all be vegetarians.

Choose The High Road

We don't have to go the low road with inherited weaknesses whether they are spiritual, mental or physical. Even if our parents were not interested in the spiritual things, we can realize for ourselves that this is the way to find the life more abundant. We can live according to our highest potential. Who wants to sit at home and feed on sympathy all his life? Perhaps the greatest advantage we find in an inherited weakness, a very serious inherited weakness, is that we are led to the spiritual path much sooner in life than we perhaps would be otherwise. Then we learn all the sooner that we can be rich in happiness and friends and in what we give forth to others.

By living close to God and nature, we can bring love streaming into these minds and bodies of ours. I am convinced that the most difficult conditions—cancer, heart disease, tuberculosis and the others—will respond well to love.

Beauty is a healing agent that most doctors tend to overlook. We all love things that are beautiful — clear blue skies, green trees, colorful flowers, magnificent waterfalls, fine works of art, music, poetry and other lovely things. We can change our own home so that we love each room

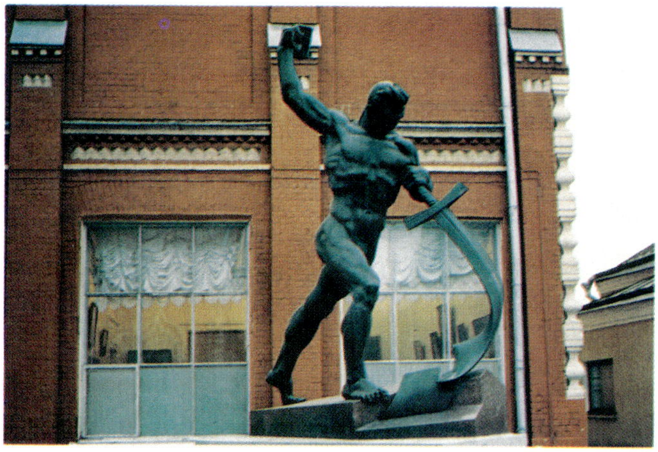

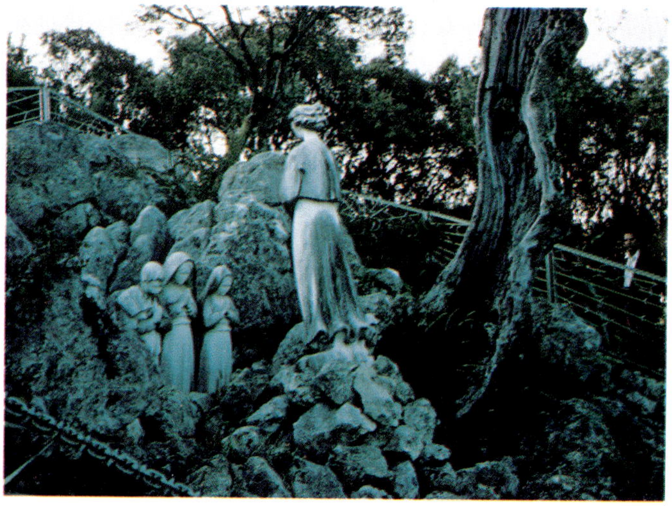

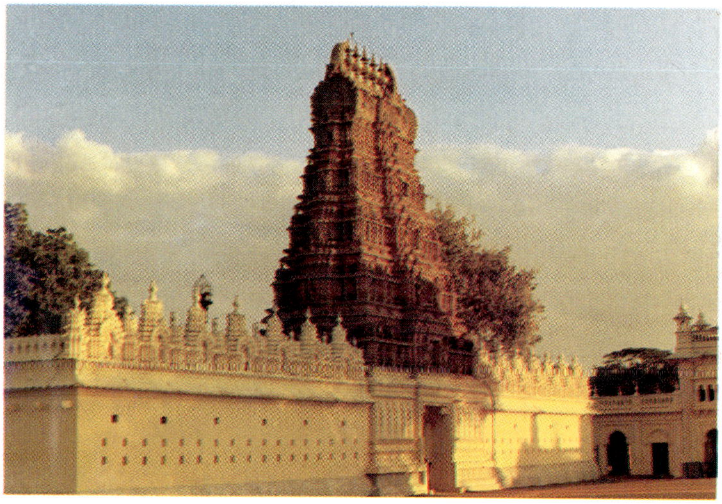

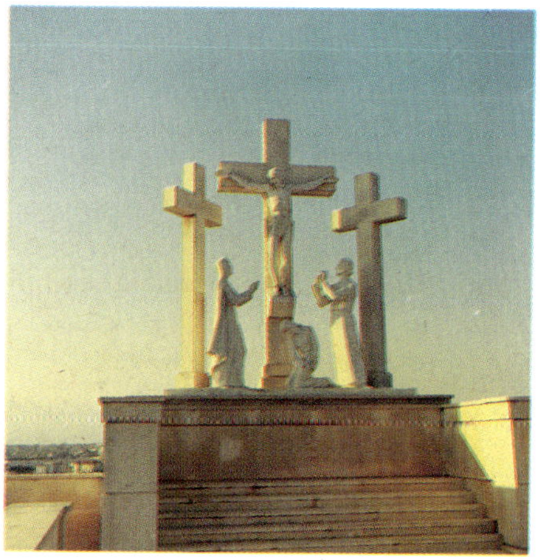

Top: Here is a sculpture illustrating the biblical principle of beating swords into plowshares, making war no more. Center: These statues commemorate the visit of Mary, the mother of Jesus, to the three children at Fatima, Portugal. Bottom: Monuments represent the deep spiritual undercurrents in all mankind.

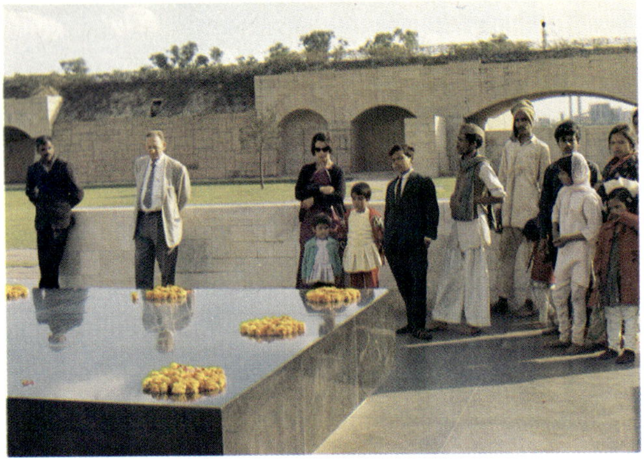

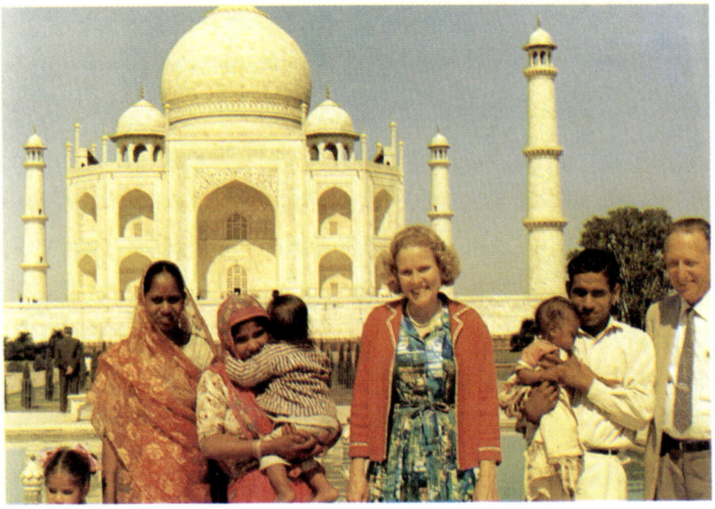

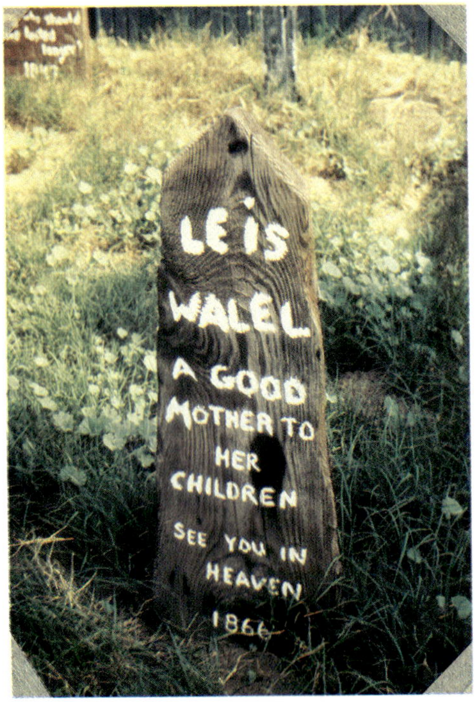

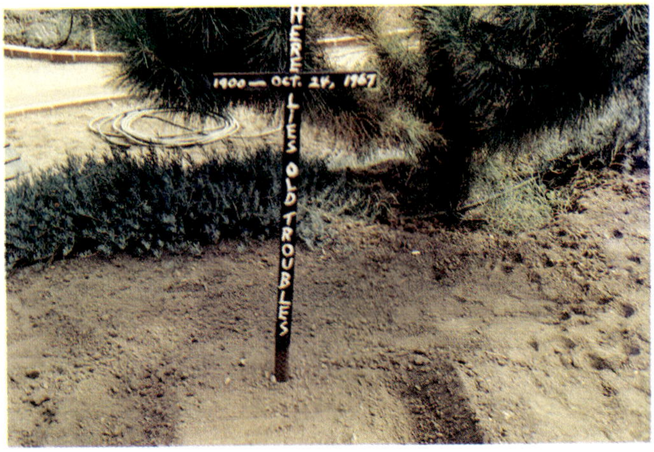

Top: This is Gandhi's tomb, very simple. A simple man, Gandhi was one of the great men of his time in moving the world. Center: An Indian family before the Taj Mahal with Dr. & Mrs. Jensen. While they may not have the riches of the prince of the past, they have riches of mind. Bottom Left: A grave marker in Boot Hill Cemetery. Bottom Right: Some 60 people joined me one morning in writing down all our troubles, and we dug a grave and allowed all of our past to pass away.

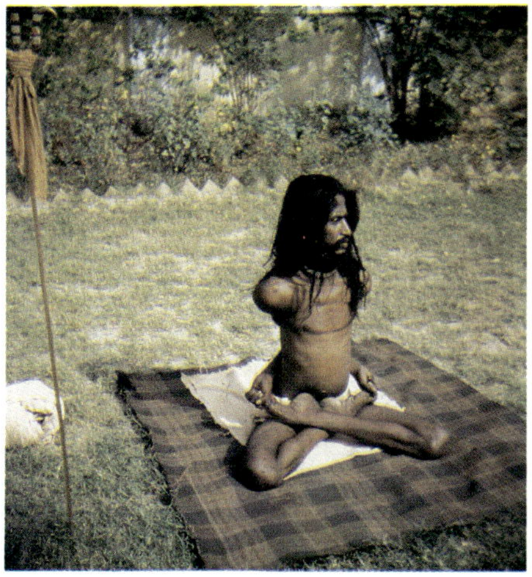

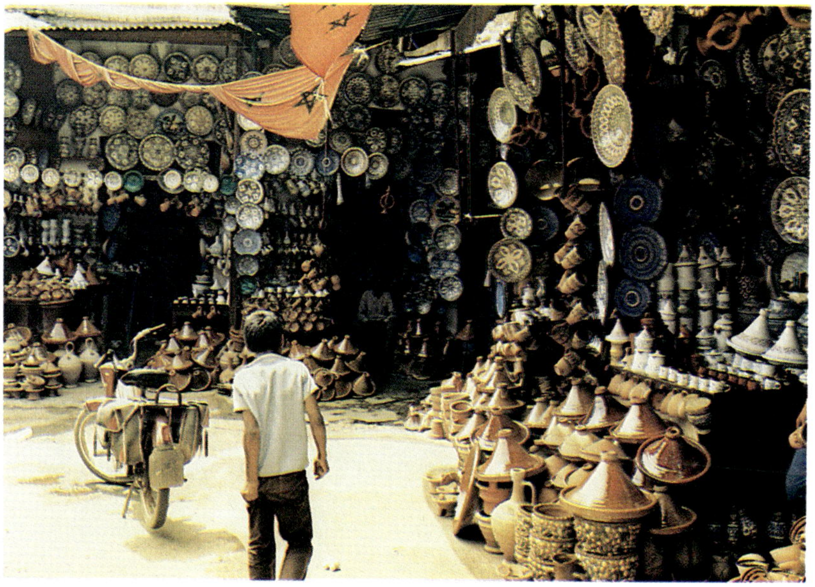

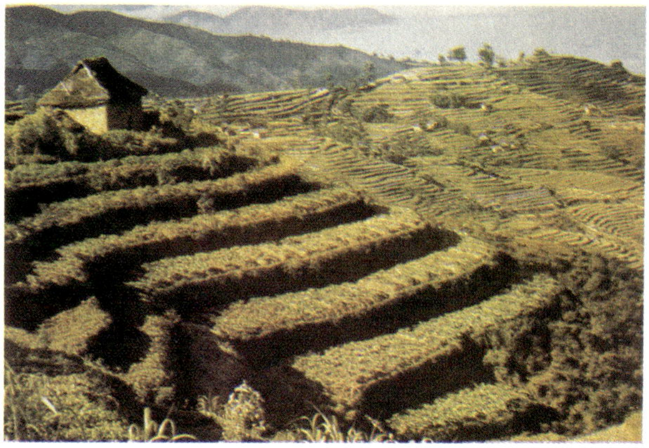

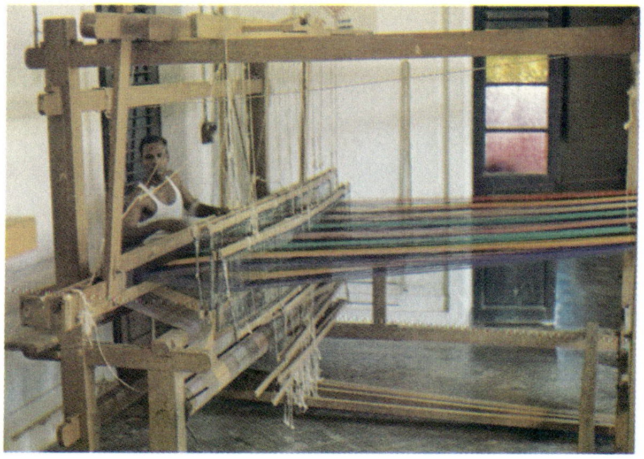

Top Left: This extreme form of yoga takes many years to master. Top Right: During my world travels, I once saw a sign on a wall which said, "Your prayer is your work." Center: Mountain terraces in India. Bottom: A weaver plies his trade. Textiles are among the greatest exports of India.

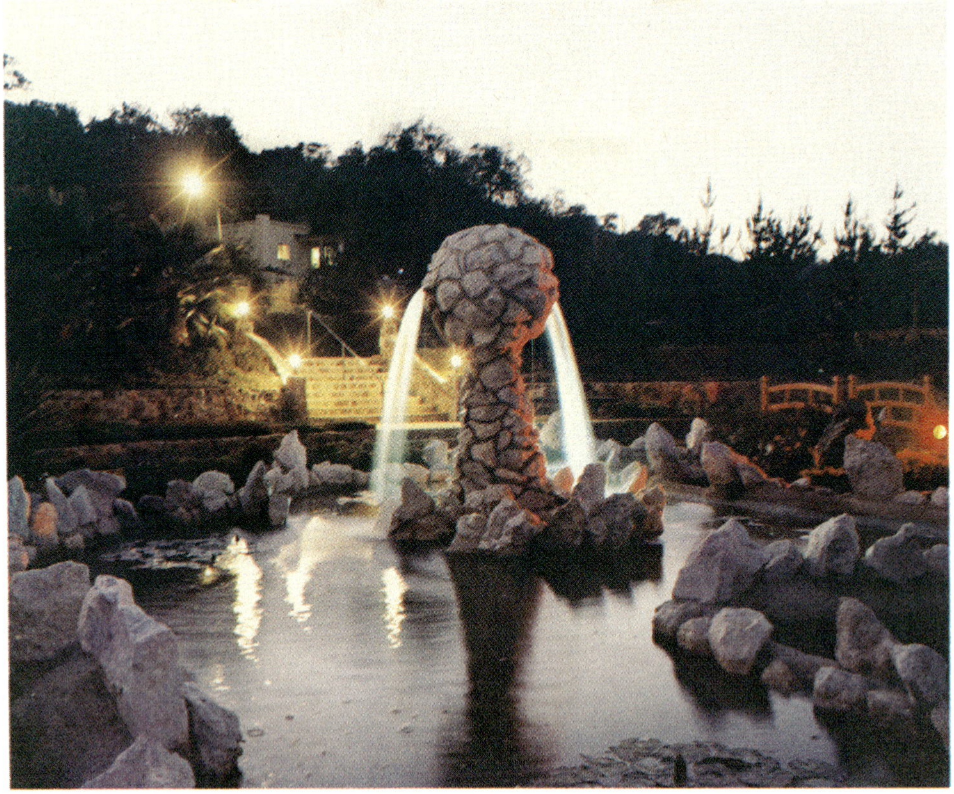

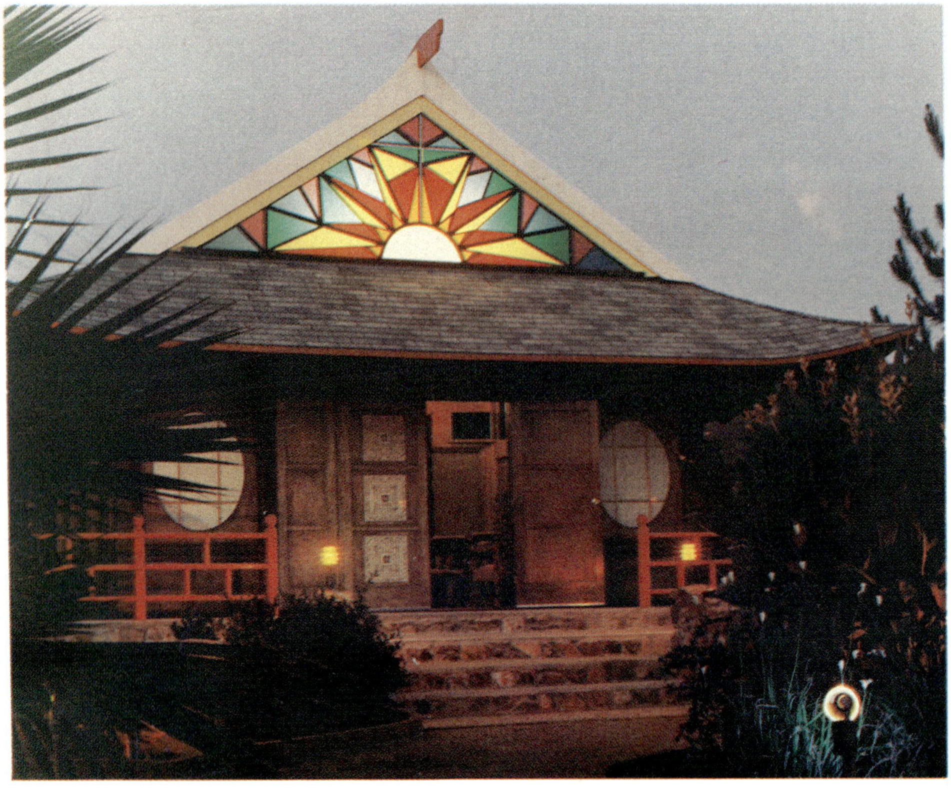

These are pictures of my Ranch before it was sold. The feeling of serenity was healing to the spirit and soul. The hungers of man must be met by many different "foods" of many different kinds. Many people are hungry for music, color, love, quietness.

— the colors, the carpets, the wall decorations, the furniture, everything. To become a beautiful person, we cultivate a beautiful mind. Then beauty will be flowing into our bodies. Then beauty will be attracted to us.

We can live so that nearly everything that goes into our memories from now on will be loving and beautiful. Our heartbeat will change, our kidney functions will change, our glands will change and even our bowel movements will become harmonious. We want to breathe a deeper breath. We want the liver to produce more bile. We would be thankful if better circulation helped the blood remake, rebuild, rejuvenate the cells of the body a little faster.

If we want this to happen, we are not going to eat as many cooked foods as we have in the past. We're going to make sure that at least sixty percent of our food intake is raw. We're going to make sure that we have at least six vegetables, two fruits, one starch and one protein every day so that our whole body is fed well. We are going to avoid cooking in oils and grease. We are going to clean out our pantry and cupboards and stock them with foods that enhance beauty, wisdom and spiritual upliftment.

Enlighten Your Outlook

I think one of my greatest experiences was having a class on spinal work with a blind instructor. He would put sandpaper of varying degrees of coarseness or fineness on the spine to help us develop our tactile sense so highly that when we encountered the different conditions of the spine with different people, we would know exactly how to adjust with precisely the right amount of force. Because of his blindness, he was able to teach us things that an instructor with normal vision wouldn't know.

This instructor gave me quite a surprise one day. I walked into his office unannounced, and he said, "Hello, Bernard." How could he do that? "No one turns the handle of the door quite the way you do," he explained. After a while he could tell it was me coming even before I reached the door. He said there was a certain spirit to my step that he could always discern as I was climbing the stairway to his office. I wonder sometimes how much we could develop each of our senses if we really tried.

Every physical handicap we have is compensated for by the development of other faculties. Helen Keller, born deaf and blind, could ride in a car through a city she was familiar with and know which block the car was passing because of certain combinations of odors and fragrances that she recognized.

We see this process of compensation come out very vividly when surgeons operate to remove varicose veins. The blood uses the alternate pathways to excellent advantage, and circulation continues unhindered. In the body, when one road is closed, another is opened. In India, they have found ways of developing nerve centers in the cheek to allow blind people to discern what is around them.

By accepting what we are and what we have, we can begin to discover what wonders these bodies of ours are. We can begin to develop our talents, realizing that challenge brings out the best in a person. It isn't how a man falls that counts, but how he gets up. Enlighten your outlook and understand that all obstacles are there for a purpose.

We must realize that our loving Father in heaven never "short-changes" anyone in this life. It is our outlook that needs to change. Rather than pity or sympathize with someone who has inherited a serious "handicap," we should respect and admire them, because God has loved them enough to give them a special lesson to learn. The wise teacher gives the hardest assignments only to the best students. We must always remember that the true riches of life are within, and there is a special reward for the person who overcomes.

We cannot escape our genetic inheritance but we can make the best of it. It is a blessing, and we must be thankful for the gift of life.

There is a humorous aspect to inheritance that I came across in this little verse that I'd like to share with you, titled "Carbon Copy."

His mother's eyes,
His father's chin.
His auntie's nose,
His uncle's grin.

His great-aunt's hair
His grandma's ears,
His grandpa's mouth,
So it appears. . .

Poor little tot,
Well may he moan,
He hasn't much
To call his own.

— Richard Armour

You know, the most important job we have as parents is to bring out the best in our children, no matter what their strengths and weaknesses are. I realize this is not easy, but we must not neglect to teach and encourage them in the right way of living at every opportunity. If we start early and persist in showing them what is right, mainly by setting a good example, it will be a blessing to them throughout their lives.

Children Learn The Most Important Lessons At Home

It is good to teach the spiritual values to our children. It is good to teach them to let go of the negative mental thoughts and replace them with the positive thoughts. And it is good to teach them to appreciate the godly foods, the foods that build a strong and healthy body. By giving our children a strong and positive inheritance in the home, we give them a good start in overcoming their weaknesses; we can show them that there are better ways than the ways of this world.

We must realize that we do not "own" our children — nor do they "own" us. They are God's children, no less or more than we are. We must not feel that we have to sacrifice our own happiness and goals to fulfill their every need, desire or want. We have our own jobs to do in this world, our own purposes to fulfill, and it is necessary to harmonize the process of child rearing with the achievement of our own goals. We don't ever want to hear our children say, "Poor mother — she gave up everything to take care of us kids," or "Poor father — he compromised his career to make sure we had everything we wanted." This is not being a good example to our children. Never behave in such a way that your children say, "Poor mom," or "Poor dad."

Let your children see you at your best in life. We are passing through this life, and if our children do not see us attempting to lift our souls, if our children do not see us living the life more abundant, then we are not setting the proper examples for them. If we bypass our opportunities for the sake of our children, we are, in effect, showing them that we really do not believe in the principles we are teaching them. Instead, we are sowing seeds of doubt in their minds. Then they may well do the same when they grow up. Do we want them to do this? No. We want them to seek the higher path, and to do this we must seek the higher path ourselves. Let them bear witness to the joy and peace you find in this way and include them in your sharing expression of these things. By doing this you will be planting the seeds of wisdom — and these seeds will grow and bear good fruit.

Certain thoughts are prayers.
There are moments when,
Whatever be the attitude of the body,
The soul is on its knees.
— Victor Hugo

From Chief Seattle, 1854:

"This we know: the earth does belong to man; man belongs to the earth. All things are connected like the blood which unites the body, like the blood which unites one family. All things are connected.

"Whatever befalls the earth befalls the sons of earth. Man did not weave the web of life. He is merely a strand in it. Whatever he does to the web, he also does unto himself."

Chapter 30

The Sacred Valley

Awake, harp and lyre; I will
awaken the dawn.
— Psalm 108:2

I have traveled all over the world and I am most thankful for the opportunity of carrying out my searching, my dreaming, my visions. A man who never had a dream, never had a dream come true.

Many years ago I had a vision of visiting a faraway place that could only be reached during a few weeks of each summer, because for the rest of the year ice and snow covered the surrounding mountains and obliterated all paths and entrances into this isolated valley. Coming into this valley you could see tropical fruits, knee-deep streams of pure sparkling water, lush green grass growing at its fullest — a life of ease. It reminded me of the valley spoken of in *Lost Horizon*.

Everyone seems to seek a Sacred Valley.

We once visited a place called Vilcabamba, some seventy-five miles from Loja, Ecuador. To me, Vilcabamba is a paradise of health. This valley is called the Sacred Valley, and the name suits it. Here the people have no heart trouble. Elderly women are able to run for blocks without getting tired. Men in their nineties still build furniture. A man 140 years of age still worked in the fields. The people are self-sufficient with the beautiful growth of foods for their needs. They grow their own herbs and drink the kind of cool delicious water that we would expect to find in a Sacred Valley. The people are unbelievably refreshed from the baths they take in the river; it seems like new life comes to them. Many a heart case has gone to Vilcabamba from Quito and other parts of Ecuador for recuperation and refreshment, and everyone that I have talked to received marvelous benefits.

We All Search For Utopia

Man is prone to chase rainbows. Many would leave their families, leave their jobs and homes, leave their country to climb the highest mountains or to explore the broad rivers that wind deep into tropical jungles. They are seeking the pastures of heaven on this earth, peace for the mind, body and soul.

If we are soil-minded, we seek a better soil. If we are diet-minded, we seek more natural foods. If we are climate-minded, we seek the right altitude, temperature and humidity. If we are a dentist, we are tooth-conscious. If we are an optometrist, we are eye-minded. If we are medicine-minded, our outlook is entirely different than if we are nature-minded. Some seek quiet relief from civilization, freedom from neighbors and relatives. Many just cry out for freedom.

Is it rest we need for the weary-minded? Is it a change we need for the physical heart problems?

Knowledge and wisdom can bring the Sacred Valley close to you, wherever you may be. Essentially, a Sacred Valley is an idea, a within-ness; it is the secret place of the Most High. We are forever seeking peace, harmony and contentment on the outside. Find it within yourself. Plow your ground until it provides beauty and abundance. Let the sparkling rivers of contentment flow, and draw life-giving water from it for all that you plant. Plant seeds that will bring a rich harvest of joy, of happiness and of good feelings. Establish harmony with everything you feel, smell, taste or see. If you stand on poor ground, it will ensnare your feet like quicksand and drain your vitality. If you stand on Holy Ground, you will have the strength to carry on through all eternity. Your every moment, your every feeling — these fleeting things create the life you live. When you live close to God, you draw life to yourself. When you live with fear and discontent, you draw death to yourself. You don't need to search for a utopia to live a life of joy.

Utopia Is Right Here — Now!

The Sacred Valley is a utopia within, where all thoughts that feed you are like the minerals that make a plant strong and healthy and beautiful. Colors, love, beauty, compassion — all are elements of the spirit that are indispensable for any human "plant" to feel good with. We must expand in consciousness to include all the virtues of saints so that we may become one with God. Patience, service and endurance are what will carry a good program to the end. It is necessary to dispense with chasing. One of these days you will have to settle down in some spot we call home. This settling down usually comes after we discover that the chasing we do is the very thing that prevents us from finding what we seek. And the effort of the chase is what is killing us. The purpose of life is to enjoy what we have, not what we could ultimately find or what the neighbor has.

It is solid, Holy Ground that we are seeking. It is not high or low ground, nor just a greener pasture. It is not just life or longevity. It is life well-lived that we want.

Many of us spend 100 years seeking and then all at once come to realize that we have been in a Sacred Valley all the time. It came when we looked to the Great Within. Realization of the Great Within gives us the necessary peace and knowing. Living in the secret place of the Most High is living in a Sacred Valley. It is the king's domain that lies within. Where do you think it is?

After traveling to the far ends of the earth, or maybe just exploring your own city, you will always be able to find plenty that is wrong as long as you deal with humankind and temporal things. We get so busy changing, moving, rearranging and doing over what man has done before. No wonder we get weary and fatigued! It seems that all of us have to go through the temporal way and the mortal way before we decide to end our seeking and accept the eternal values that were with us all the time. To try to make heaven out of man's knowing and out of earthly things leads to contamination, resentment and confusion. But to live with the King of Utopia is to live in your Sacred Valley for all time, and it is something to behold forever!

The Beauty Of The Rose

All the different kinds of experiences we go through leave an impression on our faces, in our hearts, in our inner beings. Every experience is a stirring movement to start us on our way to a more heavenly path, which we can enjoy in the days to come.

As we look to the rose that is planted as the seed, we see it going through the lowliest experiences, forcing its way up through the mud, reaching out with its roots for water and nutrients, spreading its first tiny leaves to the sun. Just to become a rose, to go on and express itself, to fulfill its destiny, we find it takes continuous experience and growth. But the destiny hidden within the very seed is fulfilled in that beautiful expression of the full blooming rose.

In the people often sitting before me, with

their burdens and cares of the day, with fears and problems of their homes and their bodily health, I see marked facial expressions, forceful gestures. They are tense and emotional; their heart activity may be irregular; their outlook is low and dismal. At this moment, truly, I can see the seed of a rose in each one of them. I recognize within you that rose-to-become, that wonderful potential that will one day unfold its delicate petals and reveal its delicate color, its beautiful full bloom, to the whole world. The start is being made at this moment.

Let us grow and fulfill our destiny. The seeds of experience, care, problems, troubles are the soil from which all roses grow. Be still, and realize that God is growing the seed and will guide your roots to the right nutrients as He lifts you ever upward to the light of the sun.

Be thankful in knowing that there is only one direction and that you will soon be in the light. See that as you work with the proper Gardener and with the proper care that a new day will soon be here. Begin to take on the beauty-consciousness that a rose expresses. See this within you. People are looking to you for that beauty within you. They should know you for that beauty. You should know yourself for the beauty that is possible within you. The many stages through which we go in our growth are the times when we branch out, add a few more leaves and become a better climber than ever.

All we need is the awareness that it is possible to have this beauty-consciousness within us. All we need is time to develop it. The moment it has been reached, you are that finished rose.

The beauty of the rose is always there. It just takes a recognition within, a knowing that we can become that beauty, so that it can also become part of our outer expression. You walk differently if you know you are that beautiful rose. Your very countenance will be different if you know there is beauty within. The hardened lines of your face will soften. You will be lovelier in your greeting and you will bring out the beauty of other people in their greetings.

Most people are lovers of beauty. That which is expressed from the heart of beauty can be worn on anyone's face. This beauty you will wear may change the lives of many people you meet to one of more beauty. The color of your temperament is expressed as part of this beauty within. The tension you bring back to yourself from others is produced from what started within you. When you are expressing the beauty of a rose, you not only help your neighbor but you express the better life for yourself. You are a more nearly finished rose. You will be blessed wherever you go. You will be wanted. You will be needed. No door will be closed to you. Surely you will be good to yourself. Your whole body will be less tense, less confused and less chaotic.

Look at a flowering rose long enough to take on its beauty. Plant it within yourself. . . nourish it. . . help it to grow. There is a rose in everyone.

To Be A Living Flower

We all have the potential of becoming more masterful in our expressions and technique. Surely within our very soul we have the privilege of becoming greater than that from which we started. Certainly from the very low spots, there is a place on high to which we can look. We are like the flower, knowing that in our upward travel and our life growth we can come out of the dust of the earth, out of the blackness, out of the mud. We can be surrounded by the darkest cloud and still look upward.

The flower is always seeking its light from above. The flower knows where to look for light — always above itself. Some have greater problems in their growth life; some are not so symmetrically designed as others; but the inherent spirit of all is to look upward and turn a lighted face to the source from which its light came in the beginning.

If the flower did nothing but bring color to those who are in remorse or in sorrow; if it did nothing but bring joy to those who are unhappy and downtrodden; if the flower did nothing but bring happiness to the sickroom, surely it would be worth its living.

To become the light of a rose, we must be all that it is possible to be, and not meet situations with resentment, resistance and stubbornness. We must live above these frailties. The rose itself is not interested in overcoming the black cloud or in overcoming the dust of the earth. It wants just to become its sweet self — a beautiful rose. Its life uplifts others because in its very self it represents the Light that brought it here. It is one with the Light that brought it here. For us to become one with the Light, we have to become all that is expected of us.

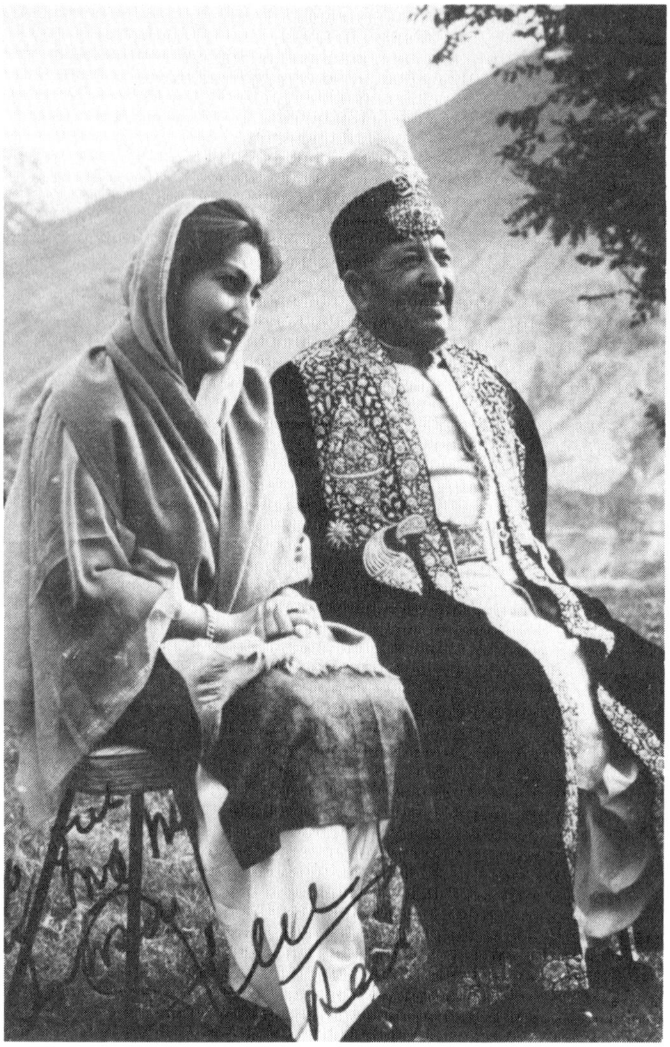

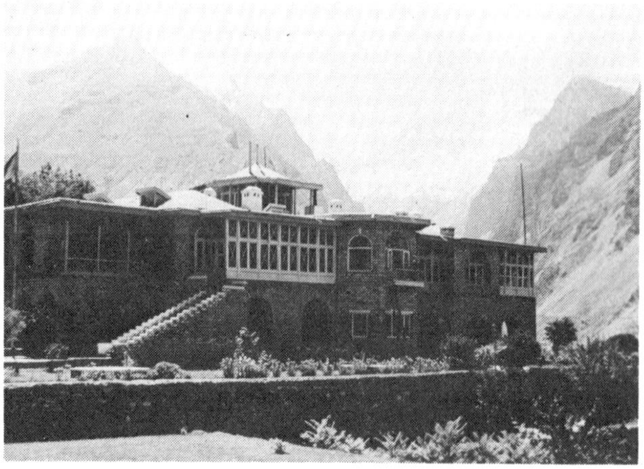

Top Left: The Mir and Rani of Hunza. Top Right: The Mir's palace where we stayed nine days. Bottom Right: This 120-year-old man from Hunza, in perfect health, worked in the fields every day. As we were leaving the Hunza Valley, the Mir gave me a hug and said, "What you have done for me in the last nine days amounts to more than most friendships do in a lifetime." The Mir valued friendship more than anything else.

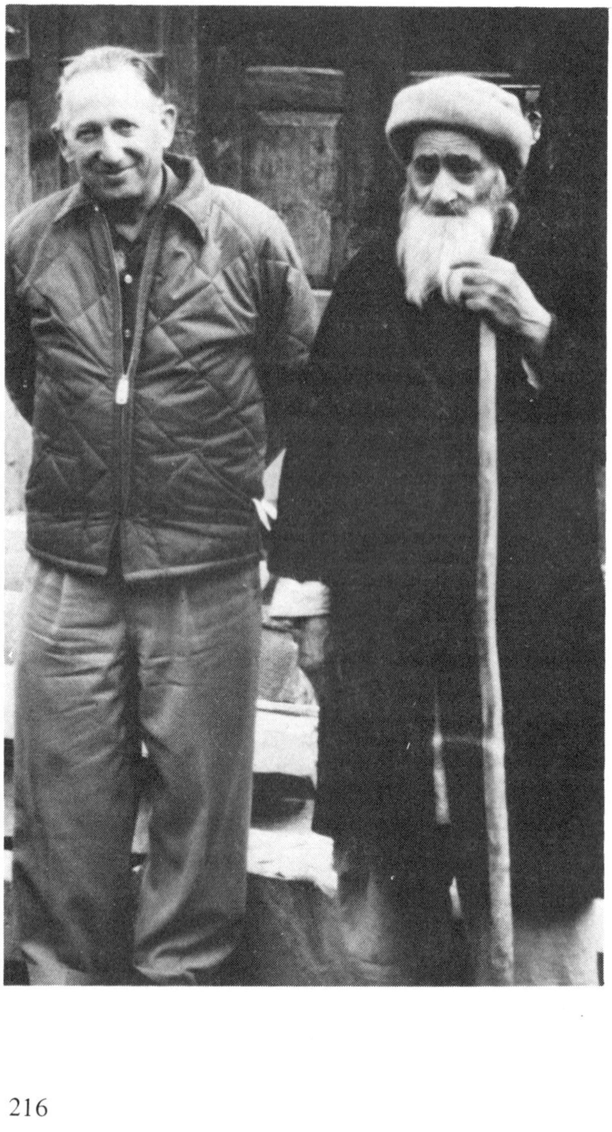

Chapter 31

A Few Parting Words With You

You are the hub of the wheel. The world is built around You! There is no world without You. It takes many people just like You to make the world but You are the one who represents your world.

When we stop and think about it, most of our vocabulary is drawn from the outer world, the material world. We don't have a pure language of the spirit by which spirit can express itself. Yet, when we speak from our heart and soul, we recognize that the real language of man begins there.

It is very difficult to find the right words to express what has meant so much to me. I really want to have all I have, to know all I know, but it is so hard to put in writing.

Words can cut to the quick or words can heal. Yet, to find words for events that occur in the twinkling of an eye, with the flick of a finger, in the echo of a footstep or the warmth of a handshake—these are things that defy expression in words. It is said, "It is the spirit that quickeneth; the flesh profiteth nothing." Perhaps it is the very quickness and subtlety of spirit that makes it so elusive to the writer.

Life expresses through us "from the inside out." So often we try to heal the outside without looking to the inside. We have to look to the other dimension of healing, the other dimension of development, the other dimension of expression—that of spirit. Man must learn to follow his "real self" and know that life is more than any symptom or external circumstance.

It is the spiritual "space" within us that we really have to find. In this space, healing begins, joy comes in and the true self makes its home. In this space, we find the "life more abundant" from which every need can be satisfied.

The great search of man has been to find this inner self, to find the true essence of man.

It Always Works

We have all had our troubles. No doubt you could sit down and tell me of things you have gone through in your life. I am sure you haven't escaped death in your family. I am sure you have lost money because of circumstances or due to unscrupulous persons.

I am sure you have met with many reverses—that you have been sick—that you know what it is to have things taken away from you—to be discouraged, disgruntled and heartbroken.

But take heart from this little story. Within these pages and between these lines you may find the one thing that can make you the richest person in the world.

What Are Riches?

Where is this rich feeling? Does it come from money? Is it found in material possessions? Does income create a feeling of security and abundance?

To me, the secret is found in this one little sentence: "Seek first the riches within—the source from which come the 'riches of Persia.'" It is all a matter of attitude (or consciousness).

The man who has only $10,000 may feel like a poor man if he once had $1,000,000. But the man who has never before had more than a couple hundred dollars and now possesses $10,000 may literally "be sitting on top of the world."

My First Patient—and Opportunity

Over 50 years ago, after a serious personal tragedy, I established my first office. It was Saturday afternoon.

A little old man drove up in an electric automobile. He stopped the car, got out, and—with a cane—stumbling because of poor eyesight—came into my office.

It was only a minute until the door opened. "I understand," said the little old man, "that you can make a certain diagnosis for me." "Yes," I replied, "I can do that for you."

"And what will the charges be?" he asked.

"Since it's Saturday afternoon and I'm not busy, I will not charge you anything." I replied.

"Well," he said with a twinkle in his eye, "I can't lose anything on that proposition, can I?"

When I had finished with the little old gentleman, he seemed delighted, expressing his appreciation again and again. He said he had not realized that anybody would give so much in so short a time. Actually, I had given him exactly the same service I would have given regardless of how much money was involved.

I Gained A Friend

"Surely," said the little old man, "surely you will let me pay you for your services."

"No," I answered, "I agreed to charge you nothing—and that's the price. I'm sticking to my bargain."

"Well," he said, in his soft little voice, "I have been saving a brand new Washington one-dollar bill for some time and I want you to have it."

At the time, it never occurred to me that this little gesture on his part was the beginning of a series of events which would actually change my life.

I did, however, recognize his gesture as something that had its beginning in my mind. That's a strange, but true, fact—everything that comes back to you must first go out from you. The good things of life are just the good things returning to you. There is more than just poetic beauty to the little sentence that reads: "As you sow, so shall you reap." This is the way it works—and "it always works."

Certainly if I had been offered one dollar for my services, I would have felt offended. But it was not a case of "value received" at all. I had given and given freely. But the little old gentleman, out of the fullness of his heart, felt like he wanted to show his appreciation. The gesture was there. That was the thing that mattered. His attitude lifted me.

I talked to my new-found friend—talked of this and of that. Before I knew it I was telling him about a new loaf of bread that I had developed—a loaf of bread made of all natural materials. I had just one loaf of this bread left, so I asked him to accept it as a gift from me, which he did. But, and he flashed his friendly smile again, "I have been saving this brand new quarter," he said, "and I want you to have it."

There was his return gesture again. There was life giving back to me the same attitude which I had sent out. There was proof again that it always works.

"If It Works—"

As my friend started to go, he asked me for suggestions as to improving the condition of his eyes.

While I was not an eye specialist, I had some ideas on care of the eyes which I gladly passed on to him.

As he went out the door, he said: "Thank you for those suggestions. I appreciate your advice. If it works, you will hear from me."

Naturally the incident slipped my mind. But a few days later, as I opened the mail, there was an envelope containing only a small card and a new Washington one-dollar bill. In scrawled handwriting, on the same card, were these words: "It Works."

In another few days, I received another telephone call asking for more advice on another matter. This advice, too, I gave freely and without obligation, for by now, this friendly little soul was a part of me.

"If it works," he said, "you will hear from me."

After that, once or twice a week, I would receive a telephone call or a personal visit from him. A friendly greeting, a request for some advice, and a cheery "if it works, you will hear from me."

Then a few days of silence.

Then came a letter containing a brand new, crisp Washington one-dollar bill, and the little card with the not too steady handwriting and the two magic words: "It works."

I wonder if you can appreciate fully the real value which I received from these little cards?

Today in a secret file, I have an envelope containing forty-eight Washington one-dollar bills. And in the same envelope, there are forty-eight little cards, on each one of which is written: "It works."

Riches Beyond Compare

Yes, it works. But there is a formula which you must follow. And you must follow it to the letter. First, you must give of yourself—fully, freely, unstintingly and without thought of reward or compensation. It can't be done any other way. Wanting the money first before you earn it, is simply wishful thinking. And if life did deliver your pay to you first, you wouldn't enjoy it half as much!

Today I am the richest man in the world for I know that "if it works, I will hear from life."

I know that I could start a business in the middle of the desert with only my mind and my hands, provided I did something worthwhile, something that followed life's formula, something "that works."

The "riches of Persia" come only to those who have "the riches of Persia" working within themselves.

A closed hand never receives.

An open hand is a working hand—a giving hand.

But when you keep your hands open to give, they are also open to receive.

Yes, It Always Works

There will be times when you are discouraged—when you feel that you are being taken advantage of—that life is not dealing fairly with you.

When those times overtake you, remember my story of the little old gentleman, who—to me—represents life itself.

Give of yourself; give all you have. In this way, you will keep yourself rich through a full realization of the things you have to give; you will be able to count your blessings as they go from you; and you will be surprised how they have multiplied when they return!

I will never spend those forty-eight one-dollar bills.

The principle that brought them to me is worth millions. I will never be poor as long as I remember how and why I received them.

Indeed, no man will ever be poor who remembers to "do a job that earns life's riches instead of working only for the dollar."

I have thanked my Creator a thousand times for the privilege and the blessing of meeting this little old gentleman at a time in my life when I needed him so much. His voice saying: "You will hear from me if it works," was like the voice of life speaking through him, showing me the way to the real riches of life. He taught me that life has a way of rewarding those who use her laws. He taught me no matter who you are, or where you are, or in what circumstances—if you will give of yourself, and give all you have, life will reward you.

This is a law of life itself—and, it always works!

The Riches Within

You have no doubt heard about the riches of Persia, the rich mines of Africa, the rich oil fields of Texas, the riches of Rockefeller, but have you heard about the true riches of man?

Man is the custodian of riches, and to know their value, he must know it first from within himself. He knows the power within himself. He has the creative power to duplicate. He has the consciousness to extend himself into all the world.

Man is the first natural scientific machine made. All other equipment comes out of man's consciousness. All that will ever become, first is in the inner consciousness of man. To realize the heights or depths of accomplishment of which man is capable through assumption, is to realize the scope of man's potential capacity.

What we assume, we are. I can accept, I can assume, I can believe and I can know, and this I know; I know I am gloriously rich.

To assume that I have all that the Father has, in both heaven and earth, is to assume a great deal. To know that we live in a heavenly kingdom and to know that it is for us, is to accept a lot. By walking in an expanded consciousness, by reaping the harvest that is already here, by realizing that "all that I have is thine," surely I am the richest man in the world. When we have the capacity to realize the richness of spiritual appreciation, the richness of companionship, happiness divine, gleeful laughter and thankfulness for eternal gifts, then we awaken to the real virtues of life. It takes experience to grow, to expand and progress. Above all, it is important to be able to feel, for to have felt your experience deeply within is to finally live in another world. You cannot say the real things in life, those things that really mean the most, until you feel it.

Richness is a state of awareness.

This is truly an awakening when it strikes you, and it came to me while on a little trip to Boston many years ago. I hired a taxi for the day and made a round-the-city tour of places of interest.

My first stop was the Bunker Hill Monument. When the car I was riding in stopped there, a boy, from a group of youngsters 5 to 8 years old who were playing about the grounds, made a wild dash in our direction. The taxi driver apparently knew what was coming, for he said, "Listen to this; it is a real speech."

The boy thrust his head through the open window of the cab and said, "You are now at the site of Bunker Hill Monument, 271 feet high. It was here that the order was given "Do not shoot until you see the whites of their eyes'"—and he went on and gave a lengthy speech. After finishing, he, of course, expected to collect whatever I felt like giving him. I handed him a small token and visited the monument without any further thought.

My next visit was to the home of Paul Revere. Here, I was met by another group of boys, one of whom reached me first and got the job of telling about this historic place. This young boy came to the window and said, "You are now at the site of Paul Revere's home. He was the village smithy who was the coppersmith, the ironsmith and the tinsmith. He was the one who made the false teeth that George Washington wore. That is why you never see a picture of George Washington smiling, because he was afraid his iron teeth would fall out." He went on and gave quite a story of this remnant of the old colonists. The exaggerated Boston brogue which he was affecting and his voice, speech and manner of speech changed entirely when I started asking questions.

When I asked him how long it took him to learn the speech, he answered, "Two weeks." When I asked him why he was giving it, he replied that he was earning money to go to a summer camp. I found out that the vacation would cost ten dollars, but he said he did not care whether he received more money or not because he had ten dollars fifteen cents. He already had what he needed. After a pleasant little chat with this young fellow. I asked him, "What does the average person pay you after you give your speech?" He answered, "All the way from five to fifteen cents." I gave him fifty cents, feeling that the extra money could go to making his vacation a little more pleasant. I was on *my* vacation having a glorious time and felt like giving him that little extra.

I proceeded through the Revere house, not thinking any more about my talk with the boy, but when I returned to the car, the driver told me I had made a young fellow very happy and related what had transpired. He said the little fellow went over to his young companions and claimed he had just been talking to a rich man. "He must have been rich because he gave me fifty cents," he told them. The other boys doubted this because they thought I looked no different from anyone else who had come there, so the boy, to get proof, went back to the taxi driver and asked, "Wasn't that a rich man? He must have been because he gave me fifty cents." The cab driver agreed, saying, "Yes, he is a rich man from the West, in fact, he is a multi-millionaire." The boys had quite a beehive discussion on this before I came out and looked me over carefully while I was getting into the car. After the cab driver's account of what had taken place, I was silent for some time.

In the eyes of these boys, I was a millionaire—yes, a multi-millionaire. These boys saw me as rich.

They saw something different than what they were accustomed to seeing and the only thing that made the difference was the token of exchange. This boy only shared his feelings with the others and they likewise assumed that I was rich. The assumption which took form in the minds of these boys can take place in the mind of anyone. Our assumptions and the claiming of our good which takes place within us make us rich or make us poor—yes, multi-rich or multi-poor. My token of exchange is my success and my happiness. It is the way of my world. It is my work for the higher good of man.

When I appreciate the equipment with which I was born: the realization that I am a child of God, that I am a complete inventory of all that is found within nature, that I was built whole to express and to receive all that is good and that I am made up of kindness, joy, freedom and love, and know I have the privilege of sharing all this—I am truly gloriously rich!

All Roads Lead To You

God has made you the hub and the center of the world in which you live.

You are the center from which all things develop.

You have within you the privilege of seeing any kind of world you wish.

You can put on glasses which qualify and refine the world's expression, actions and reactions, you can see things in beauty, see them in joyful activity, see them in the hands of the Divine.

You and God share the act of Creation, He creates beauty.

You may share it and represent it for him or you can drop to the lower spheres of living where things can become horrible, terrible, mixed-up and confused. If you become attracted to these things you will automatically represent them.

You can look at the world through rose colored glasses or the glasses can be green with envy, speckled with dirt so that you see spots on everyone at whom you look. Your glasses may be blue, dark and dreary, or they can carry a very light tint that will bathe everything with a peaceful softness that illuminates and shows all things are working for your good.

You may possess health if you recognize that you alone are responsible to yourself for keeping your mind alert, for giving your body the proper exercise, choosing proper foods, seeking proper company, breathing proper air, believing in the proper God, a God of love, harmony and contentment.

You are the one to decide whether you live with the downcast or the uplifted.

You are the one to choose melancholy or ease of mind.

You must make your agreement with the finer things with which you want to live; knowledge and culture are here for our higher good. Reach for it!

You must realize that even though you may be covered with darkness there is always a light shining that says: "Be still and know." It tells you to stand where you are and be somebody—to be in the image and the likeness of God.

You look for the healing.

You must recognize that deep within you the beginning of all feelings of recognition and awareness exists.

You must recognize your oneness and completeness as one of the Trinity, the Father, the Christ and you.

You must recognize that good health is your responsibility and is necessary for your complete Trinity with the Father. It is to love thy neighbor as thyself.

You may forget but the Divine and His creation never forgets. He has made the lily of the field. He remembers the fallen sparrow. He seeks you even to the marrow of your bones. Surely if we are unhappy, if we feel neglected it is our lack of faith and our lack of holding on to the one thing that never leaves us, ***Our Father***.

You have the privilege and the power within you to mold one with God or stand alone. What will it be?

Credo

This Credo, composed in Paris in 1928 by Romaine Rolland and Edmond Bordeaux Szekely for the International Biogenic Society, is very important to me, something I believe in very much.

We believe that our most precious possession is Life.

We believe we shall mobilize all the forces of life against the forces of death.

We believe that mutual understanding leads toward mutual cooperation; that mutual cooperation leads toward peace; and that peace is the only way of survival for mankind.

We believe that we shall preserve instead of waste our natural resources, which are the heritage of our children.

We believe that we shall avoid the pollution of our air, water and soil, the basic preconditions of life.

We believe we shall preserve the vegetation of our planet: the humble grass which came fifty million years ago, and the majestic trees which came twenty million years ago, to prepare our planet for mankind.

We believe we shall eat only fresh, pure, natural, whole foods, without chemicals and artificial processing.

We believe we shall live a simple, natural, creative life, absorbing all the sources of energy, harmony and knowledge.

We believe that the improvement of life and mankind on our planet must start with individual efforts, as the whole depends on the atoms composing it.

We believe in the Fatherhood of God, the Motherhood of Nature and the Brotherhood of Man.

I would like to close what we have shared together in this book by presenting a poem that has meant a great deal to me.

BY THE TOUCH OF THE MASTER'S HAND

'Twas battered and scarred, and the
auctioneer
Thought it scarcely worth his while
To waste much time on the old violin,
But he held it up with a smile.
"What am I bidden, good folk?" he cried,
"Who'll start the bidding for me?"
"A dollar—a dollar—then two, only two
"Going for three"—but no—
From the room far back, a grayhaired man
Came forward and picked up the bow,
Then, wiping the dust from the old violin,
And tightening the loosened strings,
He played a melody pure and sweet
As a caroling angel sings.
The music ceased and the auctioneer,
With a voice that was quiet and low,
Said, "Now, what am I bid for the old
violin?"
And he held it up with the bow.
"A thousand and who'll make it two?
"Two thousand and who'll make it three?
"Three thousand once—three thousand
twice—
"And going—and gone," cried he.
The people cheered, but some of them cried,
"We do not understand"
"What changed its worth?" Quick came the
reply,
"The touch of the Master's hand."
And many a man with life out of tune,
And battered and scarred with sin,
Is auctioned cheap to a thoughtless crowd,
Much like the old violin.
A mess of pottage—a glass of wine,
A game and he travels on;
He is going once—and going twice—
He's going—and going—gone.
But the Master comes, and the foolish crowd
Never can quite understand
The worth of a soul, and the change that's
wrought
By the touch of the Master's hand!

Bibliography

This partial list of books from my library is to help the sincere person get started on the path.

The Master Key—L. W. deLawrence
Healing: The Divine Art—Manly P. Hall
The Secret of the Ages—Robert Collier
The Bible
The Book of Mormon
A Course in Miracles
The Shroud of Turin—Ian Wilson
The Essene Gospel of Peace—Edmond B. Szekely (trans.)
Lessons in Truth—H. Emily Cady
The Prophet—Kahlil Gibran
The Science of Mind—Ernest Holmes
Isis Unveiled—H. P. Blavatsky
The Aquarian Gospel of Jesus Christ—Levi
The Art of Spiritual Healing—Joel Goldsmith
The Ministry of Healing—Ellen G. White
Life Understood—F. L. Rawson
The Temple Not Made With Hands—Walter C. Lanyon
Thrust in the Sickle—Walter C. Lanyon
Quiet Talks with the Master—Eva Bell Werber
The Voice of the Master—Eva Bell Werber
Peace Within Yourself—Joseph Murphy
The Book of Health and the Science of Truth—George Burnell
The Living Path—Lloyd Douglas
Spiritual and Mental Healing—Murdo MacDonald Bayne
Tertium Organum—P. D. Ouspenski
Self Reliance and Other Essays—Ralph Waldo Emerson
The Wisdom of the Oversoul—Paul Brunton
The Impersonal Life
Love or Perish—Smiley Blanton, MD
Think and Grow Rich—Napoleon Hill
The Dynamic Laws of Healilng—Catherine Ponder
The Prospering Power of Love—Catherine Ponder
The Science of Light—Walter Russell
The Message of the Divine Iliad—Walter Russell
Hidden Power for Human Problems—Frederick Bailes

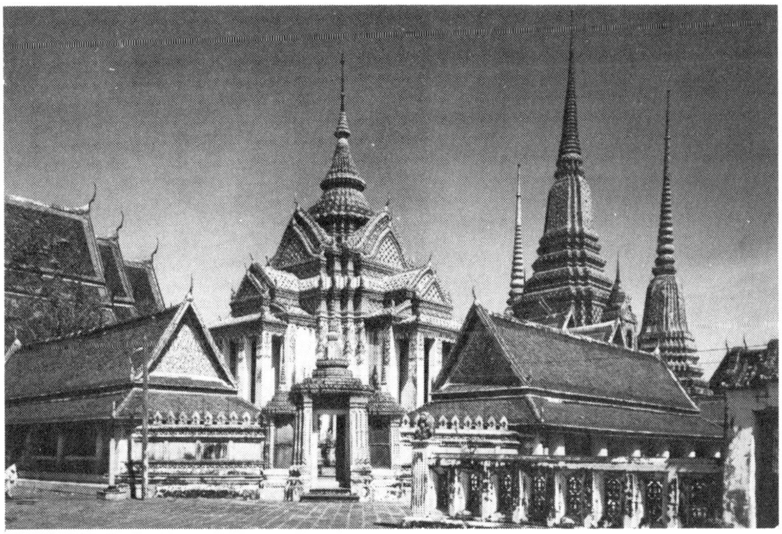

Where is beauty? All around us. But it starts in the mind and eye of the beholder.

For Your Good Health

While we have to take care of the mental and spiritual levels of man, Dr. Jensen teaches that we must also take care of the physical temple.

Build a library of right living with Dr. Jensen's books, tapes and attractive wall charts explaining the natural way to happy, healthy living. If they are not available in your local bookstore, write for our free catalog and price list to: Dr. Bernard Jensen, Route 1, Box 52, Escondido, CA 92025.

The "Man" Series by Bernard Jensen, Ph.D.

FOOD HEALING FOR MAN, Volume 1

A fascinating primer of nutrition and food facts for everyone, especially those getting started and working in the nutritional field. ***Food Healing for Man*** shows the role deficiencies play in disease and brings out the restorative power of a properly balanced regimen of whole, pure and natural foods. Chock-full of practical tips in growing, selecting, buying, drying, freezing, preparing and serving foods that prevent disease and build the best of health.

Dr. Jensen tells the story of the great pioneers in nutrition; reveals the truth about food additives, refined carbohydrates and modern food processing; shares many delightful recipes, health cocktails and menus; offers money-saving tips on food buying. Full of fascinating facts about current health-related research. **(Illustrated, Index, 448 pages)**

THE CHEMISTRY OF MAN, Volume 2

This volume, an in-depth study for students and professionals, presents the most neglected story of tissue replacement which can only come from good nutrition. Now, at last, a deep study of Dr. Jensen's phenomenal success in healing with foods in his sanitariuim work is available. The research of V. G. Rocine, Dr. Jensen's greatest teacher, on balancing biochemical deficiencies through nutrition, is revealed along with Dr. Jensen's practical applications at his sanitariums over the past 50 years. The major chemical types of man and their temperaments are discussed in detail, along with their relation to nutrition, health and disease.

Lists of symptoms for each biochemical deficiency and for some excesses are provided. Learn how to replace needed minerals depleted by poor diets and inappropriate lifestyles. This book is a must for those who would like to have a more advanced understanding of how true healing can come from nutrition. **It should be in every library and college. (Illustrated, Index, 640 pages)**

Charts. Beautiful color charts on Body Systems, Nervous System, Vitamins-Minerals-Herbs.

COMING SOON!

SLENDERIZING NATURALLY—BE FIT AND SLIM. If you have tried fad diets and gained all those lost pounds back, this is the book for you, the natural way to lose excess weight and keep it off. Dr. Jensen offers new insights on understanding how weight loss and gain happen and how the mind and brain respond to dieting, along with a diet plan and natural eating regimen to help you reach and stay at your natural weight.

FOOD PLANNING FOR FAMILY NUTRITION. This little book will delight those who need help getting started in selecting, preparing and cooking foods to keep the whole family healthy. Easy to understand, this book is especially for the beginner.

Video Teaching Tapes. Bring Dr. Jensen's lectures right into your home, clinic or classroom with this series of VCR tapes, now in final stages of production.

The "Man" Series: The Chemistry of Man, Food Healing for Man and The Healing Mind of Man will soon be joined by:

The Healing Essence of Man, Volumes I and II. The story of the finer forces of the vibratory realm and their relation to health and healing. Foods, Vital Force, Herbs, Nutrition, Iridology, Love, Sex, Children, Lilght, Color, Sound, Music, Radionics, Homeopathy, Kirlian Photography and much, much more! Many beautiful color illustrations.

COMPLETE YOUR LIBRARY!

Other Books by Dr. Jensen:

Breathe Again Naturally: How to Deal with Catarrh, Bronchitis, Asthma
Nature Has A Remedy
World Keys to Health and Long Life
Survive This Day
Blending Magic
Creating A Magic Kitchen
Doctor-Patient Handbook
Joy of Living and How to Attain It
Overcoming Arthritis/Rheumatism
Vital Foods for Total Health
You Can Feel Wonderful
You Can Master Disease
Health Magic Through Chlorophyll
A New Lifestyle for Health & Happiness (My System)
Tissue Cleansing Through Bowel Management

CASSETTE TAPES BY DR. JENSEN

(60-90 minutes: Inspirational)

Chemical Story
Building a Better Way to Eat
Replacement Therapy
Regularity Management
Divine Order
Seeds
Natural Healing
Key to Inner Calm
Breathing Exercises
Pathways to health
Arise and Shine

Now retired from active practice, Dr. Jensen offers a few Rejuvenation seminars and the Ultimate Tissue Cleansing classes several times each year. Write for details.

Dr. Bernard Jensen
Route 1, Box 52
Escondido, CA 92025

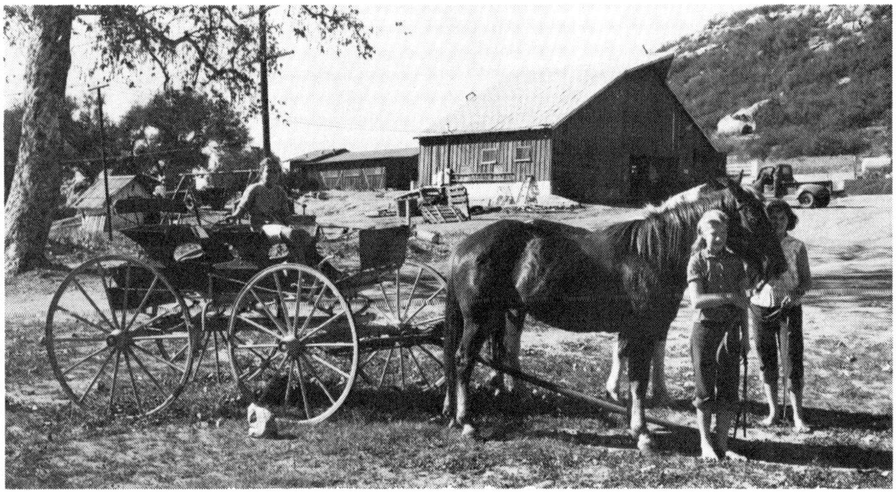

Ranch living, out in the country, provides peace and a tranquil mind.